COMPLETE PHLEBOTOMY

EXAM REVIEW

Pamela B. Primrose, PhD, MT(ASCP)

Program Chair of Medical Laboratory Technology/Phlebotomy
Professor of Medical Laboratory Technology/Phlebotomy/Life Sciences
Ivy Tech Community College
South Bend, Indiana

Contributing Editor
Tina Lewis, MT(ASCP)(AMT)

Medical Department Co-Director
Spencerian College
Louisville, Kentucky

SAUNDERS

ELSEVIER

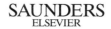

SAUNDERS
ELSEVIER

3251 Riverport Lane
Maryland Heights, Missouri 63043

COMPLETE PHLEBOTOMY EXAM REVIEW   978-1-4160-5331-6
Copyright © 2011 by Saunders, an imprint of Elsevier Inc.

All rights reserved. No part of this publication may be reproduced or transmitted in any form or by any means, electronic or mechanical, including photocopying, recording, or any information storage and retrieval system, without permission in writing from the publisher. Permissions may be sought directly from Elsevier's Rights Department: phone: (+1) 215 239 3804 (US) or (+44) 1865 843830 (UK); fax: (+44) 1865 853333; e-mail: healthpermissions@elsevier.com. You may also complete your request on-line via the Elsevier website at http://www.elsevier.com/permissions.

Notice

Neither the Publisher nor the Author assumes any responsibility for any loss or injury and/or damage to persons or property arising out of or related to any use of the material contained in this book. It is the responsibility of the treating practitioner, relying on independent expertise and knowledge of the patient, to determine the best treatment and method of application for the patient.

The Publisher

Library of Congress Cataloging-in-Publication Data
Primrose, Pamela B.
  Complete phlebotomy : exam review / Pamela B. Primrose ; contributing editor, Tina Lewis.
    p. ; cm.
  Includes index.
  ISBN 978-1-4160-5331-6 (pbk. : alk. paper) 1. Phlebotomy—Examinations, questions, etc. I. Lewis, Tina, 1969- II. Title.
  [DNLM: 1. Phlebotomy—Examination Questions. 2. Phlebotomy—Outlines. QY 18.2 P953c 2011]
  RB45.15.P75 2011
  616.07'561--dc22

                                                                        2010001064

Publishing Director: Andrew Allen
Managing Editor: Ellen Wurm-Cutter
Publishing Services Manager: Hemamalini Rajendrababu
Project Manager: Deepthi Unni
Designer: Karen Pauls

Printed in United States

Last digit is the print number: 9 8 7 6 5 4 3 2 1

Working together to grow
libraries in developing countries

www.elsevier.com | www.bookaid.org | www.sabre.org

ELSEVIER   BOOK AID International   Sabre Foundation

This book is dedicated to all the students I have had the privilege of advising and teaching over the past 19 years. It has been my pleasure and joy to see you begin your journey into health care with a career in phlebotomy, choose to stay there serving the community, or to carry your phlebotomy skills forward into other health care careers.

My heartfelt thanks goes to my husband Robert for his patience, sense of humor, support, and love during the many hours I was sequestered at the computer each day.

A huge thank you to all!

Pamela Primrose

REVIEWERS

Keith Bellinger, PBT(ASCP)
Assistant Professor of Phlebotomy
School of Health Related Professions
University of Medicine and Dentistry of New Jersey
Newark, New Jersey

Kristi Bertrand, MPH, CMA(AAMA), CPC, PBT(ASCP)
Spencerian College
Lexington, Kentucky

Kim Boyd, AAS, BAAS, MS, MT(AMT), MLT(ASCP)
Assistant Professor
Amarillo College
Amarillo, Texas

Karen Drummond, CPC, CPC-H, PCS, FCS, ACS-RA, ACS-OB/GYN, CMC, CMBS-I
Stark State College
Canton, Ohio

Karen M. Escolas, EdD, MT(ASCP)
Professor
Medical Laboratory Technology Program
Farmingdale State College
Farmingdale, New York

Gail I. Jones, PhD, MT(ASCP)SC
Instructor
Department of Biology
Texas Christian University
Fort Worth, Texas

Donna R. Kirven, BPPVE, CPTI(CA), PBT(ASCP), NCPT(NCCT)
Phlebotomy Education, Training, and Outreach
  Coordinator
Laboratory Education Department
John Muir Health
Walnut Creek, California

Carole A. Mullins, BS, MT(ASCP), MDA, CLDir(NCA)
Southwestern Michigan College
Dowagiac, Michigan

Cathy Robinson, MSA, MT(ASCP), CLS-G
Phlebotomy Coordinator
Allied Health Department
Instructor, Clinical Laboratory Technology Program
Louisiana State University at Alexandria
Alexandria, Louisiana

Anne T. Rodgers, MT(ASCP), PhD
Professor of Medical Technology, Retired
Hendersonville, North Carolina

Judith D. Symons
Medical Assistant
Geisinger Medical Center
Danville, Pennsylvania
Adjunct Instructor
McCann School of Business
Pottsville, Pennsylvania

PREFACE

The health care industry is growing, government oversight and regulatory policies are increasing, accreditation agencies are requiring hospitals and laboratories to provide patient care that focuses on a higher level of quality and safety, and, in turn, the necessity of qualified, competent health care workers has become more important than ever before. Many hospitals and laboratories require formal training and/or certification, registration, or licensure as minimum qualifications for entry-level phlebotomy positions. Certification or licensure indicates to employers that a phlebotomist has met the educational and/or experiential requirements as set forth by accreditation agencies in the field.

Complete Phlebotomy Exam Review was conceived and developed with the intent to go beyond traditional examination review books by offering more than just a series of review questions. This book provides a concise yet detailed review outline for each phlebotomy content area in addition to more than 1000 review questions, answers, and referenced rationales to aid students in their study, allowing them to assess their knowledge level and application and evaluation skills.

Who Will Benefit from This Book?

Whether students are just beginning the study of phlebotomy through a formal program or self-directed study, preparing to take a certification or licensure exam, or refreshing their knowledge, *Complete Phlebotomy Exam Review* encompasses and meets the needs for each stage of student learning. The outline at the beginning of each chapter is perfect for use in a formal program setting. It allows students to follow along during lectures without having to take copious notes, instead making small notations as necessary. Use of the Certification Preparation Questions and Answers and Rationales sections following each outline allows students to test their understanding, reinforce the correctness of each answer, and learn why other choices are incorrect. For those seeking self-directed study or preparing for certification or licensure exams, *Complete Phlebotomy Exam Review* can be used

as a companion to a phlebotomy textbook or it can be used as a single resource that provides a quick, concise review of the content prior to testing students' knowledge in the Certification Preparation Questions section.

In essence, *Complete Phlebotomy Exam Review* is an easy-to-use tool that will enable students to put knowledge and practice together in a way that supersedes all other review books by providing understanding and reinforcement of phlebotomy concepts immediately followed by the opportunity for practical application of those concepts in the assessment section of each chapter.

Organization of the Book

Complete Phlebotomy Exam Review provides a thorough review of each phlebotomy content area in the same progression as most phlebotomy textbooks, beginning with an introduction to phlebotomy, the health care setting, safety, and infection control; phlebotomy basics that include medical terminology and anatomy and physiology; routine, special, and non-blood specimen collection; special populations; specimen handling, transport, and processing; and professional issues, such as quality assurance/control, legal issues, and point-of-care testing. It addresses each of the content areas delineated in the various certification and licensure content outlines. Each chapter begins with a detailed outline for review of the content area followed by questions, answers, and rationales. Although rationales are referenced by page number to *Phlebotomy: Worktext and Procedures Manual*, second edition, by Warekois and Robinson, they can also be easily matched to any textbook by referring to the chapters covering similar content.

Distinctive Features and Learning Aids

The distinctive features of *Complete Phlebotomy Exam Review* differentiate it from other phlebotomy review books:
- Progression of study from basic to more complex topics
- Companion book for phlebotomy textbooks

- Suitable for all levels of student: beginning students in formal programs, self-study students, and those preparing for certification or licensure
- Detailed content outlines for each chapter precede assessment questions, answers, and rationales
- Review questions offer a variety of styles ranging from simple knowledge–level questions to more complex comprehension, application, analysis, synthesis, and evaluation questions
- Scenario questions that cover important situations that phlebotomists may encounter in practice allow students to integrate and apply all the knowledge they have acquired
- Over 1,000 different questions—no repeat questions as in other review books
- Mock certification exam and an additional 150+ practice questions
- Online repository of questions on Evolve that can be used to create practice exams based on content areas in which students need more practice
- Up-to-date information on phlebotomy certification and licensure requirements and contact information for eight agencies
- Chart for anticoagulants and mode of action
- Chart for tube top color, additive, test, department
- Chart for clot activators and other additives
- Chart for CLSI order of draw standards
- Strategies for developing a plan of study, progression of study, retention of information, and having efficient and effective study sessions
- Test-taking strategies for multiple-choice question exams.
- Tips on overcoming test anxiety
- Tips for Certification Day!

Ancillaries

For additional practice, visit the Evolve website at http://evolve.elsevier.com/Primrose/phlebotomy/ and create practice exams based on areas of weakness and take mock exams using all the questions in the book plus more than 150 additional questions.

Acknowledgments

Many people were involved in the conceptualization of this book and determining what would make it stand above all the other review books in the marketplace. The converging of all of these ideas has culminated in the production of *Complete Phlebotomy Exam Review*. My appreciation goes to Tina Lewis for her contributions to the later chapters. Many thanks also to my editor, Ellen Wurm-Cutter, for giving me the opportunity to join this project, and for all of her direction and support to me as a new writer, in addition to all of her hard work in getting the book ready for production. My deepest gratitude and thanks to all.

I would also like to acknowledge Robin Warekois and Richard Robinson for the use of the introductory paragraphs of their text, *Phlebotomy: Worktext and Procedures Manual,* second edition.

Pamela Primrose

Navigating the Certification/Licensure Process

CERTIFICATION

Certification of a phlebotomist is evidence to health care employers that a person has met the educational and training requirements set forth by the certifying agency. Furthermore, successfully passing a certification exam is testament to the fact that the person has demonstrated competency of the established standards for knowledge and skills in phlebotomy.[4,7,13,23,25]

Some confusion exists regarding the completion of an accredited, approved, or structured phlebotomy program that culminates in a certificate. This certificate documents completion of a training program by the institution that provided the education or training. It does not confer certification to the individual. Certification is a credential that is awarded by certifying agencies through successful completion of a certification exam, thereby demonstrating proficiency in a particular area of practice; in this case, phlebotomy.

Phlebotomists who have successfully completed an accredited or approved training program or who have documented work experience as a phlebotomist are eligible to take a certification exam. Specific requirements for eligibility are set forth by each certifying agency and are delineated on each agency's website.[4,7,9,25,29] Required standards in skills and knowledge may include the following: knowledge of health care providers in the medical field, interaction as a team, and the role of the phlebotomist; organizational structure of the hospital and laboratory; anatomy and physiology, medical terminology and pathology as it relates to phlebotomy; phlebotomy equipment and techniques for blood and nonblood collections; specimen processing and handling; point-of-care testing; quality assurance, quality control, and quality improvement; regulatory agencies; safety and infection control; interpersonal relations; and legal and ethical issues pertaining to phlebotomy.[3,7]

LICENSURE

Regulations governing health care workers within each state change over time so it is important to know the laws that govern phlebotomists in the state for which you are seeking employment. In the state of Nevada, phlebotomists are classified as laboratory assistants (employed in a licensed clinical lab) or office assistants (employed in a physician's office). Both are required to be licensed by the state of Nevada. Licensure for laboratory assistants requires a high school diploma or GED plus 6 months of training in a licensed clinical laboratory OR successful completion of a certification exam. Licensure of office assistants simply requires the signature of the office physician in addition to a high school diploma or GED. This process differs from licensure requirements of phlebotomists in other states. California and Louisiana are currently the only states that require licensure of phlebotomists who are working in health care facilities. Each of these states has specific requirements and regulations governing the education, training, and certification of phlebotomists. Certification for licensure approval also requires successful completion of either a state examination or an approved certifying agency exam. If you are planning on working as a phlebotomist in either state you will need to meet their eligibility requirements for licensure.[6,11,22]

Contact information for licensing agencies in California and Louisiana are:

- California licensure information:
  https://secure.cps.ca.gov/cltreg/pt_faq.asp
  Contact Laboratory Field Services for eligibility or board approval questions: 510-620-3800
  Online application questions: email CPS at clsinfo@cps.ca.gov or call 916-263-3624, option 4
- Louisiana Credentialing Agency
  Louisiana State Board of Medical Examiners
  630 Camp Street
  New Orleans, LA 70130
  http://www.lsbme.org
  Contact information for the licensing agency in Nevada is:
- Nevada Department of Health and Human Services
  Health Care Quality and Compliance
  Bureau of Licensure and Certification Medical Laboratories
  http://health.nv.gov/HCQC/Forms/ClinicalLabPersonnelCert.pdf
  702-486-6515

CERTIFICATION AGENCIES

There are many organizations that offer examinations for phlebotomy certification. Reputability and national recognition levels vary among the agencies. When choosing a certifying agency it is important to research which agencies are recognized by the health care institutions for which you are seeking employment in your particular geographical region. It is also important to compare the requirements and benefits of each agency in order to select the one that best fits your needs.[13]

The Center for Phlebotomy Education (http://www.phlebotomy.com) identifies several key factors you should keep in mind when choosing a certifying agency.[12] Does the agency:
- Have national recognition?
- Have good standing with the Better Business Bureau?
- Engage in ethical business practices?
- Base its instruction materials and examinations on current CLSI practices?
- Require examination of all applicants that they certify?
- Require continuing education to maintain certification status?

Several certifying agencies (in alphabetical order) that meet these criteria and that also meet state approval for California and Louisiana licensure are listed below:[11,22]

American Certification Agency
PO Box 58
Osceola, IN 46561
www.acacert.com
574-277-4538

American Medical Technologist
710 Higgins Road
Park Ridge, IL 60068
www.amt1.com
847-823-5169 or 800-275-1268

American Society for Clinical Pathology
33 W Monroe, #1600
Chicago, IL 60603
www.ascp.org
312-541-4999 or 1-800-267-2727

National Center for Competency Testing
7007 College Boulevard, Suite 705
Overland Park, KS 66211
www.ncctinc.com
800-875-44040

National Healthcareer Association
7 Ridgedale Ave., Suite 203
Cedar Knolls, NJ 07927
www.nhanow.com
973-605-1881 or 800-499-9092

In addition to the aforementioned certifying agencies, Louisiana has also approved the following certifying agencies for Louisiana licensure:[22]

American Society of Phlebotomy Technicians
PO Box 1831
Hickory, NC 28603
www.aspt.org
828-299-0078

International Academy of Phlebotomy Sciences
629 D'Lyn Street
Columbus, OH 43228
Phone: 614-878-7751

National Phlebotomy Association
1901 Brightseat Rd.
Landover, MD 20785
www.nationalphlebotomy.org
301-386-4200

Certifying agencies (in alphabetical order) that meet the state approval criteria for Nevada:

American Medical Technologist
710 Higgins Road
Park Ridge, IL 60068
www.amt1.com
847-823-5169 or 800-275-1268

American Society for Clinical Pathology
33 W Monroe, #1600
Chicago, IL 60603
www.ascp.org
312-541-4999 or 1-800-267-2727

CREDENTIALS

On successful completion of a certification or licensure examination you will be awarded a certificate that documents your achievement as proof to employers that you have met the requirements set forth by the certifying agency or licensing agency. Most of the certifying and licensing agencies require completion of a specified number of continuing education credits or units per year or within a specified time period in order to maintain certification or licensure. Some certifying agencies also offer continuing education programs and award CEUs upon completion of each competency activity or unit of study. These requirements are explained on each agency's website and information for CEUs is usually disseminated along with the credentialing certificate.[5,7,9,23,26,27]

If you have been out of the field for some time and are contemplating reentering, it is always wise to update your skills by retaking a phlebotomy course and/or getting recertified if your certification credentials have lapsed. This documents you are current in the field and makes you more marketable to employers whose applicant pool will also include recent completers of phlebotomy programs.

GETTING CERTIFICATION OR RECERTIFICATION

Getting certified requires that you research the certifying agencies to see what each agency's specific requirements are for eligibility and finding one that is a match for your training program or work experience and your needs. You should be aware of the certifying agency's deadlines for application. Once you have selected your certifying agency you will need to complete their application process by doing the following:[1,4,7,9,26,27]

- Verifying your academic education: high school graduation diploma; official college transcripts
- Verifying your work experience if required
- Verifying the training program
- Getting required signatures and/or other required documentation
- Completing the online application or mailing in a downloaded application
- Paying the assessment fee
- Scheduling the examination date and selecting the examination site

THE EXAM

Just as there are a number of certifying agencies, there are also a number of different types of exams offered. The traditional paper and pencil exam is still available as an examination option at several certifying agencies. There are a few agencies that also require a practical component as a part of their certification process whereby the individual must physically demonstrate venipuncture procedures. Many certifying agencies offer computer-based knowledge examinations that offer the convenience of multiple examination sites, faster scoring of the exam, and immediate notification of pass/fail at the conclusion of the exam or within a few days time. [1,4,7,9,25,27,29]

Most certifying agencies have *Exam Content Outlines* posted on their websites or which are available for purchase. These outlines reflect phlebotomy categories of routine venipuncture, dermal punctures, special procedures, equipment, nonblood specimens, complications, safety, legal issues among others. Procedures are based on the Clinical and Laboratory Standards Institute (CLSI) standard procedures and protocols.[2,4,7,9,29]

Exam questions are based on levels of difficulty and taxonomy categories of knowledge, comprehension, application, analysis, synthesis, and evaluation of required standards in skill and knowledge of phlebotomy as previously discussed. The importance of being able to answer questions at a higher taxonomy level allows for the recognition of those who have grasped the depth of knowledge to ensure competency and safety in the practice of phlebotomy.

- **Knowledge** questions assess the ability to recall or remember facts.
- **Comprehension** questions assess the ability to not only recall facts but to explain, classify, or identify facts, ideas, or concepts.
- **Application** questions determine the ability to use information. Facts are recalled and understood but are now required to be applied to a real situation to interpret, solve, or identify the impact of those facts on a situation.
- **Analysis** questions require the ability to interpret, compare, and contrast the information presented to determine the correct answer.
- **Evaluation** requires the ability to appraise, judge, evaluate, and support the information as it relates to a situation.

Is it important for you to know which questions fall into these taxonomy levels? No; but what is important is that you are prepared beyond the basic recall or knowledge level so that you can correctly answer questions that require higher levels of thought processes. You can achieve higher levels of critical thinking by practicing the review questions as presented in this book.[15]

Computer adaptive testing (CAT) is the format of computer-based knowledge testing offered by the ASCP. All questions are criterion referenced to the content outline for the phlebotomy exam. This type of testing format is driven by the ability level of the student answering the questions. When the question is answered correctly the next question presented has a slightly higher degree of difficulty. The degree of difficulty increases as each question is answered correctly and then drops to an easier level when a question is incorrectly answered. Questions in the test bank are calibrated or given a weighted value based on the level of difficulty. The resultant score is calculated on the number of questions answered correctly and their weighted value. The more difficult questions that are answered correctly the higher the score. Passing the exam requires that a person demonstrate competency at higher cognitive levels than just straight recall thereby ensuring that an appropriate level of knowledge is held by the examinee for competent and safe practice.[8]

STRATEGIES FOR DEVELOPING A PLAN OF STUDY

Determine Your Style of Study
Engaging in productive study for your selected certification exam requires that you determine what works best for you in terms of when, where, and how to study. No two people are the same when it comes to studying, and what works for one person may not work for you.[16] Some people are auditory learners and learn much faster by hearing the information. Others are visual learners and need to see information in written or illustrated format. Some are kinesthetic learners who like to do a physical activity such as tapping fingers or a foot and or write things out, or move around as they learn. There are those who prefer study groups and learn much more quickly through discussion. Once you decide which method is most effective and conducive to your learning and retention of information, you need to focus on that particular preference and complement it with other techniques.[24]

Positive Attitude
It is said that the biggest difference between people is their attitudes. Some people love to learn, and for others learning is a complete drudgery. Those in between the loving or drudgery attitudes view learning as a requirement along the road to success. Keeping a positive mindset uses a mental attitude that expects success in one's endeavors. Do not let negative thoughts and actions deter you from achieving your goal of certification. A positive attitude toward your review session changes the chemistry of your brain by producing more dopamine, the neurotransmitter that makes you feel good. A positive mindset will keep you motivated in your study and will improve your performance on your certification exam. Expect success in your study and preparation for the exam. Expect success when you take the exam. Visualize success. Success is within your reach![24,31]

Three C's
Martin's study skills booklet presents numerous tips on being a successful student that have stood the test of time. He states that being proactive in your study preparation not only requires knowing your style of study and having a positive mindset but also requires three "C's": commitment, control, and challenge to put your style of study into action and to promote positive thinking.[24]

Commitment
You need to make a positive commitment to yourself to prepare for the exam, be enthusiastic in your study, praise yourself for your successes along the way, and dream of success on your certification exam.[24]

Control
You need to control your mind and keep it focused as you study. Set goals and priorities for your study plan. Develop a strategy for dealing with distractions and problems that might impede your study time and progress. How will you handle interruptions by phone calls, children, and non-essential demands on your time? Be honest with yourself about what is realistic for you in terms of your plan and don't be afraid to tweak it as you go.[24]

Challenge
Be optimistic as you approach each study session. Do your very best and you will see improvement and success as you progress through your course of study. Don't be discouraged when it seems as if you are not progressing as well as you had anticipated. View this as a challenge and an opportunity to learn and add to your knowledge base. Each review session will improve your ability to retain, comprehend, apply, and analyze your phlebotomy study materials.[24]

Plan Your Study
Before you think about the process of studying for the certification exam, you must develop a study schedule. The value of a schedule is that it allows you to manage your time effectively so that you can meet the needs of your lifestyle and commitments. Your schedule should include work hours, doctor's

appointments, grocery store and errand runs, children's schedules, and time for you so that you can see where you have time to incorporate your study hours. Your study time should not be at the end of the day when you are exhausted and your mind is weary. Set times of 1 to 3 hours at the most for when you are most energetic and alert so that you can efficiently and effectively review the material. It may be necessary to temporarily delete some activities from your schedule and delegate them to someone in your support system in order to make time for study. Once your schedule has been set you need to follow it. If you find that it is not meeting your needs you can always revise it accordingly. But the important thing is to have blocks of time scheduled for uninterrupted study that are realistic for you. Equally important is that you plan and implement your study schedule well in advance of the date of your certification exam so that you have plenty of time to cover all of the review material and practice exams.[16]

THE PROCESS OF STUDY

An effective study process must include where to study, when to study, what to study, and how to study in order to have a productive study session.[16]

Where to Study

In reality you can study anywhere; however, some places are more conducive to study than are others. The place you choose should be free of distractions such as a television, telephone, or children. It may be at home in a secluded room away from the family or you may choose to go to the library or some other setting. Whatever setting you select should be comfortable for you in terms of seating, lighting, temperature, and noise level.[16]

When to Study

The issue of when to study has been set by your study schedule. However, it is important to keep in mind that you should schedule your study for times when you are rested and alert. So do not wait until the day's and night's activities are over to begin your study. Some people are morning people and some are night people. At what time of the day do you feel your energy and performance are highest? Do not schedule your study at times when you find yourself too tired to retain any information; try to schedule them at your peak performance times if possible. Physical and emotional exhaustion will derail your study.

Do not let unimportant things push your study time off schedule.[16,20]

What to Study

This review book is an excellent means of reviewing all the content that is included in the certifying agencies' Exam Content Outlines. The chapter outlines provide a quick review of phlebotomy topics to assess your strengths and weaknesses. If you need further clarification or more in-depth review of particular topics you can use your textbook and notes to supplement your review as well. The review questions for each chapter of this review book provide various taxonomic levels of questions to test your level of retention of knowledge (recall), comprehension, application, analysis, synthesis, and evaluation of phlebotomy practice. Each question has an explanation for the correct answer as well as insight into the other choices and why they are incorrect. As you go through the review questions mark your selected answer and check to see if you were correct; you can then circle the incorrect questions and go back to the outline to review the areas in which you had difficulty. The mock test and the Evolve website provide further practice for various types of questions that may be encountered on a certification exam.

In addition to this review book, some of the certifying agencies offer practice exams for purchase to provide further study, review, and practice.

STRATEGIES FOR RETENTION OF INFORMATION

Retaining information once you have studied it requires effort on your part. The following brain-compatible learning principles will help to refine your study habits and retention. Carolyn H. Hopper's book, *Practice College Learning Strategies* (2007) presents the following tips for study:

Intent to Remember

As you study and review you may find your mind wandering. Learning is different from attention. But if you do not pay attention you will not learn. Your intent to remember requires using concentration techniques such as a concentration check sheet to help you stay focused. When your mind starts to wander simply put a check mark on the sheet. By doing this each time you lose concentration and focus you will program your mind to pay attention to what you are studying. You can also put a rubber band on your wrist and snap it each time you lose focus. Another technique is to talk out loud as you read and answer the questions or recite information from the outlines included in the review book.[14]

Meaningful Organization

Trying to remember a large block of information is difficult, but if you break it down into smaller, more manageable blocks, the information is easier to remember. Use the subheadings in the outlines or in your textbook to categorize information as you review. Some people alphabetize items and make up groupings of letters to organize and retain information. Another method of organizing information for memory is the use of first-letter mnemonic devices whereby the first letter of each item to be remembered is used to make a word, phrase, or sentence. Two types of mnemonics that are typically used are acronyms and acrostics. Some mnemonics are well known but you can make up your own to help you remember as you study.

- *Acronyms* are formed from the first initials of words contained in a phrase to form a pronounceable word. Examples include NICU for neonatal intensive care unit; PASS for fire extinguisher use where P = Pull, A = Aim, S = Squeeze, and S = Sweep.
- *Acrostics* are usually in the form of a poem where the first line of the poem begins with the first letter of the item to be remembered. They can also be a phrase where the first letter of each word in the phrase is a cue for remembering it. The most commonly remembered acrostic is Roy G Biv used for remember the colors of the rainbow: R = red, O = orange, Y = Yellow, G = Green, B = Blue, I = indigo, and V = violet.

There is no right or wrong way to use these memory techniques or mnemonics. Use your creativity to come up with something that works for you. If a device is not useful to you then do not use it as a study technique. Only use those memory devices that will help you remember the information in a meaningful way. In order to form a sharp memory the information needs to be encoded accurately into your memory by whatever means works for your style of learning, strengthened as well as maintained over time, and then triggered by an association or cue.[14]

Strengthening Neural Connections
Recitation

If you read and then recite in your own words what you have learned when reviewing the chapter outlines, you are using the intent to remember, you get immediate feedback, you demonstrate understanding, and you are using a different part of your brain in the process. The more senses that are engaged in the learning process, the stronger the neural trace. Saying the information out loud in your own words serves to strengthen the synaptic connections in the brain. You may find using flashcards or having a study partner may be useful in this process.[14]

Mental Visualization

Approximately 90% of sensory input into the brain is visual, so it stands to reason that the majority of people remember what they see much better than what they hear or read. Visualizing mnemonics, writing what you recite, making charts, diagrams, or association images as you study serve to improve retention of the material.[14]

Association

Association as it applies to memory principles is the process of encoding and retrieval of information. New information must be consciously encoded because optimal learning occurs when the neural networks of the brain work in synchrony. Associating your review of phlebotomy content areas with information you already know about phlebotomy will help you to better comprehend, apply, synthesize, and evaluate the information. For example knowledge about the tourniquet can be associated with routine venipuncture, site selection, preanalytical sampling errors, complications, and so on.[14]

Solidifying Neural Pathways
Consolidation

The brain requires time for new information to become solidified in memory. Consolidation of information into long-term memory takes time to develop pathways of connectivity and recall. Reinforce the acquisition of knowledge through your preferred learning style (i.e., auditory, visual, or kinesthetic). Reinforce learning as many times as it takes for you to be able to recall it without fail. The number of times material needs to be studied varies with individuals. The length of study time for reinforcing learning may take seconds to hours depending on the individual and the information. As you study you will find content that you know very well that has already been solidified. There will be other areas of content that you cannot recall as quickly or as completely and those are the areas that need further reinforcement and consolidation into your long-term memory.[14]

Distributed Practice

Learning is optimized when distributed practice is put into play. Taking a 10-minute break after each hour you study to go back and review what you have just learned allows time for the brain to consolidate information. It has been shown that short sessions of review and study promote the growth of dendrites and neural connections exponentially. That means when you divide the information into smaller sections and take breaks from continuous learning by stopping every hour to review you will dramatically improve your retention and recall.[14]

STRATEGIES FOR EFFICIENT AND EFFECTIVE STUDY SESSIONS

There are several strategies that you can use to provide efficient and effective study.

Divide the Content

Assess the amount of time (i.e., days, weeks, months) that you have between now and your exam date. Divide the chapters by days or weeks into manageable sections of material to be covered for each study session and enter the topics or chapters on your schedule for each day. This will serve as a guide and keep you focused during your study session. Your goal is to complete the assigned content area by reviewing the outline, notes, book, and review questions as necessary. You may know some topics better than others and will require less study time for these. As you divide the content, assign the easier topics to the shorter blocks of study time and those that require more study to the longer blocks of time.

Practice Review Questions

It is presumed by certifying agencies that you are already well-versed in phlebotomy because you have completed a training program or have worked in the field as a phlebotomist. A quick review of the outline at the beginning of each chapter in this review book should suffice to refresh your memory on the content contained in each section. At this point it is important that you learn how to successfully answer various types of multiple-choice questions that may be asked on the certification exam. Simply memorizing factual knowledge and answering simple recall questions will most likely not be enough to deliver a passing score. Certification exams are designed to probe beyond the mastery level of simple recall. You must be able to actively apply, analyze, synthesize, and evaluate the information in the questions in the exam. By practicing the multiple-choice questions in the review book your will get experience practicing these types of questions. So be sure to complete the review questions for the chapter that you are reviewing during that session. Go back and check your answers, read the rationales for each answer, and mark the questions you answered incorrectly. Examine the questions and the correct answers, looking for the connections that make them correct. Review the outline material pertaining to that question or refer to your textbook or class notes. As you progress through the book make note of the areas or topics that you are weak in and then make a point to go back to those areas for further study and review.

Review, Re-Review, and Review Again

As previously discussed in Distributed Practice, repetition embeds information into long-term memory. So as you study each section and progress, you should go back and review previously studied material. If you have learned the content well, the review will go much more quickly than a first review. To quote Vince Lombardi: "Practice doesn't make perfect; perfect practice makes perfect."[10] Perfect practice entails keeping to your schedule, reviewing the outlines, practicing review questions, reviewing content areas in which you are weak, and practicing review questions again. The value of practicing review questions is that you will become more adept at analyzing what a question is asking, which choice best answers the question, and why the other choices are incorrect.

The Importance of Breaks

During longer periods of study it is important to take breaks and get up and move around so that you can refresh your mind and be more productive in your study. Short breaks away from your study room to get a refreshment or stretch help you to relieve the stress and fatigue of study. Do not forget to go back to resume your study! If it is not feasible to wander out of your study space to take a break for fear of becoming captive to family or friends' activities then make sure that you have refreshments available in your study area.[21,34]

Ready for the Practice Exam and Evolve

Once you have completed your review of the chapter outlines and review questions and are confident in your grasp and understanding of the material, it is then time to take the Mock Exam at the end of the book. There are an additional 150+ questions on the Evolve website that will also further test your knowledge and understanding. Again, it is important to note the questions that are incorrect so that you can go back and review specific areas of weakness.

Study on the Go

Carry your review book with you in the car, to your appointments, work, or other places. You never know when you might be able to squeeze in some time for review.

TEST-TAKING STRATEGIES

Knowing strategies on how to approach a test and the questions contained therein will help you remain relaxed and in control as you take your certification exam. The following tips are worth learning and applying as you review for the exam and will be second nature when you are ready to take the certification exam. Again perfect practice builds confidence and aids in attaining a successful score on the exam.

- Read all instructions carefully. If you do not understand an instruction ask the proctor for clarification.
- Most exams are timed. So be sure to pace yourself so that you will have time at the end of the exam to go back and review. Monitor the time periodically throughout the exam. Do *not* panic as time ticks down— remain in control. If you find you are moving too slowly, make the necessary adjustments to increase your pace. The more questions you answer the better your score will be and the better your odds of achieving a passing score.
- Answer each question even if you are unsure. Guessing gives you 20% to 25% chance of getting the question correct versus a 0% chance if you do not answer it. You can temporarily skip a question and come back to it later but answer to the best of your ability first. Do **NOT** however, spend too much time on questions you do not know the answer to because that wastes precious time. As you progress through the rest of exam questions your memory may be triggered, thus allowing you to correctly answer questions you may have skipped.

Tips for Taking Multiple-Choice Exams

The best way to ensure that you select the correct answer in a multiple-choice exam is to *know* the right answer. So pre-exam preparation is your key to success. The following tips will assist you in reading, interpreting, and answering the questions on your certification exam, but nothing is better than knowing the information and being able to comprehend, apply, synthesize, and analyze that information.

- Multiple-choice questions are made up of two parts: the stem and the choices[19,30,32]
  - **Stem**: is the statement or question
    - Read the stem as if it were a stand-alone statement.
    - Anticipate the word or phrase that would correctly complete the statement and then compare the choices to the one you anticipated.
    - Read EACH choice before selecting your answer even if one matches your answer because there may be a choice that is better.[19,30,32]
  - **Choices:** are known as distracters or foils[19,30,32]
    - Four or five options are usually presented to complete the stem statement or question.
    - The correct choice will be the option that completely satisfies the thought expressed in the statement or question.
    - Choosing the correct option requires reasoning ability on the part of the test taker. Relate each option to the statement or question to see which one logically completes the expressed statement or question.
    - Use information in previous questions to answer questions you that you do not know.[19,30,32]
  - **Strategies** for selecting the correct answer
    - *Choose the BEST* answer available. There may not be a perfect answer but there will be one that satisfies the question more accurately than the other choices.
    - *Eliminate* answers that are obviously incorrect. You can then focus on those answers that appear to be more reasonable before selecting the one that is *most* correct.[19,32,33]
    - *Mark key terms* in the question either mentally or on paper if possible.

- Identify and focus on the important information in the question and discard the rest.
- Look for the terms *not, except, but*: they change the meaning of the statement or question.
- Examine options that appear similar, and compare them to each other and to the question to see which one is more correct.
- Look for grammatical construction between the question and the answers. If the statement ends in "an" then the answer begins with a vowel—all choices may not begin with a vowel. Also watch for agreement between the subject and the verb or predicate.[19,32,33]

- *Avoid* choosing answers that contain words that are unfamiliar or seem odd to you. If you studied thoroughly, you should recognize the terminology presented in the questions.
- *Do not panic* if you are presented with a question that you did not expect to see. Use all of your knowledge about phlebotomy and the terminology to decide on a reasonable answer.
- *If you draw a blank* you have options before moving on to the next question. Try slowly rereading the question with each distracter to see which one fits best. If you are still unsure then skip the question and go back later. Succeeding questions may trigger your memory.
- *If more than ONE answer seems correct*: Some strategies to help you eliminate answers that are incorrect are as follows:[19,32,33]
  - Ask if the answer completely addresses the question. If it is only partially true or only true under specific conditions then it is probably not the correct answer.
  - Do you have to make an assumption for the answer to be true? Is making that assumption obvious to everyone who would take the exam? If not then the answer is probably incorrect.
  - Is it a trick question? No. Certification exams will not ask trick questions. Be sure to read and interpret the question at face value. Do NOT read into the question. Only your knowledge and the skills you have acquired are needed to answer the questions. You may need to do an analysis or synthesis of the scenario within the question to arrive with the correct answer but it will not be a trick.
  - As a last resort, if you cannot choose between two plausible answers don't use the one that feels wrong to you. This tip is useful to some students but remember it is NOT infallible.[19,32,33]

- *Do NOT be afraid to change your answer.* The first answer selected is often correct but *IF* upon reflection it appears to be incorrect, **change it.** Studies conducted over the past 70 years demonstrate that students who change dubious answers usually end up with higher scores. A 2005 study reported in *Journal of Personality and Social Psychology* revealed that students who changed their answers went from a wrong answer to a right answer 51% of the time; went from a right to a wrong answer 25% of the time, and went from a wrong to a wrong answer 23% of the time.[17,33]
- *Review the test* after you have completely finished. Many times you will catch some mistakes or you may find better answers once you have gone through the entire test.[19,32,33]

TEST ANXIETY

Most people experience some anxiety before or during an exam, but if the anxiety level negatively affects your performance on the exam it needs to be addressed. Text anxiety is actually performance anxiety and can result in butterflies in the stomach, a stomachache, a tension headache, or the person may feel shaky, sweaty, nauseated, have heart palpitations, etc.[18] There are several tips for minimizing, alleviating, and learning to cope with anxiety:

- Be prepared for the exam. Begin your review well ahead of time so that you have adequate time to cover all of the material and practice exam style questions. Follow the suggestions for developing a plan of study, retention of information, and developing efficient and effective study sessions. Nothing reduces anxiety more than knowing that you are well prepared and confident in your knowledge and skills.

- Approach the exam with confidence.
- Personalize your success on the exam:
  - Visualize success as you answer each question
  - Logically assure yourself that you are well prepared
  - Use positive self-talk before and during the exam[18]
- View the exam as an opportunity to demonstrate your skill and knowledge and receive the reward of certification for all your hard work.
- Strive to achieve and maintain a relaxed state of concentration.
  - Relax by taking slow, deep breaths: you are in control
  - Do not think about being afraid before or during the exam
  - Stay focused on the questions and answers step by step[18]
- Use positive reinforcement by acknowledging that what you have done and what you are doing is the very best you can do.
- Expect to have *some* anxiety— it can be a good thing:
  - Use it as a reminder that you want to perform to the best of your ability
  - Use it to provide positive energy, *not* stress
  - Keep it manageable by streaming it into positive action and thoughts during the exam: change positions, stretch, breathe
- Visualize your success![18]

TEST-TAKING TIPS FOR CERTIFICATION DAY!

There are a number of strategies that will make your certification day much easier:[18]

- Know where you are going. Do a practice run to the examination center you have selected so that you know exactly where you are going and how long it will take you to get there. Driving the route at the time of day that you will be going will give a more accurate estimate of your travel time. Be sure to add some extra travel time in case there are unexpected delays such as an accident, weather-related delays, or car trouble.
- Get a good night's sleep before the test.

- Set your alarm and a back-up alarm so you do not oversleep and then have to rush to get to the testing center on time. This will reduce your stress and anxiety levels.
- Eat a good breakfast or lunch before you go. Be sure to eat some protein and do not eat a lot of carbohydrates as they will make your sleepy.
- Check to make sure that you have the required items to take the exam, such as a photo ID, pencils, calculator, cough drops, and tissues. Make sure you organize them the night before. If you do not have a photo ID make sure to get a state ID or other form of ID in advance of your test date.
- Bring earplugs if you are distracted by noises. There may be other testers in the same room taking a different type of exam in which they are continuously typing. The clicking of computer keys can be very distracting to some test takers.
- Wear layers of comfortable clothing so that you are prepared if the room is too warm or too cool.
- Arrive early so you can get acclimated to the environment of the testing center.
- Choose a computer or desk that is located in an area where you will feel the most comfortable.
- Stay relaxed. Your nerves may start to kick in but take a few deep, relaxing breaths before you begin.[18] You have studied, you are prepared, and you can successfully do this! Keep a **POSITIVE** attitude throughout the exam!

REFERENCES

1. American Certification Agency, (2009): Recertification: Phlebotomy Technician. Retrieved June 12, 2009, http://www.acacert.com
2. American Certification Agency, (2009): Examination Requirements. Retrieved June 13, 2009, http://www.acacert.com/exam_requirements.htm
3. American Medical Technologists, (2008): AMT Registered Phlebotomy Technician (RPT) Certification Examination Construction Parameters. Retrieved June 13, 2009, http://www.amt1.com/files/RPT%20Competencies.pdf
4. American Medical Technologists, (2009): Certification Process. Retrieved June 12, 2009, http://www.amt1.com/page.asp?i=160
5. American Medical Technologists, (2009): Continuing Education. Retrieved June 12, 2009, http://www.amt1.com/page.asp?i=180
6. American Society for Clinical Laboratory Scientists, (2009): Personnel Licensure. Retrieved June 12, 2009, http://www.ascls.org/jobs/grads/personnellicensure.pdf

7. American Society for Clinical Pathology, (2009): Get Certified: Certification by the ASCP Board of Registry. Retrieved June 12, 2009, http://www.ascp.org/FunctionalNavigation/certification/GetCertified.aspx

8. American Society for Clinical Pathology, (2009): Computer Adaptive Testing. Retrieved June 12, 2009, http://www.ascp.org/FunctionalNavigation/certification/GetCertified/ComputerAdaptiveTestingCAT.aspx

9. American Society of Phlebotomy Technicians, (2009): Welcome to the American Society of Phlebotomy Technicians. Retrieved June 13, 2009, http://www.aspt.org

10. Brainy Quote, (2009): Vince Lombardi Quotes. Retrieved June 13, 2009, http://www.brainyquote.com/quotes/quotes/v/vincelomba138158.html

11. California Department of Public Health Department, (2009): Phlebotomy Certification. Retrieved June 12, 2009 from http://www.cdph.ca.gov/programs/lfs/Pages/Phlebotomist.aspx

12. Center for Phlebotomy Education, (2009): Directory of Phlebotomy Certification Agencies. Retrieved June 12, 2009, http://www.phlebotomy.com/Certification-Agencies.cpe

13. Dilulio R: The science of credentialing scientists. *Clinical Lab Products.* 2006.

14. Hopper C: Memory Principles. In Hopper C: *Practicing college learning strategies.* Boston, 2007, Houghton Mifflin.

15. Huitt W: Bloom et al's taxonomy of the cognitive domain, *Educational Psychology Interactive.* Valdosta, Ga, 2004, Valdosta State University.

16. Kizlik R, (2009): Effective study skills: How to study and make the most of your time. Retrieved June 13, 2009 from http://www.adprima.com/studyout.htm

17. Kruger J, Wirtz D, Miller DT: Counterfactual thinking and the first instinct fallacy. *Journal of Personality and Social Psychology,* 88:725, 2005.

18. Landsberger J, (2009): Study Guides and Strategies: Overcoming test anxiety. Retrieved June 14, 2009, http://www.studygs.net/tstprp8.htm

19. Landsberger J, (2009): Study Guides and Strategies: Multiple choice tests. Retrieved June 14, 2009, http://www.studygs.net/tsttak3.htm

20. Landsberger J, (2009): Study Guides and Strategies: Organizing for test-taking. Retrieved June 14, 2009, http://www.studygs.net/tstprp6.htm

21. Landsberger J, (2009): Study Guides and Strategies: Time management. Retrieved June 13, 2009, http://www.studygs.net/timman.htm

22. Louisiana State Board of Medical Examiners, (2009): Licensure > Clinical Laboratory Personnel. Retrieved June 12, 2009, http://www.lsbme.la.gov/ClinicalLaboratoryPersonnel.htm

23. Madsen Myers K, Certification, professional competency, and licensure. *NAACLS News.* 87,4–7 Chicago: NAACLS, 2004.

24. Martin D, (1991): How to be a successful student. Retrieved June 13, 2009, http://www.marin.cc.ca.us/~don/study/2positive.html

25. National Center for Competency Testing, (2009): Value of Competency Testing. Retrieved June 12, 2009, http://www.ncctinc.com/Documents/valueofcompetencytesting_0.pdf

26. National Center for Competency Testing, (2009): Certification Types. Retrieved June 12, 2009, http://www.ncctinc.com/Certifications/CertificationTypes.aspx

27. National Healthcare Association, (2009): Certified Phlebotomy Technician. Retrieved June 12, 2009, http://www.acacert.com

28. National Credentialing Agency for Laboratory Personnel, (2009): Tips and Guidance. Retrieved June 13, 2009, http://www.nca-info.org/study/materials.asp

29. National Phlebotomy Association, (2009): A Non-Profit Organization for Education and Certification of Phlebotomists. Retrieved June 13, 2009, http://professional.captus.com/npa/default.htm

30. Netwind Learning Center, (2009): A+ certification test-taking tips. Retrieved June 14, 2009, http://www.netwind.com/html/a-test-taking.html

31. Peale N. *The power of positive thinking.* New York, 1952, Simon and Schuster.

32. Shippensburg University, (2008): Learning center: Study skills: Tips for taking multiple choice exams. Retrieved June 14, 2009, http://webspace.ship.edu/learning/studyskills/MC%20Exam%20Tips.pdf

33. Social Psychology Network, (2009): Tips on taking multiple choice tests. Retrieved June 14, 2009, http://www.socialpsychology.org/testtips.htm#preparing

34. Suite101.com, (2006): Study Break Tips for Exam Week. Retrieved June 13, 2009, http://collegeuniversity.suite101.com/article.cfm/healthy_procrastination_habits_

CONTENTS

INTRODUCTION TO PHLEBOTOMY

Pamela Primrose

INTRODUCTION

Phlebotomy is the practice of drawing blood. The term phlebotomy is a Greek derivative of *"phlebotomas"* or phlebot—meaning vein—and -otomy, meaning to make an incision or cut. The modern phlebotomist is a trained professional with a wide variety of job skills and personal characteristics, including communication skills, organizational skills, and compassion. After initial training, the phlebotomist may become certified by one or more professional organizations. Continuing education courses keep the phlebotomist up-to-date on the latest changes in techniques and regulations in the field. The phlebotomist must also be aware of important legal issues, including patient confidentiality and informed consent.

CONTENT OVERVIEW

Modern Phlebotomy

I. Job skills
   A. Technical phlebotomy skills
   B. Highly organized
   C. Detail oriented
   D. Interpersonal skills
   E. Able to handle stress
II. Job duties
   A. Correctly and positively identify the patient.
   B. Choose the appropriate equipment for obtaining the sample.
   C. Select and prepare the site for collection.
   D. Collect the sample, ensuring patient comfort and safety.
   E. Label the sample correctly and transport it to the lab in a timely manner, using appropriate handling procedures.
   F. Public relations—liaison between the lab and patients, visitors, staff
   G. Beyond these responsibilities, phlebotomists must also:
      1. Adhere to all safety regulations.
      2. Effectively interact with both patients and health care professionals.
      3. Keep accurate records and be knowledgeable about the computer operations of the lab.
      4. Develop other health care skills.
III. Personal characteristics
   A. Dependability—on time, minimal absences, completes tasks efficiently
   B. Honesty and integrity—admission of errors
   C. Positive attitude—patients, co-workers, others
   D. Empathy and compassion—sensitive to needs, reassuring
   E. Professional detachment—balance of sympathy, understanding, and professional distance
   F. Professional appearance—clean, conservative
   G. Assertiveness—express needs without violation of others
   H. Interpersonal skills—verbal/nonverbal communication and listening skills
   I. Telephone skills—prompt, accurate recording, reporting, and receiving messages

Professional Organizations and Standards

I. Accreditation or approval from a professional organization
   A. Administration of program meets and documents established requirements
      1. Classroom experiences
      2. Clinical experiences
   B. National agencies granting accreditation or approval
      1. American Allied Health Professionals (AAAHP)
      2. American Medical Technologists (AMT)
      3. American Society of Phlebotomy (ASPT)
      4. National Accrediting Agency for Clinical Laboratory Sciences (NAACLS)
      5. National Healthcareer Association (NHA)
      6. National Phlebotomy Association (NPA)
      7. State accreditation
         a. California
         b. Louisiana
II. Certification
   A. Individual has demonstrated proficiency in a particular area of practice

B. Certification examination agencies
  1. AAHP
  2. AMT
  3. ASPT
  4. NPA
  5. ACA—American Certification Agency for Healthcare Professionals
  6. ASCP—American Society for Clinical Pathology
  7. NHA—National Healthcareer Association
III. Licensure
  A. Permit that grants the bearer permission to perform a particular service or procedure.
  B. Requirements of education and experience meet standards set by licensing agency
  C. Examinations
    1. State licensure examination
    2. National certification examination
      a. Accepted in lieu of the state licensure examination
      b. Given *reciprocity* by some states— state accepts license from another state as valid without reexamination or accepts successful completion of a national examination in lieu of a state examination
  D. States requiring phlebotomy licensure
    1. California—first state to require licensure of phlebotomists
    2. Louisiana
    3. Nevada
      a. Phlebotomists classified as laboratory assistant in licensed clinical lab
        i. 6 months' training in licensed lab or certification by ASCP or AMT
      b. Phlebotomists classified as office assistant in physician's office
        i. Physician signs off on licensure application form only
IV. Continuing education
  A. Maintain a certain number of continuing education units to remain certified
  B. Provide update on new information and refresh skills used less frequently
  C. Programs
    1. Onsite at health care facility
    2. Professional agencies: ASCP, AMT, ASCLS, ASPT, NPA
V. Professional organizations—disseminate information to professionals and provide continuing education opportunities.

A. Journals
B. Workshops
C. Seminars
VI. The California Plan
  A. Educational requirements specific for state
  B. Certification examination agency approved by state

Legal Issues in Phlebotomy
I. Informed consent and the patient
  A. Information on treatments and their risks
  B. Understands treatments and their risks
  C. Agrees to procedure
  D. Right to refuse any medical treatment or procedure—informed nonconsent
  E. Types of consent
    1. Expressed consent—verbal and/or written
    2. Implied consent—by action; emergency situations when unable to give consent
    3. Consent of minors—requires parental consent; guardian consent
      a. Exception is emancipated minor
      b. State laws delineate rights of minors in health care matters
    4. HIV consent—typically patient signature is required
      a. Purpose, meaning, use, limitations
II. Confidentiality
  A. Never discuss patients with co-workers not involved in patients' treatment.
  B. Health Insurance Portability and Accountability Act (HIPAA) covers privacy of protected health information (PHI)

CERTIFICATION PREPARATION QUESTIONS

1. The first state to enact legislation mandating licensure of all phlebotomists:
   a. Louisiana
   b. Tennessee
   c. Florida
   d. California

2. Visible signs of professionalism include:
   a. Multiple earrings in each ear
   b. Well-groomed and conservative hairstyle
   c. Excessive body art
   d. Obscured employee identification badge

3. Maintaining confidentiality includes all of the following *except*:
   a. Logging off the computer
   b. Discussion of patients in the hallway
   c. Discussion of patients on need-to-know basis
   d. Filing patient records

4. The role of the phlebotomist includes public relations and involves which of the following?
   a. Being a liaison between the laboratory and the patients, visitors, and staff
   b. Promoting good public relations between the laboratory and patients, visitors, and staff
   c. Executing phlebotomy procedures with knowledge, skills, and professional patient interaction
   d. All of the above

5. Phlebotomy duties include which of the following?
   a. LIS maintenance
   b. Give injections
   c. Start intravenous (IV) lines
   d. Transport specimens to the laboratory

6. Agency or agencies that approve(s) phlebotomy training programs:
   a. American Association of Allied Health Professionals (AAAHP)
   b. National Accrediting Agency for Clinical Laboratory Sciences (NAACLS)
   c. American Society for Clinical Laboratory Science (ASCLS)
   d. Clinical and Laboratory Standards Institute (CLSI)

7. The documentation of workshop/conference participation required to demonstrate current knowledge in the field and renew certification is called:
   a. Registration/certification
   b. Standard essentials
   c. Continuing education units
   d. Reciprocity

8. Proper telephone etiquette includes all of the following *except*:
   a. Answering the phone promptly
   b. Recording information and verbally verifying it
   c. Requesting the caller to call back later
   d. Speaking slowly and clearly

9. The term "phlebotomy" is derived from the Greek word *"phlebotomas"* that literally means:
   a. Draw blood from vessels
   b. Cut a vein
   c. Puncture an arterial vessel
   d. Remove a portion of the vein

10. Job skills required in phlebotomy include:
    a. Technical skill
    b. Interpersonal skills
    c. Organizational skills
    d. All of the above

11. Reciprocity refers to:
    a. Recognition and acceptance of licensure granted by another state
    b. Reexamination using the same examination from state to state
    c. Governing medical practice acts
    d. Conforming to a specified standard

12. When answering a phone call the phlebotomist must adhere to telephone etiquette, which includes all of the following *except*:
    a. Maintaining patient confidentiality
    b. Identifying the department and self
    c. Complying with the institution's protocols
    d. Never taking a message, always giving an answer

13. Continuing education is important for phlebotomists and other health care professionals for purposes of all of the following *except*:
    a. Receiving updates on new information, regulations, and techniques
    b. Validating competencies
    c. Refreshing skills used infrequently or learning new skills
    d. Meeting recertification or relicensure requirements

14. The difference between certification and licensure is:
    a. Certification and licensure both document evidence of proficiency and grant permission to perform a service or procedure
    b. Certification grants permission to perform a service or procedure, whereas licensure documents evidence of proficiency in practice

c. Licensure grants permission to perform a service or procedure, whereas certification documents evidence of proficiency in practice
d. Only certification addresses both documentation of proficiency and granting permission to perform a service or procedure

15. The *primary* responsibility of the phlebotomist is to:
    a. Collect blood specimens
    b. Input physician orders into the laboratory computer
    c. Perform waived testing
    d. Assign accession number and process all specimens

16. Personal characteristics of a phlebotomist should include all of the following *except*:
    a. Professional detachment
    b. Assertiveness
    c. Honesty and integrity
    d. Aggressiveness

ANSWERS AND RATIONALES

1. **Answer: D**
   Rationale: California established a set of state regulations that governed the education, training, and licensure of phlebotomists. A phlebotomist is able to apply to the state for licensure to practice phlebotomy once the state educational requirements are met.
   Text Reference: pp. 6-8

2. **Answer: B**
   Rationale: First impressions are the ones remembered. Appearance is a significant factor in a phlebotomist as viewed by the patient, co-workers, and the public.
   Text Reference: p. 5

3. **Answer: B**
   Rationale: Confidentiality includes keeping all patient records and information protected from unauthorized persons. On leaving a workstation, all health care workers must log off. Discussion of patient information should only be done between persons involved in the direct care of the patient on a need-to-know basis. These conversations should

never occur in hallways, elevators, waiting rooms, cafeterias, etc.
Text Reference: pp. 8-9

4. **Answer: D**
   Rationale: All of the above is the correct answer. The phlebotomist is often the first and only person patients see from the laboratory. The impression left by the phlebotomist may extend to the entire facility and the quality of care received during that time.
   Text Reference: p. 3

5. **Answer: D**
   Rationale: The duties of the phlebotomist vary depending on where they are employed. Primary responsibilities of the phlebotomist include blood draws and transportation of specimens to the laboratory. Other responsibilities may include taking blood pressures, collecting nonblood specimens, instructing patients on how to collect nonblood specimens, point-of-care testing, quality control procedures, and maintenance on point-of-care instruments. It is not in the phlebotomist job description to start intravenous (IV) lines, give injections, or perform LIS maintenance. Computer operations would include logging specimens, making labels, registering patients, etc.
   Text Reference: p. 4

6. **Answer: B**
   Rationale: American Society for Clinical Laboratory Science (ASCLS) is a professional organization for laboratory personnel. The National Accrediting Agency for Clinical Laboratory Sciences (NAACLS) accredits or approves training programs. The Clinical and Laboratory Standards Institute (CLSI) develops standards and guidelines for use in clinical and laboratory testing. The American Association of Allied Health Professionals (AAAHP) certifies phlebotomists.
   Text Reference: p. 7

7. **Answer: C**
   Rationale: Workshops and seminars are offered by professional agencies at various conferences and through online continuing education program subscriptions. Many employers also provide onsite continuing education programs to provide health care

workers opportunities to earn credits required for renewal of certifications and licenses. Continuing education credits are awarded for each event attended or each online study completed. Copies of records for continuing education credits can be sent to certifying agencies as proof of continuing education.
Text Reference: p. 6

8. **Answer: C**
Rationale: Phone calls should be answered promptly. One should speak slowly and clearly, accurately recording information, and verbally restating it for verification. Callers should never be told to call back later. If the information requested is not available or an answer is not readily available, the caller should be informed that will receive a return call as soon as possible.
Text Reference: p. 5

9. **Answer: B**
Rationale: The literal translation of *"phlebotomas"* means opening or cutting a vein.
Text Reference: p. 3

10. **Answer: D**
Rationale: A wide variety of job skills is required in phlebotomy and includes technical, interpersonal, and organizational skills.
Text Reference: p. 3

11. **Answer: A**
Rationale: Reciprocity refers to the state process whereby a professional license obtained in one state may be accepted as being valid for practice in another state. The practice of reciprocity exists per agreement between states and does not require reexamination. It also refers to the state granting petitioners a license on successful completion of a national examination in lieu of a required state examination.
Text Reference: p. 6

12. **Answer: D**
Rationale: All laboratory personnel, including the phlebotomist, are to identify themselves and their departments on answering the telephone. Compliance with the institution's protocols for phone calls, along with

protecting patient confidentiality, are vitally important. If the phlebotomist does not know the answer to the question and cannot place the caller on hold then a message must be taken, along with caller identification and the phone number for a call-back if necessary.
Text Reference: p. 5

13. **Answer: B**
Rationale: Continuing education allows phlebotomists to receive updates on new information, regulations, and techniques and to refresh skills that are not routinely used or learn new skills. In addition, many certification and/or licensure agencies now require the completion of a specified number of continuing education hours within a specified time period to maintain certification or licensure.
Text Reference: p. 6

14. **Answer: C**
Rationale: Certification is evidence that an individual has demonstrated proficiency in a specified area of practice. Licensure is a documented permit that is issued by a government agency, municipality, or state that grants permission to perform a service or procedure.
Text Reference: p. 6

15. **Answer: A**
Rationale: The principal function of a phlebotomist is to obtain blood specimens per the physician's request for clinical analysis in the laboratory.
Text Reference: p. 3

16. **Answer: D**
Rationale: Phlebotomists need to be honest and have great integrity. They should be connected to their patients through empathy and compassion but should maintain a proper modicum of professional detachment so as not to become emotionally involved with their patients. Assertiveness is necessary when working in stressful environments where everyone is overloaded. Although a fine line may distinguish between assertive and aggressive behavior, aggressiveness may embody tones of hostility that have no place in health care.
Text Reference: pp. 4-5

HEALTH CARE STRUCTURE

Pamela Primrose

INTRODUCTION

Although phlebotomists may be employed in a variety of health care settings, including health maintenance organizations, clinics, urgent care centers, nursing homes, or physician office laboratories, most phlebotomists work in the hospital clinical laboratory. The various departments within the clinical laboratory are all involved in the analysis of patient samples, whether they are blood, urine, or other body fluids or tissues. All clinical labs must meet standards set by a variety of national organizations to be certified.

CONTENT OVERVIEW

Hospital Organization

The medical staff is overseen by the chief of staff, and the central administration of the hospital is the responsibility of the hospital administrator. There are four branches of support personnel:

I.   Fiscal services
   A. Admissions
   B. Medical records
   C. Billing
   D. Accounting
   E. Other financial aspects
II. Support services—physical plant
   A. Cleaning
   B. Maintenance
   C. Security
   D. Food service
   E. Purchasing
   F. Human resources
III. Nursing services
   A. Direct patient care
   B. Titles of nursing staff
     1. RN—BS or associate degree
     2. LPN—technical certificate
     3. CNA—career development certificate—customized training
     4. PCT/PCA—usually CNA certification plus additional skills
     5. Ward clerk or unit secretary

C. Hospital departments—dependent on size of hospital
     1. ER—emergency department
     2. OR—operating room
     3. ICU—intensive care unit
     4. CCU—coronary care unit
     5. Nursery—newborns
     6. Pediatrics—discharged newborns returning due to illness, children, teens
     7. Labor and delivery
     8. Nephrology—renal
     9. Inpatient floors—medical, surgical, psychiatric
     10. Other—gastroenterology, oncology, orthopedics, etc.
IV. Professional services
   A. Includes departments that provide specialized services at physician request such as:
     1. Pharmacy—prepare and dispense drugs
     2. Physical therapy—physical treatment for rehabilitation after injury or illness
     3. Occupational therapy—adaptive aids or compensatory strategies for daily living for people with physical or mental impairment
     4. Respiratory therapy—respiratory disorders
     5. Radiology—radiographs, CT scans, MRI scans, PET scans, fluoroscopy
     6. Nuclear medicine—radioisotopes often used as tracers to perform tests and treat disease
     7. Radiation therapy—x-rays or high energy radiation to treat cancer
     8. Clinical laboratory
       a. Anatomic and surgical pathology—analyzes cells and tissues
       b. Clinical pathology—analyzes blood and body fluids

Introduction to the Clinical Laboratory

I.   Personnel
   A. Pathologist—physician who heads up the laboratory and analyzes tissues and fluids.
   B. Laboratory manager—directs administrative functions of lab

C. Manager of information services (MIS)—manages all information
D. Laboratory information services (LIS) coordinator—manages laboratory computer information—interfaces, reporting, errors, etc.
E. Section supervisor—supervises personnel, monitors instrument/equipment maintenance and test results
F. Medical laboratory scientist (MLS) (BS degree)—runs analyses; new designation for MT/CLS is MLS
G. Medical technologists (MTs) (BS degree)—run analyses same as MLS but MT is the older designation for those who were registered prior to 2004, and is the current designation for other certification agencies such as AMT
H. Medical laboratory technicians (MLTs) (associate's degree)—runs analyses
I. Phlebotomists (certification)—collects specimens for analysis
J. Note: Medical technologists who were certified by ASCP prior to 2004 are not required to participate in a certification maintenance program. If they do not participate their credential will remain MT (ASCP). If they do complete a certification maintenance program their designation changes to MLS (ASCP)^{CM}. This does not affect those who are certified as MT by AMT.

II. Departments of the anatomic and surgical pathology area
A. Cytology
  1. Processes and stains cells in body fluid or tissue
  2. Examines for cancer cells or other disease
B. Histology
  1. Prepares tissue samples from autopsy, surgery, or biopsy
  2. Stains slides for pathology review of cellular morphology
C. Cytogenetics
  1. Examines chromosomes for evidence of genetic disease

Departments and Functions of the Clinical Pathology Laboratory

I. Hematology
A. Analyzes blood for evidence of diseases affecting the blood-forming tissues and the cells produced by those tissues
B. Includes tests for diagnosis of leukemia, anemia, infections, genetic diseases of blood (i.e., sickle cell anemia, etc.) (see Tables 2-1 and 2-2 on page 15 of textbook)
  1. CBC
  2. Sickle cell test

II. Flow cytometry
A. Identifies cellular markers on the surface of WBCs
B. Determines lymphocyte subclasses on AIDS patients—CD4/DC8 ratios—to track health of patients
C. Classifies malignancies to aid in treatment plans

III. Coagulation and hemostasis—sometimes housed within hematology
A. Measures clotting factors and platelets
B. Performs tests on citrated plasma
C. Diagnoses a variety of clotting disorders (i.e., hemophilia)
D. Monitors anticoagulation therapy of stroke, heart attack, thrombophlebitis patients
E. Includes two primary tests (see Box 2-1 on page 16 in textbook)
  1. APTT—monitors heparin therapy
  2. PT—monitors warfarin (Coumadin) therapy

IV. Chemistry
A. Tests chemical components of blood
B. Uses small amounts of blood for testing on automated, advanced, and complex instrumentation
C. Monitors amount of blood drawn for patients requiring frequent blood analysis
D. Includes the examples of chemistry tests listed in Table 2-3, page 17 of the textbook
  1. Basic metabolic panels (BMPs)
  2. Chem 7
  3. Renal panels
  4. Glucose

V. Sections in chemistry
A. Electrophoresis
  1. Separates chemical components of blood
  2. Analyzes hemoglobin, enzymes, other proteins
B. Toxicology
  1. Analyzes plasma levels for drugs and poisons
  2. Therapeutic drug monitoring
  3. Identifies illegal drugs
  4. Detects lead and other toxic substances
C. Immunochemistry
  1. Uses antibody testing to identify a wide range of substances in blood such as thyroid function, cardiac and cancer markers, fertility/reproductive markers, etc.

a. RIA—radioimmunoassay
   i. Antibody linked to radioactive molecule
b. EIA—enzyme immunoassay
   i. Antibody linked to an enzyme

VI. Specimen collection for chemistry
   A. Serum
      1. Clear red-top
      2. Red-top
      3. SST
      4. Red/gray
      5. Orange
      6. Gray/yellow
   B. Plasma
      1. Sodium or lithium heparin
      2. Sodium fluoride
      3. EDTA (*toxicology*)
      4. Sodium citrate
      5. ACD
   C. Terms associated with serum/plasma
      1. Icteric—dark yellow due to bilirubin
      2. Lipemic—cloudy due to fats/lipids
      3. Hemolyzed—pink to red tinge due to breakage of RBCs

VII. Microbiology—bacteriology
   A. Culture and sensitivity (C & S) of pathogenic organisms
   B. Specimens include blood, urine, throat swabs, sputum, feces, body fluids, wounds
   C. Other departments with microbiology
      1. Mycology—study of fungi
      2. Parasitology—study of parasites
      3. Virology—study of viruses

VIII. Urinalysis and clinical microscopy
   A. Assesses kidney disease and metabolic disorders (i.e., UTIs, damage from diabetes, etc.)
   B. Includes urinalysis—physical, chemical, and microscopic analyses of urine; tests are as listed in Table 2-4, page 18 of textbook.

IX. Serology or immunology
   A. Evaluates immune responses through detection of antibodies (proteins) that bind to antigens (infective agent)
   B. Includes RPR, rheumatoid factor, C-reactive protein, and among others, as listed in Table 2-5, page 18 of textbook.

X. Blood bank or Immunohematology
   A. Performs testing on blood for transfusions using plain red-top and EDTA tube (purple or pink)
      1. Blood type—ABO, Rh (others)
         a. Identify antigens on surface of patient and donor RBCs
      2. Compatibility testing—no clumping of RBCs in testing of patients serum and donor cells
   B. Prepares blood from *autologous donations* (self-donations) for patients to use during their own surgery
   C. Performs Coombs test (DAT) direct antigen test on newborns—assess risk of hemolyestic disease of the newborn
   D. Processes donated blood into components
      1. Packed cells—RBSs, WBCs, platelets without plasma
      2. Fresh frozen plasma—factor deficiencies, plasma exchange, limited usage
      3. Platelets—patients with bleeding or platelet disorders
      4. Cryoprecipitate—patients with clotting disorders

XI. Molecular diagnostics (cytogenics)
   A. Performs genetic and biochemical techniques
      1. Diagnoses genetic disorders
      2. Analyzes forensic evidence
      3. Tracks disease
      4. Identifies microbiologic pathogens
      5. Analyzes chromosomal DNA at the molecular level
   B. Analyzes DNA in blood, body fluids, skin, hair, other body tissues
   C. Requires special tubes and handling to keep free from contamination
   D. Includes tests for HIV, cystic fibrosis, paternity

XII. Phlebotomy—Refer to Chapter 1, Content Overview

XIII. Referrals
   A. Handles and ships tests not performed at laboratory to a reference lab, an independent lab that analyzes specimens from other health care facilities
   B. Includes newer tests and those requiring special equipment/instrumentation
   C. Provides information for physicians' inquiries

Standards and Accreditation for the Clinical Laboratory

I. Clinical Lab Improvement Act 1988 (CLIA '88)

A. Mandates regulation of all facilities performing patient testing
II. Clinical and Laboratory Standards Institute (CLSI) formerly known as National Committee for Clinical Laboratory Standards (NCCLS)
   A. Sets standards and guidelines for all testing
   B. All labs performing patient testing are required to have a CLIA certificate valid for 2 years (four types)
      1. Certificate of waiver for waived tests (8 waived tests) (i.e., performed in physicians' offices)
      2. Certificate for moderately complex testing and waived tests
      3. Certificate for moderately complex testing, complex testing, and waived testing
      4. Registration certificate or interim certificate allows labs to test until HCFA can judge lab's compliance and then issue full-fledged certificate
   C. Labs must meet standards to be eligible for accreditation of laboratory
III. The Joint Commission
   A. Evaluates laboratories every 2 years for accreditation
   B. Accredits other health care facilities and entities
IV. College of American Pathologists (CAP)
   A. Inspects and accredits labs every 2 years
   B. Provides proficiency testing programs for laboratories

Other Health Care Settings
I.   HMO (health maintenance organization)
II. PPO (preferred provider organization)
III. Urgent care centers
IV. POL (physician office lab)
V.   Reference laboratory
VI. Nursing home

CERTIFICATION PREPARATION QUESTIONS

1. A clinical laboratory worker who has completed a 4-year degree in the field of clinical laboratory sciences.
   a. Medical laboratory technician
   b. Medical laboratory scientist
   c. Clinical laboratory technician
   d. Phlebotomist

2. The laboratory is typically overseen by a (an):
   a. Hospital administrator
   b. Chief of staff
   c. Assistant administrator
   d. Pathologist

3. The department that uses x-rays and other high-energy radiation versus radioisotopes for the treatment of cancer is:
   a. Respiratory therapy
   b. Nuclear medicine
   c. Radiation therapy
   d. Radiology

4. The hospital organization branch that provides services at the request of the physician that aid in the diagnosis and treatment of patients:
   a. Professional services
   b. Nursing services
   c. Support services
   d. Fiscal services

5. Support services are responsible for:
   a. Nursing personnel
   b. Laboratory personnel
   c. Admissions and medical records
   d. Cleaning, maintenance, security, food service

6. A patient in need of supportive oxygen therapy would require the services of:
   a. Occupational therapy
   b. Respiratory therapy
   c. Pharmacy
   d. Physical therapy

7. The professional service that helps to prepare a patient recovering from a stroke to be able to return to their home:
   a. Physical therapy
   b. Nursing services
   c. Occupational therapy
   d. Support services

8. A patient coming to the hospital for a prescribed *treatment* of a cancerous tumor would report to:
   a. Physical therapy
   b. Radiation therapy
   c. Respiratory therapy
   d. Nursing services

9. A patient suffers an MI at a large metropolitan hospital and is admitted to which department within the hospital?
   a. ICU
   b. CCU
   c. PEDS
   d. ECG

10. A newborn baby who you had previously performed a capillary puncture on for newborn screening before discharge has been readmitted to the hospital and needs a blood draw. You will find this newborn in which hospital division?
   a. Medical
   b. Pediatrics
   c. Nursery
   d. ER

11. The phlebotomist has orders to draw a K^+ on a patient awaiting dialysis and proceeds to the following division:
   a. Nephrology
   b. Medical
   c. Pneumonology
   d. Nuclear medicine

12. The *main* division of the laboratory that analyzes cells and tissues is:
   a. Clinical pathology
   b. Anatomic and surgical pathology
   c. Clinical laboratory
   d. Clinical microscopy

13. Departments of clinical pathology include all of the following *except*:
   a. Immunology
   b. Molecular diagnostics
   c. Cytogenics
   d. Referrals

14. The phlebotomist works in which *division* of the clinical laboratory?
   a. Anatomic/surgical area
   b. Outpatient center
   c. Urgent care center
   d. Clinical pathology

15. The basic purpose of the hematology department:
   a. Chemical analysis of blood
   b. Analysis of the formed elements of the blood

   c. Analysis of cellular markers on WBCs
   d. Analysis of metabolic disorders of the blood

16. The basic purpose of the chemistry department:
   a. Analysis of the chemical components of the blood
   b. Process and stain cells in body fluids or tissue samples
   c. Examine chromosomes for evidence of genetic disease
   d. Identify pathogenic microorganisms in patient samples

17. The phlebotomist returns to the lab with a specimen for cross-match or compatibility testing and delivers it to:
   a. Immunochemistry
   b. Molecular diagnostics
   c. Immunohematology
   d. Immunology

18. The clinical laboratory is usually but not always under the supervision of a(an):
   a. Pathologist
   b. Director of nursing
   c. MLS/MT supervisor
   d. HMO

19. A blood bank is also referred to as:
   a. Immunohematology
   b. Immunology
   c. Serology
   d. Hematology

20. This test will be delivered to immunology for testing:
   a. CBC
   b. BUN
   c. RPR
   d. AST

21. The phlebotomist has received a specimen for chromosomal studies and delivers it to which laboratory department:
   a. Immunochemistry
   b. Molecular diagnostics
   c. Cytology
   d. Cytogenics

22. Coagulation testing includes which of the following?

a. CBC
b. PTT
c. BNP
d. ALT

23. You are a phlebotomist in a small rural hospital and have just returned to the lab with a STAT specimen for electrolyte analysis. Which department will you deliver the specimen to?
a. Hematology
b. Immunology
c. Immunochemistry
d. Chemistry

24. The phlebotomist has just completed centrifuging specimens for the chemistry department and notes that one of the tubes is cloudy and pinkish-red. This specimen is:
a. Icteric
b. Lipemic and icteric
c. Lipemic and hemolyzed
d. Hemolyzed and icteric

25. The phlebotomist is processing specimens received for lead testing and is preparing them to be delivered to which department?
a. Toxicology
b. Chemistry
c. Immunochemistry
d. Electrophoresis

26. The chemistry department is made up of all of the following department sections *except*:
a. Electrophoresis
b. Immunochemistry
c. Toxicology
d. Flow cytometry

27. The phlebotomist returns to the laboratory with a CBC and delivers it to:
a. Chemistry
b. Cytology
c. Immunology
d. Hematology

28. The required specimen for the occult blood test is:
a. Serum
b. Feces

c. Plasma
d. Synovial fluid

29. The phlebotomist is drawing which of the following tests for a patient being screened for diabetes mellitus?
a. BUN
b. Micro-albumin
c. Glucose
d. Hemoglobin

30. A newborn is born with severe anemia and the phlebotomist has collected a specimen for a direct antibody test (Coombs) to be delivered immediately to:
a. Hematology
b. Blood bank/immunohematology
c. Serology/immunology
d. Urinalysis

31. The phlebotomist is working in specimen processing and has received a wound culture. The specimen will be placed in the tray that will be delivered to:
a. Chemistry
b. Hematology
c. Microbiology
d. Serology

32. This department performs CT, MRI, and PET scans:
a. Occupational therapy
b. Radiology
c. Pharmacy
d. Respiratory therapy

33. You have an order for a maternal panel that includes ABO Rh blood typing that will be performed in:
a. Blood bank
b. Hematology
c. Immunology
d. Coagulation

34. The phlebotomist collected a STAT D-dimer on a patient in open-heart recovery and will deliver it for immediate testing to:
a. Blood bank
b. Immunology
c. Coagulation
d. Chemistry

35. While working the second shift, a courier drops off several PAP smears to be examined for the presence of canceous cells. You will log these specimens in and deliver them to:
    a. Histology
    b. Hematology
    c. Flow cytometry
    d. Cytology

36. Urinalysis testing includes all of the following *except*:
    a. Physical
    b. Microscopic
    c. Chemical
    d. Volume

37. A physician calls the laboratory requesting the procedure for a patient who wishes to donate his own blood before his surgery. This type of donation is known as:
    a. Heterogeneous donation
    b. Autologous donation
    c. Homogeneous donation
    d. Xenogenous donation

38. Blood and body fluid testing is performed in which *division* of the laboratory?
    a. Cytology and chemistry
    b. Anatomic/surgical and clinical pathology
    c. Clinical pathology
    d. Chemistry and hematology

39. A health maintenance organization (HMO):
    a. Does not employ phlebotomists
    b. Functions as a full-service outpatient clinic
    c. Provides walk-in services, no appointments
    d. Functions as an independent laboratory analyzing samples from other labs

40. The phlebotomist is working in specimen processing and notices that one of the specimens is a dark yellow color after centrifugation and states that the specimen is:
    a. Icteric
    b. Lipemic
    c. Hemolyzed
    d. Clear

41. The most common microbiology tests are:
    a. Culture and sensitivity (C & S)
    b. Throat cultures
    c. PT/PTT
    d. Ova and parasite (O & P)

42. Electrolytes is a commonly ordered test and includes all of the following *except*:
    a. K^+
    b. Cl^-
    c. Ca^{++}
    d. Na^+

43. Standards and guidelines for laboratory patient testing are set forth by:
    a. CLIA
    b. CLSI
    c. JCAHO
    d. CAP

44. Accreditation of laboratories is a function of which of the following?
    a. CLSI and JCAHO
    b. JCAHO and CAP
    c. CAP and CLIA
    d. CLIA and CLSI

45. Phlebotomists may be employed in a variety of health care settings that include all of the following *except*:
    a. POL
    b. PCT
    c. Urgent Care Centers
    d. PPO

46. The Clinical Lab Improvement Act of 1988 functions to:
    a. Provide a set of standards for accreditation of laboratories
    b. Mandate regulations of all facilities that performs patient testing
    c. Analyze samples from other health care facilities through a network of labs
    d. Provide laboratory inspections for accreditation every 2 years

47. The phlebotomist is called to the ER for blood work on a patient suspected of having an MI. One test that will most likely be drawn is:
    a. Bilirubin
    b. RA
    c. Troponin
    d. Retic

48. In order for a laboratory to receive Medicare and Medicaid reimbursement, the laboratory must be:
    a. Licensed
    b. Approved

c. Accredited
d. Registered

49. The analysis of DNA samples is performed in:
    a. Cytology
    b. Flow cytometry
    c. Clinical microscopy
    d. Molecular diagnostics

50. Mycology is the study of:
    a. Bacteria
    b. Parasites
    c. Viruses
    d. Fungi

ANSWERS AND RATIONALES

1. **Answer: B**
   Rationale: The educational requirement for the medical technologist (MT) and the medical laboratory scientist (MLS) is a 4-year bachelor of science degree. The title depends on which national certification examination was taken and passed (i.e., the AMT examination confers the MT title and ASCP confers the MLS title). The MT designation was conferred by ASCP prior to October 2009.
   Text Reference: p. 14

2. **Answer: D**
   Rationale: The laboratory is typically overseen by a pathologist. The pathologist is one who studies the theory or cause of disease through analysis of tissues and fluids and may also oversee the clinical laboratory. The hospital administrator oversees the four branches of support personnel. Each of these branches is overseen by an assistant administrator.
   Text Reference: p. 13-14

3. **Answer: C**
   Rationale: The radiation therapy department uses radiant energy to treat cancer using x-ray or high-energy radiation sources. Radiology uses various forms of radiant energy to image the internal organs and structures of the body. Respiratory therapy provides treatment for respiratory disorders. Nuclear medicine injects radioisotopes (i.e., tracers) into the blood in various test procedures and then tracks them to reveal the structure and function of internal organs.
   Text Reference: p. 13

4. **Answer: A**
   Rationale: Professional services personnel provide services at the request of physicians that aid in the diagnosis and treatment of patients. Support services include all aspects of the physical plant of the hospital. Nursing services provide direct care to all patients. Fiscal services oversee admissions, medical records, billing, accounting, and other financial aspects of the hospital.
   Text Reference: p. 13

5. **Answer: D**
   Rationale: Support services are responsible for all aspects of the physical plant, including cleaning, maintenance, security, food service, purchasing, and human resources. Nursing services provide direct care to patients. Laboratory personnel works mostly in the laboratory department, including phlebotomists. Fiscal services oversees admissions, medical records, billing, accounting and other financial aspects of the hospital.
   Text Reference: p. 13

6. **Answer: B**
   Rationale: Respiratory therapy provides treatment for those suffering from respiratory diseases. Blood gas analysis and/or breath sounds would indicate whether patients need oxygen therapy or breathing treatments.
   Text Reference: p. 13

7. **Answer: C**
   Rationale: Occupational therapists assess patients' physical or mental abilities and needs in order to design optimal adaptive aids or compensatory strategies to help them perform tasks of daily living. Physical therapy services work with patients to restore or improve function and mobility, relieve pain, and prevent or limit permanent physical disabilities.
   Text Reference: p. 13

8. **Answer: B**
   Rationale: Radiation therapy is the department that treats some forms of cancer using x-rays or other types of high radiant energy to destroy tumors. Physical therapy is

the department that assesses patients before and after treatment to devise exercises, stretching programs, and other physical treatments that aid in the rehabilitative process after injury or illness. Nursing services provide direct care to patients. Respiratory therapy provides treatment for respiratory disorders.
Text Reference: p. 13

9. **Answer: B**
Rationale: CCU is the coronary care unit within a hospital and treats patients with heart-related illnesses. ICU is the intensive care unit, which provides comprehensive and continuous care for patients who are critically ill with nonheart–related illnesses. Smaller rural hospitals may not have a CCU unit and in that case patients would be placed in the ICU. PEDS is the pediatric unit for children. ECG is the medical abbreviation for electrocardiogram, a test to record the electrical activity of the heart to aid in the diagnosis of heart disease.
Text Reference: p. 13

10. **Answer: B**
Rationale: Newborns are typically in the nursery until they are discharged. If a newborn has been released from the hospital and needs readmission they are placed in pediatrics or the pediatric ICU, not the nursery, because they have been outside in the general population and could have become contaminated with "germs." Infection control requires that those babies be isolated in peds away from the nursery. The baby has been admitted and therefore would not be found in the ER. Children are placed in pediatric divisions away from the adult population and therefore would not be admitted to the medical floor.
Text Reference: p. 13 and Outline

11. **Answer: A**
Rationale: Nephrology deals with the diagnosis and treatment of kidney disease. Patients needing dialysis suffer from severe renal failure that is permanent or potentially reversible depending on the cause. Pneumonology deals with the diagnosis and treatment of respiratory diseases. Nuclear medicine uses radioisotopes

in certain test procedures and in treatment of disease. The medical floor of a hospital houses adult patients with a wide range of diseases and complex medical diagnoses.
Text Reference: p. 13 and **Content Overview**

12. **Answer: B**
Rationale: Anatomic and surgical pathology is one of two main divisions within the clinical laboratory, the other being clinical pathology, which analyzes blood and other body fluids. The clinical laboratory is the term that encompasses both clinical pathology and anatomic and surgical pathology. Clinical microscopy is part of urinalysis and refers to any procedure that requires microscopic examination for identification.
Text Reference: pp. 14, 18

13. **Answer: C**
Rationale: Cytogenics is a subdivision of the department of anatomic and surgical pathology. Immunology, molecular diagnostics, and referrals are all departments within clinical pathology.
Text Reference: p. 14

14. **Answer: D**
Rationale: The phlebotomist works in the clinical pathology area of the clinical laboratory. Anatomic/surgical analyzes the characteristics of cells and tissues. The reference lab is an independent laboratory that analyzes samples from other health care facilities. Urgent care centers are outpatient clinics that provide walk-in services to patients who cannot wait for scheduled appointments with their primary health care providers.
Text Reference: pp. 14, 20

15. **Answer: B**
Rationale: The primary function of the hematology department is to analyze blood for evidence of diseases affecting the blood-forming tissues and the cells produced by those tissues (i.e., RBCs, WBCs, and platelets).
Text Reference: p. 14

16. **Answer: A**
Rationale: The purpose of the chemistry department is to perform a wide range of tests on the chemical components of blood. Chromosomes are analyzed in molecular

diagnostics. Microbiology isolates and identifies pathogenic organisms in various samples. Cytology processes and stains cell that are either shed in body fluids or removed from tissue via needle aspiration, etc.
Text Reference: p. 16

17. **Answer: C**
Rationale: Immunohematology or the blood bank performs compatibility testing to ensure that the patient's immune system does not reject the donor blood. Immunochemistry uses antibodies in testing procedures to detect a wide range of constituents in blood. Immunology or serology evaluates the patient's immune response through the detection of antibodies. Molecular diagnostics uses genetic and biochemical techniques to diagnose genetic disorders, analyze forensic evidence, track disease, or identify pathogenic microorganisms.
Text Reference: p. 19

18. **Answer: A**
Rationale: A pathologist is a physician who has undergone specialized training in laboratory analysis of body fluids and tissues and usually supervises the clinical laboratory. The director of nursing supervises nursing staff. The MLS/MT supervisor is usually in charge of one or more departments within the clinical laboratory or supervises a particular shift. The HMO is the major provider of health care and function as full-service outpatient clinics with many medical specialties housed in a single building.
Text Reference: p. 14

19. **Answer: A**
Rationale: The blood bank department is referred to as immunohematology and deals with blood used for transfusions. Immunology is another name for the serology department and analyzes blood for antigens and antibodies. Hematology deals with blood counts and differentiation of cell types.
Text Reference: pp. 14-19

20. **Answer: C**
Rationale: CBC is performed in hematology. BUN and AST are performed in chemistry. RPR is performed in serology/immunology.
Text Reference: pp. 15, 17

21. **Answer: D**
Rationale: Cytogenics is the department that analyzes chromosomes to diagnose genetic diseases such as trisomy Down syndrome. Molecular diagnostics is the department that uses genetic and biochemical techniques to analyze chromosomal DNA at the molecular level for diagnosis of genetic disorders (i.e., cystic fibrosis). Immunochemistry uses antibodies to detect a wide range of substances in the blood. Cytology processes and stains cells that are shed into body fluids or removed from tissues.
Text Reference: pp. 14, 19

22. **Answer: B**
Rationale: The PTT is used to assess heparin therapy and general coagulation status of a patient and is performed in the coagulation department. BNP and ALT tests are performed in the chemistry department. A CBC is performed in the hematology department.
Text Reference: p. 16, Box 2-1

23. **Answer: D**
Rationale: Electrolytes is a test for potassium (K^+), chloride (Cl^-), sodium (Na^+), and bicarbonate (HCO_3^-) that is performed in the chemistry department.
Text Reference: p. 17

24. **Answer: C**
Rationale: Icteric refers to a dark yellow appearance of serum due to the presence of bilirubin. Lipemia refers to cloudiness or turbidity due to the presence of lipids, and pink-red refers to hemolysis of RBCs.
Text Reference: p. 17

25. **Answer: A**
Rationale: Toxicology performs testing on specimens for lead and other toxic substances, poisons, and illegal drugs along with therapeutic drug monitoring.
Text Reference: p. 16

26. **Answer: D**
Rationale: Chemistry is a department that has several different department sections that include, but are not limited to, electrophoresis, immunochemistry,

and toxicology. Larger laboratories may have several other sections as well. Flow cytometry is a special analytical technique used in hematology, immunology, or in anatomic pathology to identify cell markers.
Text Reference: pp. 15-16

27. **Answer: D**
Rationale: Complete blood count (CBC) is performed in the hematology department. The chemistry department performs a wide range of tests on the chemical components of blood. Cytology processes and stains cells from body fluids and tissues. Serology or immunology evaluates the patient's immune response through the detection of antibodies and/or antigens.
Text Reference: p. 15

28. **Answer: B**
Rationale: Occult blood testing is performed on feces as a screen for colorectal cancer. Serum and plasma are both liquid portions of blood, but serum is found in nonadditive or SST blood tube after centrifugation, and plasma is found in an anticoagulant blood tube after centrifugation. Synovial fluid is found in the freely moveable or synovial joint cavity space.
Text Reference: p. 18

29. **Answer: C**
Rationale: Glucose levels are evaluated to diagnose or monitor diabetes. BUN is blood urea nitrogen and is used to assess kidney function. Micro-albumin is used to assess kidney disorders after diagnosis of diabetes mellitus or hypertension, etc. Hemoglobin determines the amount of hemoglobin in the blood as a whole and determines oxygen-carrying capacity of blood. It is useful in the diagnosis of anemia and blood loss.
Text Reference: p. 17, Table 2-3; p. 15, Table 2-1

30. **Answer: B**
Rationale: Direct antibody test (Coombs) is performed in immunohematology or the blood bank and is used to assess the risk of hemolytic anemia in newborns.

Urinalysis analyzes urine to assess kidney and metabolic diseases. Immunology evaluates the patient's immune response through the detection of antigens and antibodies. The hematology department analyzes blood for evidence of diseases affecting the blood-forming tissues.
Text Reference: p. 19

31. **Answer: C**
Rationale: Microbiology isolates and identifies pathogenic microorganisms in patient samples. Microbiology consists of the study of bacteria, fungi, parasites, and viruses. The chemistry department performs a wide range of tests on the chemical components of blood. Serology or immunology evaluates the patient's immune response through the detection of antibodies. The hematology department analyzes blood for evidence of diseases affecting the blood-forming tissues.
Text Reference: p. 18

32. **Answer: B**
Rationale: X-ray procedures and other imaging techniques such as CT, MRI, and PET scans are performed in the radiology department. The occupational therapy department assists mentally and physically disabled patients in developing adaptive or compensatory strategies to perform daily living skills. The pharmacy prepares and dispenses drugs and serves as a consultant to physicians. The respiratory therapy department aids in the treatment and management of lung disorders.
Text Reference: p. 13

33. **Answer: A**
Rationale: Blood typing and compatibility testing are performed in the blood bank or immunohematology department. The hematology department analyzes blood for evidence of diseases affecting the blood-forming tissues. The immunology department analyzes blood for antigen or antibodies to assess the patient's immune response. The coagulation department primarily monitors anticoagulant therapy (i.e., Coumadin and heparin).
Text Reference: p. 19

34. **Answer: C**
Rationale: D-Dimer testing is used to detect fibrin degradation products. This test is performed in the coagulation department and is useful in diagnosing disseminated intravascular coagulation (DIC). The chemistry department performs a wide range of tests on the chemical components of blood. The blood bank department deals with blood used for transfusions. The microbiology department isolates and identifies pathogenic microorganisms in patient samples.
Text Reference: p. 16, Box 2-1

35. **Answer: D**
Rationale: Cytology processes and stains cells that are present in body fluids or in tissue samples obtained through needle aspiration, etc. The Pap smear test is one of the most common tests performed in cytology. Hematology analyzes blood for evidence of diseases affecting the blood-forming tissues. Histology prepares tissue samples from autopsy, surgery, or biopsy procedures for microscopic examination. Flow cytometry is a specialized analytical procedure that is used to identify cellular markers on the surface of WBCs.
Text Reference: p. 14

36. **Answer: D**
Rationale: The urinalysis department is used to assess prerenal, renal, and postrenal disorders through the analysis of the physical, chemical, and microscopic components of urine. Although urine specimens are assessed for adequate volume when received into the lab for testing, this is a part of the physical assessment of the routine urinalysis test.
Text Reference: p. 18

37. **Answer: B**
Rationale: Autologous donation is the term used for patients who donate their own blood for use at a later time for themselves. The term heterogeneous refers to multiple or dissimilar constituents and thus is not a term associated with self-donation. Homogeneous is a term that refers to having common properties throughout but is not identified as coming from self-donation.

Xenogenous donation is from a source other than the patient.
Text Reference: p. 19

38. **Answer: C**
Rationale: The lab is divided into two main areas: (1) the anatomic and surgical pathology area that analyzes the characteristics of cells and tissues; (2) the clinical pathology area that analyzes blood and other body fluids.
Text Reference: p. 14

39. **Answer: B**
Rationale: An HMO is a corporation that is financed by insurance premiums, has physicians and professional staff who are affiliated with the corporation, and provides curative and preventive medicine to its members. HMOs typically function as full-service outpatient clinics.
Text Reference: p. 20

40. **Answer: A**
Rationale: The appearance of serum is normally a clear, pale-yellow fluid. Icteric refers to the dark yellow color of serum due to excess bilirubin in the blood. Lipemic refers to cloudy serum due to the presence of lipids, and hemolyzed refers to serum/plasma that is a pink- to reddish-tinged color due to ruptured RBCs.
Text Reference: p. 17

41. **Answer: A**
Rationale: The most common microbiology tests are culture and sensitivity (C & S) tests, which detect and identify microorganisms and determine the most effective antibiotic therapy.
Text Reference: p. 18

42. **Answer: C**
Rationale: Electrolytes include sodium (Na^+), potassium (K^+), chloride (Cl^-), and bicarbonate (HCO_3^-).
Text Reference: p. 17, Table 2-3

43. **Answer: B**
Rationale: The Clinical and Laboratory Standards Institute sets the standards and guidelines for patient testing. Laboratories that meet these standards are then eligible

to receive accreditation by one or more agencies such as The Joint Commission and CAP. The Clinical Lab Improvement Act of 1988 (CLIA '88) established standards for laboratory testing that serve to ensure the accuracy and reliability of patient test results and to determine if labs are meeting the standards as set forth. The Joint Commission and College of American Pathology (CAP) are two organizations that grant accreditation to laboratories.
Text Reference: p. 20

44. **Answer: B**
Rationale: The Joint Commission and CAP are both agencies involved in the accreditation of laboratories. CLSI is the agency that sets the standards and guidelines that must be met for a laboratory to be eligible for accreditation.
Text Reference: p. 20

45. **Answer: B**
Rationale: Phlebotomists may be employed in a variety of health care settings that include HMOs, PPOs, urgent care centers, POLs, reference laboratories, and nursing homes. PCT is the designation of a patient care technician.
Text Reference: pp. 12, 20

46. **Answer: B**
Rationale: CLIA '88 mandated that the regulation of all facilities that perform patient testing except human research studies come under the auspices of the Centers for Medicare & Medicaid Services (CMS). The intent and purpose were to ensure quality laboratory testing.
Text Reference: p. 20

47. **Answer: C**
Rationale: Troponin levels are drawn to assist in the determination of the occurrence and timing of when a patient may have suffered a myocardial infarction. Bilirubin is a test used to assess the overall health standard of a patient along with liver health; RA is a test used to assist in the diagnosis of rheumatoid arthritis. Retic is used to evaluate bone marrow response to various conditions that would result in decreased marrow activity.
Text Reference: pp. 15-18

48. **Answer: C**
Rationale: Accreditation is a requirement for laboratories and health care facilities to receive Medicare and Medicaid reimbursement.
Text Reference: p. 20

49. **Answer: D**
Rationale: Molecular diagnostics uses DNA samples to diagnose genetic disorders, analyze forensic evidence, track disease, etc., through the use of genetic and biochemical techniques. Cytology processes and stains cells in body fluids and tissue samples to assess the presence of cancer or other diseases. Flow cytometry identifies cellular markers on the surface of WBCs. Clinical microscopy uses various types of microscopes to examine cells and other structures.
Text Reference: pp. 14-15, 18-19

50. **Answer: D**
Rationale: Mycology is the study of fungi; bacteriology is the study of bacteria; virology is the study of viruses; and parasitology is the study of parasites.
Text Reference: p. 18

SAFETY

Pamela Primrose

INTRODUCTION

As does any workplace, a hospital or other health care facility contains certain hazards that must be treated with caution and respect to prevent injury. These hazards include biological, physical, chemical, fire, electrical, and radioactive factors. Of particular importance is exposure to blood borne pathogens from needle-stick and other sharp-related injuries. Latex sensitivity is also a growing concern in the workplace. The Occupational Safety and Health Administration (OSHA) is the governmental agency responsible for identifying occupational exposure to blood or other potentially infectious materials and developing policies and practices to minimize those risks to workers.

CONTENT OVERVIEW

Occupational Safety and Health Administration (OSHA)

I.   Develops workplace safety regulations and revises them as needed to reflect new information and hazards
   A. Informs workers about hazards in the workplace
   B. Protects workers from harm

Types of Safety Hazards

I.   Biological hazards: infectious agents such as HIV and hepatitis
   A. Follow Standard Precautions
      1. Developed by Centers for Disease Control and Prevention (CDC) to replace blood and body fluid precautions in the hospital setting
      2. Used on all patients to prevent spread of HIV and hepatitis B while providing patient care
      3. Applies to all blood, body fluids, secretions, excretions except sweat, nonintact skin, and mucous membranes
      4. Follow handwashing guidelines and use personal protective equipment (PPE)
   B. Universal precautions
      1. Applies to blood
      2. Applies to other body fluids if visibly bloody, such as semen and vaginal

secretions, but not to feces, nasal secretions, sputum, sweat, tears, urine, saliva, and vomit unless these contain visible blood or are likely to contain blood
      3. Used in daycare settings, schools, dental offices, etc.
   C. Biohazard symbol identifies biological hazards
II. Physical hazards: wet floors, heavy lifting
   A. Observe general guidelines of safety—no running, watch for wet floors
   B. Follow proper lifting techniques using legs
III. Sharps hazards: needles, lancets, broken glass
   A. Follow all OSHA bloodborne pathogen guidelines for handling and disposal of *all* sharps
   B. Adhere to mandates of Needlestick Safety and Prevention Act of 2001
      1. Switch to safety needle devices
      2. Input from nonmanagerial employees on selection of safety devices
      3. Log all needlesticks
      4. Annual review of exposure plan
      5. Fine for noncompliance
   C. Use and engage safety engineered needles, butterflies, syringes, etc., as designed
   D. Follow protocol for all blood collection procedures
   E. Follow protocol for any mucous membrane or parenteral exposure to blood or body fluids
      1. Treatment of permucosal exposures of the mouth, nose, eyes, or of intact skin
         a. Flood with water for 15 minutes
         b. Use soap on skin exposure
      2. Treatment of percutaneous or parenteral exposure (i.e., needlestick)
         a. Encourage free bleeding of puncture site
         b. Wash with warm water and soap or chlorhexidine for 15 minutes
         c. Perform first-aid treatment as needed
      3. Incident report completed immediately after completing steps 1 or 2
         a. Ensure appropriate risk management to reduce risk of blood-borne virus transmission

     b. Document incident in case of claim of occupational injury or infection

    4. Counseling regarding management of incident per institution's protocol

     a. Assessment of risk and treatment required

     b. Blood from exposed staff person and source patient for risk assessment and baseline testing

     c. Follow-up testing

IV. Chemical hazards: preservatives and reagents (laboratory-grade chemicals)

  A. OSHA Hazard Communication Standards: Employee Right to Know

    1. Hazardous materials must be labeled—*do not* use a chemical that is not labeled

     a. Warning

     b. Explanation

     c. List of precautions

     d. First-aid measures if exposed

    2. Material safety data sheets (MSDS) must be provided for each chemical and kept on file for employee review

     a. Information about chemical

     b. Hazards

     c. Procedures for cleanup

     d. First aid

  B. Department of Transportation (DOT) label

    1. Type of hazard

    2. United Nations hazard class number and identifying number

  C. The National Fire Protection Association (NFPA) label

    1. Warns of location of hazardous material in event of fire

    2. Diamond-shaped symbol with four color-coded quadrants—placed on doors, cabinets, reagent bottles

     a. Red—flammability

     b. Yellow—reactivity warning (i.e., stability of chemical)

     c. White—other

     d. Blue—health hazards

  D. Adhere to institution's chemical hygiene plan—yearly training

    1. Safety procedures—PPE

    2. Special precautions

    3. Emergency procedures used when working with chemicals

  E. Examples of exposure in phlebotomy

    1. Hydrochloric acid—urine preservative

    2. Bleach—used to disinfect counters, etc.

  F. Precautions

    1. Never mix chemicals unless following an approved protocol

    2. Store chemicals at or below eye level

    3. Always add acid to water to dissipate heat and prevent splatter

    4. Know location of safety showers and eyewash

    5. Do not try to neutralize chemicals spilled on the skin—flush with running water for minimum of 15 minutes

  G. Exposure and spills—per facility protocol

    1. Skin exposure—safety shower or eyewash for minimum of 15 minutes

    2. Chemical spill—appropriate cleanup kits to neutralize chemical

V. Radioactive or x-ray hazards: equipment and reagents

  A. Recognize the radioactive hazard symbol—yellow background, center circle, three blades

  B. Exercise extra caution in areas where radioactive materials are in use

    1. Protocol for drawing and handling blood

    2. Pregnancy—do not enter room during first trimester

  C. Learn your institution's procedures

    1. Minimize exposure—time, dose, distance

    2. Respond to accidents

VI. Electrical hazards: high-voltage equipment— shock or fire

  A. Avoid using extension cords

  B. Report frayed cords, overloaded circuits, and ungrounded equipment

  C. Unplug a piece of equipment before servicing it

  D. If a piece of equipment is marked with an electrical caution warning, do not attempt to open it—know high-voltage symbol

  E. Know the location of the circuit breaker box for the equipment you are using

  F. Avoid contact with any electrical equipment while drawing blood

  G. In event of electrical shock

    1. Do *not* touch person

    2. Shut off power and/or if possible remove source with *nonconductive* tool (i.e., wooden broom handle)

    3. Move person to safety

    4. Call for help (i.e., code blue if required, etc.)

    5. Follow-up per institution's protocol for reporting incident, etc.

VII. Fire or explosive hazards: open flames, oxygen, and chemicals—require tetrahedron comprised of heat, fuel, oxygen, and combustion.
   A. Classes of fire per NFPA—fuel source and correspond to type of fire extinguisher (see Table 3-1 on p. 29 in textbook)
      1. Type A—wood, paper, cloth
      2. Type B—grease, oil, flammable liquids
      3. Type C—electrical equipment
      4. Type D—flammable metals
      5. Type K—cooking oils and grease
   B. Minimize risk of injury in case of fire by knowing the following:
      1. Location of and how to activate the fire alarm
      2. Location of fire extinguishers and fire blankets
      3. How to use a fire extinguisher
      4. Know the locations of emergency exits
   C. Emergency action in case of a fire
      1. NFPA acronym: RACE
         a. R—Rescue and remove patients from danger
         b. A—Activate the alarm or call fire department and alert others
         c. C—Confine or contain the fire: close windows and doors
         d. E—Evacuate or extinguish fire if possible
      2. Acronym for use of a fire extinguisher: PASS
         a. P—Pull pin
         b. A—Aim at base of the fire
         c. S—Squeeze the discharge handle
         d. S—Sweep agent across the fire
VIII. MRI hazards
   A. Powerful magnet used to create images of body
   B. Warning signs—no metallic objects or patient with metallic implants in room
IX. Latex sensitivity hazards: allergic reaction to latex in gloves or other equipment
   A. FDA requires labeling of medical gloves containing natural rubber latex or powder
   B. Prevention
      1. ID bracelets
      2. Ask patients about allergies to fruits and nuts—latex-similar proteins—chestnuts, kiwi, avocado, banana
      3. Use nonlatex gloves and tourniquets
   C. Three forms of latex sensitivity
      1. Irritant contact dermatitis—caused by residue left during manufacturing process
         a. Redness, swelling, itching within minutes to hours
         b. Remove glove and wash
      2. Allergic contact dermatitis—immune system reacts to proteins of latex
         a. True allergic response
         b. Absorption through skin—perspiration increases absorption
         c. Inhalation of glove powder
         d. Symptoms not necessarily localized
      3. Anaphylaxis
         a. Rapid, severe immune reaction
         b. Life threatening
         c. Requires emergency treatment—epinephrine injection

Emergency First Aid
I. Bleeding aid
   A. Apply direct pressure to a bleeding wound
   B. Elevate the limb
   C. Maintain pressure until medical help is available
II. Breathing aid and CPR—follow guidelines
   A. Determine if victim is conscious
   B. Position victim's head
   C. Check for breathing and pulse
   D. No breathing/no pulse—begin chest compressions 100 per minute until help arrives; mouth-to-mouth no longer required in cardiac arrest
   E. If child or adult drowning victim; drug overdose; carbon monoxide poisoning—traditional CPR—two breaths plus compressions
III. Shock prevention
   A. Recognize signs of shock—pale, cold, clammy, rapid pulse, shallow breathing, weakness; possible nausea, vomiting, expressionless face
   B. Keep victim lying down
   C. Elevate legs unless fracture
   D. Keep airway open, head to side in case of vomiting
   E. Keep victim warm
   F. Call for professional assistance.
IV. Disaster emergency plan—know institution's plan for flood, fire, earthquake, etc.

CERTIFICATION PREPARATION QUESTIONS

1. The phlebotomist withdraws the needle from the patient and accidentally sticks herself. The first course of action is to:
   a. Get prophylactic medical therapy
   b. Fill out an employee incident report
   c. Decontaminate the puncture site
   d. Ask the nurse about the patient's health status

2. Hospitals and laboratories have disaster emergency or emergency readiness plans in place that are activated in the event of a(n):
   a. Terrorist attack
   b. Fire
   c. Earthquake
   d. All of the above

3. Any time you receive a shock on touching a centrifuge you should:
   a. Have someone else touch the centrifuge to see if they too get shocked
   b. Plug the centrifuge into a different wall socket
   c. Assume it is static electricity from dry air in the laboratory
   d. Check for a frayed cord, overloaded circuit, or bad ground connection

4. The single greatest job-related risk to all health care workers and one that is especially perilous for the phlebotomist is:
   a. Radiation exposure
   b. Needlesticks
   c. Chemical exposure
   d. Pathogen exposure

5. The OSHA mandate that requires manufacturers to supply MSDS for their products comes from the:
   a. Bloodborne Pathogen Standard
   b. Hazard communication (HAZCOM)
   c. NFPA guidelines
   d. DOT regulations

6. The designation of ABC on a fire extinguisher label indicates that it can be used for which type of fire?
   a. Paper
   b. Electrical
   c. Flammable liquids
   d. All of the above

7. Three basic protection methods to protect health care workers and patients from external sources of radiation exposure include all of the following, *except*:
   a. Direction
   b. Shielding
   c. Time
   d. Distance

8. On completion of the venipuncture procedure, the phlebotomist discards the needle by:
   a. Activating needle safety device and placing needle/tube holder unit in a biohazard bag
   b. Recapping and placing needle/tube holder unit in an approved biohazard bag
   c. Activating needle safety device and placing needle/tube holder unit in an approved sharps container
   d. Recapping the needle and placing needle/tube holder unit in an approved sharps container

9. Prevention of shock includes all of the following actions, *except*:
   a. Be alert for early signs of shock
   b. Keep the patient upright
   c. Keep the patient warm
   d. Keep the patient's airway open

10. Workplace safety is regulated by:
    a. HAZCOM
    b. OSHA
    c. CDC
    d. NFPA

11. The phlebotomist was in a hurry to make aliquots of the STAT specimen that was going to two departments and simply popped the top off of the tube and a blood mist splattered her in the eye. The type of exposure the phlebotomist incurred was:
    a. Cutaneous
    b. Transdermal
    c. Permucosal
    d. Percutaneous

12. The NFPA acronym RACE stands for:
    a. Rescue, alarm, confine, extinguish
    b. Respond, activate, close, escape
    c. Report, activate, close, extinguish
    d. Remove, alarm, contain, escape

13. The Employee Right to Know law allows employees to review the:
    a. Bloodborne Pathogen Standard
    b. Standard Precautions guidelines
    c. Chemical hygiene plan
    d. Hazard Communication Standard

14. Standard Precautions is used in the hospital setting to prevent the spread of HIV and HBV during patient care and applies to all body fluids, *except*:
    a. Sweat
    b. Synovial fluid
    c. Blood
    d. Urine

15. While working in specimen processing, you notice flames shooting up from underneath one of the older centrifuges. You quickly activate RACE and grab a fire extinguisher that can be used on a _____ fire.
    a. Type A
    b. Type B
    c. Type C
    d. Type D

16. As a member of the health care team, the phlebotomist knows the importance of Standard Precautions and routinely applies them to the care of:
    a. Patients in isolation
    b. Patients known to be HIV positive
    c. Patients in protective isolation
    d. All patients

17. All manufacturers of hazardous chemicals are required to provide users of hazardous chemicals a _____.
    a. Hazard Communication Plan
    b. MSDS
    c. Biohazardous label
    d. Chemical hygiene plan

18. The acronym to assist one in remembering how to use a fire extinguisher is:
    a. RACE
    b. PASS

    c. NFPA
    d. AIM

19. The phlebotomist walks into a patient's room and finds the nurse unconscious on the floor still in contact with an electrical source. The first thing the phlebotomist does is:
    a. Press the patient's call button for assistance
    b. Grab the victim and pull her away from electrical cord
    c. Check for breathing and pulse
    d. Shut off the source of electricity

20. Safety engineering practices or controls for sharps include:
    a. Recapping needle devices
    b. Removing needles from syringes
    c. Shielded or self-blunting needles
    d. Both a and c

21. The phlebotomist is checking in supplies for the outpatient phlebotomy satellite lab. Which of the following items will have an MSDS that the phlebotomist must file?
    a. Distilled water
    b. Bleach concentrate
    c. Isopropyl alcohol
    d. b and c

22. The DOT label for hazardous substances is:
    a. Diamond shape with United Nations hazard class number and identifying number
    b. Diamond shape with four quadrant colors representing hazards in four areas
    c. Center circle with trifans in fuchsia or yellow colorations and identifying number
    d. Center circle with tricircles erased on outer edges representing hazards in three areas

23. The phlebotomist is pouring hydrochloric acid into a 24-hour urine collection container and accidentally spills some on her hand. Immediate safety protocol requires the phlebotomist to:
    a. Go to the ER for treatment of a chemical burn
    b. Wipe the acid off with a paper towel and apply a burn ointment
    c. Flush the hand with running water for a minimum of 15 minutes
    d. Run a steady stream of saline over the area for 10 minutes

24. OSHA requires that every workplace develop and train employees in a chemical hygiene plan. This plan would include all of the following, *except*:
    a. Knowledge of MSDS for chemicals used in the laboratory and clinical setting
    b. Familiarity with different hazardous labels to be affixed to specimen collection containers
    c. Procedure for acid dilutions by adding water to acid when making acidic preservative dilutions
    d. Knowledge of where to find first aid protocols for exposure to chemicals used in the lab

25. The current American Heart Association protocol for cardiopulmonary resuscitation on adults who are found unconscious with no respiration or pulse includes:
    a. 100 chest compressions per minute
    b. 2 breaths per 15 chest compressions per cycle
    c. 1 breath per 30 chest compressions per cycle
    d. 50 chest compressions per minute

26. Laboratory safety practices include all of the following, *except*:
    a. Following PPE guidelines
    b. Tying long hair back from face
    c. Avoiding hand-face contact in the work area
    d. Chewing gum in the laboratory

27. To prevent parenteral exposure to blood-borne pathogens during venipuncture procedures, the phlebotomist should *not*:
    a. Use a blood transfer device when performing a syringe draw
    b. Hold evacuated tube while transferring blood from syringe into tube
    c. Use safety needle device when performing venipuncture
    d. Use a safety butterfly collection set with a syringe

28. A phlebotomist's percutaneous exposure to bloodborne pathogens can result from which of the following:
    a. Processing specimens without wearing gloves
    b. Anchoring the vein above and below the intended puncture site
    c. Removing a contact lens from the eye in the laboratory
    d. Using a blood transfer device in conjunction with a syringe

29. First aid for victims who are bleeding include all of the following, *except*:
    a. Applying direct pressure to the site of bleeding
    b. Elevating limbs above heart level even if broken
    c. Maintaining pressure until medical assistance arrives
    d. Securing a tourniquet if bleeding cannot be stopped by direct pressure

30. A gunshot victim arrives in the emergency room (ER) just as you are arriving to draw blood from a patient. You note that the patient is in shock and observe the medical staff applying all of the following measures, *except*:
    a. Keeping the victim in an inclined position
    b. Keeping victim lying down with head to side
    c. Keeping victim lying down with legs elevated
    d. Covering the victim with blankets

31. As a phlebotomist you know that latex sensitivity can present as an issue for patients and yourself with repeated exposure to latex. You are aware that the following latex reaction(s) can occur at any time in patients and yourself:
    a. Irritant contact dermatitis
    b. Allergic contact dermatitis
    c. Anaphylactic shock
    d. All of the above

32. To prevent injury when lifting heavy items, the phlebotomist should:
    a. Bend from the waist to grasp the object
    b. Squat and lift with the legs, keeping spine erect
    c. Squat, bend over item, and hoist item upward using back muscles
    d. Spread legs shoulder width apart, bend at waist to grasp object

33. Fire or explosive hazards in the workplace include which of the following:
    a. Chemicals
    b. Radioactive chemicals
    c. Oxygen
    d. a and c

34. A color-coded, numeric system for indicating the health, flammability, and reactivity hazards of chemicals was developed by:
    a. DOT
    b. OSHA
    c. NFPA
    d. HAZCOM

35. The blue quadrant of the NFPA label lists the relative danger of a chemical in the area of:
    a. Flammability
    b. Reactivity
    c. Health
    d. Other

36. The Needlestick Safety and Prevention Act of 2001 requires employers to do all of the following, *except*:
    a. Switch to safety needle devices for all procedures using needles
    b. Solicit input from employees at the managerial level on selection of safer devices
    c. Maintain a sharps injury log on employees who suffer needlesticks
    d. Review exposure control plans annually to reflect latest updates

37. An electrical shock to the patient while having blood drawn by the phlebotomist may occur if:
    a. The phlebotomist touches the patient's pulse oximeter plugged into the wall
    b. The patient answers the hospital phone before the needle is withdrawn
    c. The patient drinks water during the blood collection procedure
    d. The phlebotomist did not dry their hands well after washing them

38. Which of the following departments requires the removal of *all* metallic objects before entering the area?
    a. MRI
    b. X-ray
    c. Nuclear medicine
    d. CCU

39. The phlebotomist stuck her hand in the centrifuge to stop it from spinning, a tube broke, and blood splashed in her eye. Immediate first aid requires:
    a. Running to the ER for emergency medical treatment

b. Using the eyewash station for a minimum of 15 minutes
    c. Performing saline lavage for a minimum of 10 minutes
    d. Allowing the eye to tear and blotting with a gauze pad for 10 minutes

40. The class of fire that is represented by wood, paper, or cloth is:
    a. Class A
    b. Class B
    c. Class C
    d. Class D

41. The phlebotomist enters the patient's room to find the patient trying to put out a fire on a blanket caused by sneaking a smoke in bed. The first thing the phlebotomist must do is:
    a. Call for assistance using the call device
    b. Remove the patient from the room
    c. Activate the alarm outside the nurse's station
    d. Put out the fire using the patient's water pitcher

42. The phlebotomist notices that the patient has some redness, swelling, and itching on the arm where the tourniquet was applied. She suspects:
    a. She tied the tourniquet too tightly, irritating the patient's skin
    b. The patient has an active case of eczema
    c. The patient developed anaphylaxis
    d. The patient developed irritant contact dermatitis

ANSWERS AND RATIONALES

1. **Answer: C**
   Rationale: In the event of an accidental needlestick with a contaminated needle, the very first course of action is to decontaminate the puncture site. The exposure incident is then reported to the supervisor and a facility incidence report must be completed. The source of the blood exposure will usually be tested; the phlebotomist would receive baseline testing, counseling, medical evaluation, and possible treatment if indicated. Depending on the facility, the employee health nurse may spearhead the review or the pathologist who oversees the laboratory.
   Text Reference: p. 25

NORTHEAST WISCONSIN TECHNICAL COLLEGE LIBRARY - 2740 W MASON ST GREEN BAY, WI 54307

2. **Answer: D**
   Rationale: Disaster emergency plans or emergency readiness plans are activated by health care facilities in the event of a terrorist attack, massive fire, earthquake, flood, etc.
   Text Reference: p. 30

3. **Answer: D**
   Rationale: If someone receives a shock from equipment, the devise should immediately be turned off by unplugging it or switching off the circuit breaker. Maintenance should be called to come and inspect the equipment for a faulty ground connection, frayed cords, overloaded circuits, etc. Never have anyone else touch the equipment to verify a shock and never just assume it is static electricity.
   Text Reference: p. 28

4. **Answer: B**
   Rationale: The single greatest risk for all health care workers is needlestick injury. The percutaneous risk of injury due to venipuncture is less than those arising from other types of procedures using needles or other sharps; however, the absolute number of needlesticks is high due to the sheer volume of venipunctures performed annually. The risk for contraction of HIV seroconversion is 0.3%, whereas the risk for hepatitis B infection is 30% to 40% if the source of the contaminated needle was positive for either of these diseases.
   Text Reference: p. 25

5. **Answer: B**
   Rationale: OSHA's HAZCOM Standard requires that manufacturers of chemicals develop and disseminate MSDS for their chemicals in the workplace. These sheets provide information regarding the identity of the chemical, its hazards, cleanup procedures for spills, and first-aid measures for exposure.
   Text Reference: p. 26

6. **Answer: D**
   Rationale: An ABC fire extinguisher is a multipurpose dry chemical fire extinguisher that can be used on paper, electrical, and flammable liquids, grease, and oil fires.
   Text Reference: p. 29

7. **Answer: A**
   Rationale: Three basic protection methods used to protect health care workers and patients from external sources of radiation include minimizing the time of exposure, maximizing the distance between the worker or patient and the x-ray tube, and using lead shielding as appropriate. Since there are times a health care worker may be in the room with a patient being x-rayed, it is important to take all necessary protective precautions. Even one step farther from the patient can cut the exposure amount by four times.
   Text Reference: p. 28

8. **Answer: C**
   Rationale: OSHA's national policy in regard to the disposal of needles and tube holders following blood drawing procedures requires the use of "a sharp with engineered sharps injury protection" (SESIP) such as safety needles that are attached to the tube holder. At the completion of the blood draw, the entire unit—needle and tube holder—are discarded into an approved sharps container. Never manually recap a needle as it may cause an accidental needlestick.
   Text Reference: p. 25

9. **Answer: B**
   Rationale: Prevention of shock includes early recognition of symptoms of shock: pale, cold, clammy skin; rapid pulse; shallow breathing; weakness; possible presence of nausea or vomiting. The patient should be kept warm and in a supine position with the head turned to the side so that the airway can remain open in the event of emesis.
   Text Reference: p. 30

10. **Answer: B**
    Rationale: The Occupational Safety and Health Administration (OSHA) regulates workplace safety. The CDC or Centers for Disease Control is the lead federal agency that protects American citizens' health and safety. NFPA is the National Fire Protection Association, and HAZCOM refers to the OSHA Hazard Communications Standards.
    Text Reference: pp. 24, 26

11. **Answer: C**
    Rationale: Permucosal exposures refer to blood or body fluid exposures to the mucous membranes of the mouth, nose, and eyes. Mucous membranes can be a point of entry for pathogenic organisms.

Parenteral refers to exposures through routes other than oral. Cutaneous refers to the skin. Percutaneous and transdermal refer to exposure through the skin (i.e., needlestick).
Text Reference: pp. 25, 46

12. **Answer: A**
Rationale: The NFPA acronym RACE stands for Rescue, Activate alarm, Confine fire, and Evacuate or extinguish.
Text Reference: p. 26 and Content Overview (earlier in this chapter)

13. **Answer: D**
Rationale: The OSHA Hazardous Communication Standard is also known as the Employee Right to Know in regard to working with hazardous materials and allows access to information on chemical hazards in the workplace. Bloodborne Pathogens Standards are OSHA guidelines that apply to all occupational exposure to blood or other potentially infectious materials. Standard Precautions are the basic level of infection control to be used for all patients and are based on the principle that all blood, body fluids, secretions, excretions with the exception of sweat, nonintact skin, and mucous membranes may contain infectious agents and thus all infection control measures and PPE are to be used. The chemical hygiene plan describes all safety precautions and emergency procedures to be used when working with chemicals.
Text Reference: pp. 26-27 and Content Overview (earlier in this chapter)

14. **Answer: A**
Rationale: Standard Precautions applies to all body fluids with the exception of sweat. Universal Precautions applies to blood, other body fluids if visibly bloody, including semen and vaginal secretions, but not to feces, nasal secretions, sputum, sweat, tears, urine, saliva and vomit unless these others contain visible blood or are likely to contain blood. See CDC guidelines
Text Reference: pp. 24, 40

15. **Answer: C**
Rationale: Type C fires are for use on energized electrical equipment such as the centrifuge. Type A fires are wood, paper, cloth. Type B fires are grease, oil, flammable, liquids. Type D fires are flammable metals.
Text Reference: p. 29

16. **Answer: D**
Rationale: Standard Precautions applies to all patients at all times to prevent the transmission of disease. As such it is not necessary to know which patients are HIV positive or which patients have hepatitis B. Special isolation cases require additional precautions in addition to Standard Precautions such as patients in protective or reverse isolation, transmission-based isolations, etc.
Text Reference: See Content Overview (earlier in this chapter)

17. **Answer: B**
Rationale: Material Safety Data Sheets (MSDS) are required for all hazardous chemicals and are to be sent to institutions that purchase these chemicals. Information contained on MSDS includes chemical information, its hazards, and procedures for cleanup and first aid.
Text Reference: p. 26

18. **Answer: B**
Rationale: The acronym PASS refers to Pull the pin, Aim at the base of the fire, Squeeze the discharge nozzle, and Sweep across the when using a fire extinguisher.
Text Reference: See Content Overview (earlier in this chapter)

19. **Answer: D**
Rationale: Electrical shock can flow from the victim to the rescuer so the victim should not be touched until the power is shut off at the source. If a nonconductive tool is available, it can be used to remove the victim from the electrical source. CPR should be initiated if required until assistance arrives.
Text Reference: p. 28 and Content Overview (earlier in this chapter)

20. **Answer: C**
Rationale: Safety engineering practices for sharps include shielded or self-blunting needles for both vacuum tubes and butterflies, and cylindrical sheaths for syringe needles. Needles should never be recapped or removed from syringes as the potential for needlesticks is greatly increased by those actions.
Text Reference: p. 25

21. **Answer: D**
    Rationale: MSDS must be provided for hazardous chemicals that require labeling, such as bleach concentrate and isopropyl alcohol.
    Text Reference: p. 26

22. **Answer: A**
    Rationale: The Department of Transportation's label for hazardous materials is a triangle displaying the type of hazard, the United Nations hazard class number, and an identifying number.
    Text Reference: p. 27

23. **Answer: C**
    Rationale: If a chemical spills on you, then proceed immediately to the sink, safety shower, or eyewash station as necessary for type of exposure and flush the affected area with running water for a minimum of 15 minutes.
    Text Reference: p. 27

24. **Answer: C**
    Rationale: When making acid dilutions always add acid to water to dissipate the heat buildup at the interface of the acid and water while gently mixing. Knowledge of MSDS and where to find them in the lab, familiarity with various hazardous labels used within the institution, and knowledge of first aid procedures for commonly used chemicals in the lab are all part of a good chemical hygiene plan.
    Text Reference: pp. 26-27

25. **Answer: A**
    Rationale: The most recent changes by the American Heart Association regarding CPR include 100 chest compressions per minute with no breaths. Recent studies have found that rapid, deep, compressions on the victim's chest until help arrives are just as effective as standard CPR for sudden cardiac arrest in adults. Standard CPR is provided on adult victims of drowning, drug overdose, and carbon monoxide poisoning.
    Text Reference: p. 29 and Content Overview (earlier in this chapter)

26. **Answer: D**
    Rationale: There is to be no eating, drinking, smoking, or chewing gum while in the laboratory setting. Keeping hair back from face, wearing PPE when required by guidelines, avoiding hand-face contact in the work area are practices that will keep workers safe from workplace hazards and exposures.
    Text Reference: p. 24

27. **Answer: B**
    Rationale: Parenteral exposure risks increase when phlebotomists hold the evacuated tube in hand while inserting the syringe needle directly into the tube. The procedure should be performed using the single-hand technique if there is no blood transfer device available. The use of safety needles and butterfly devices also serves to lessen the risk of parenteral exposures through needlesticks.
    Text Reference: p. 25

28. **Answer: B**
    Rationale: Using the two-finger stretch where the vein is anchored above and below the draw site does serve well to anchor the vein but also puts the phlebotomist at risk for a percutaneous needlestick injury should the patient jump. Nonintact skin exposures can occur if gloves are not worn during specimen processing should there be a break in the skin. Removing a contact lens from the eye in the laboratory puts the worker at risk for a mucous membrane exposure. Using a blood transfer device in conjunction with a syringe is correct protocol for transferring blood from a syringe into evacuated tubes.
    Text Reference: p. 25

29. **Answer: B**
    Rationale: Applying direct pressure and maintaining it until help arrives are appropriate measures to stop bleeding. If bleeding cannot be stopped by direct pressure, a tourniquet may be applied as a last resort with caution so as not to incur tissue damage from lack of blood flow. Bleeding limbs should not be elevated as more serious injury to a broken limb can occur upon movement without appropriate support.
    Text Reference: p. 29

30. **Answer: A**
    Rationale: Patients in shock should be kept lying down, legs elevated unless fracture

suspected, head to the side in case of vomiting, and kept warm.
Text Reference: p. 30

31. **Answer: D**
Rationale: Latex sensitivity can take on any of the three forms of reactions listed.
Text Reference: p. 30

32. **Answer: B**
Rationale: The proper form for lifting heaving objects is to squat, keep spine erect, and lift using leg muscles to bear the weight instead of the back.
Text Reference: p. 25

33. **Answer: D**
Rationale: Chemicals and oxygen present a fire or explosive hazard in the laboratory. Certain chemicals exhibit high flammability. Oxygen is a hazardous oxidizer and is an important element in the fire tetrahedron. The tetrahedron is made up of heat, fuel, and oxygen. The fourth element is combustion, a self-sustaining chemical reaction that keeps the fire burning.
Text Reference: pp. 26-27 and Content Overview (earlier in this chapter)

34. **Answer: C**
Rationale: The color-coded, numeric system for indicating health, flammability, and reactivity of hazardous chemicals was developed by the National Fire Protection Association.
Text Reference: p. 26

35. **Answer: C**
Rationale: The red quadrant lists flammability dangers; the yellow quadrant lists the reactivity warning; the white quadrant lists other dangers; and the blue quadrant lists the health dangers of a chemical on the NFPA label.
Text Reference: p. 27

36. **Answer: B**
Rationale: Safety device selection was mandated to include input from nonmanagerial employees who are the workers who will be using the needle safety devices.
Text Reference: p. 25

37. **Answer: A**
Rationale: The phlebotomist should avoid contact with any electrical equipment during the venipuncture procedure as electricity may pass through the phlebotomist and the needle, and shock the patient. Answering the phone, drinking water, or wet hands will not result in a shock to the patient.
Text Reference: p. 24

38. **Answer: A**
Rationale: Magnetic resonance imaging uses very powerful magnets to create images of the body. The magnet can pull magnetic objects across the room. Thus, all metallic jewelry and clothing items must be removed before entering the area. Patients with magnetic implants are barred from entering.
Text Reference: p. 29

39. **Answer: B**
Rationale: Immediate first aid on exposure to blood or body fluids is critical. For eye exposure, the use of the eyewash station will provide a continuous flow of water to wash blood from the mucous membranes for a minimum of 15 minutes.
Text Reference: p. 25

40. **Answer: A**
Rationale: Class A fires have wood, paper, or cloth as fuels. Class B fires have grease, oil, or flammable liquids as fuels. Class C fires have energized electrical equipment as fuels. Class D fires have flammable metals as fuels.
Text Reference: p. 29

41. **Answer: B**
Rationale: In the event of a fire, RACE must be implemented with rescue of patients being the very first course of action. R stands for rescue; A stands for activate the alarm; C stands for confine or contain the fire; and E stands for evacuate or extinguish the fire.
Text Reference: p. 29 and Content Overview (earlier in this chapter)

42. **Answer: D**
Rationale: Redness, swelling, and itching are all signs of latex sensitivity in the form of irritant contact dermatitis that can develop within minutes to hours of contact. Eczema is characterized by a scaly, itchy rash that may have areas of blisters that ooze and then crust.
Text Reference: p. 30

INFECTION CONTROL

Pamela Primrose

INTRODUCTION

The goal of infection control is to develop and maintain an environment that minimizes the risk of acquiring or transmitting infectious agents to hospital personnel, patients, and visitors. It is not always possible for you to know if a patient is infectious or is in the incubation phase of an infection. Therefore, it is important that you understand how infections occur, and that you follow infection control practices and policies to protect yourself and your patients from infectious agents. Infection control requires recognizing potential sources of transmission and breaking the chain of infection. Techniques for preventing transmission include hand hygiene, use of personal protective equipment, and use of both Standard Precautions when required and expanded precautions. By taking appropriate precautions against potentially infectious organisms, you can make the workplace safe for you, your patients, and your coworkers.

CONTACT OVERVIEW

Infection

I. Infection—an invasion and growth of a microorganism in the human body that causes disease
II. Pathogens—infectious organisms
   A. Viruses
   B. Bacteria
   C. Fungi
   D. Rickettsiae
   E. Protozoa
   F. Helminths
III. Health care–associated infections (HCAIs) or nosocomial infection
   A. Direct contact
   B. Failure of hospital personnel to follow infection control practices such as hand hygiene
IV. Common infectious organisms—refer to Table 4-1, p. 35 of textbook

Chain of Infection

I. The chain of infection requires a continuous link among three primary elements: the source, the means of transmission, and susceptible host

Means of Transmission

I. Infectious agents can spread by five different means:
   A. Contact transmission—most frequent and important for HCAIs
      1. Direct contact—person to person
      2. Indirect contact—person and fomite
   B. Droplet transmission
      1. Greater than 5 μm in size
      2. Propelled short distance (3 feet) then fall
      3. No special ventilation required
      4. Modes
         a. Coughing
         b. Sneezing
         c. Talking
         d. Liquid splashes
         e. Aerosols
   C. Airborne transmission
      1. Airborne or droplet nuclei/dust
      2. Smaller than 5 μm
      3. Remain suspended for long periods then inhaled
      4. Special ventilation and air handling equipment required
         a. HEPA filters
         b. Microbe examples: *Mycobacterium tuberculosis*, varicella-zoster (chickenpox)
         c. Environmental organisms: *Aspergillus*, anthrax
      5. Modes
         a. Sneezing
         b. Coughing
         c. Singing/talking
         d. Aerosol procedures (i.e., suctioning, bronchoscopy)
   D. Common vehicle transmission
      1. Results in multiple cases of disease
      2. Modes
         a. Food—salmonellosis, listeriosis
         b. Water
         c. Medications
         d. Devices
         e. Equipment

E. Vector transmission
1. Carrier agents not harmed by organism
2. Mode—arthropods
   a. Insects (i.e., mosquitoes—malaria, yellow fever)
   b. Ticks—Lyme disease, Rocky Mountain spotted fever

Breaking the Chain of Infection

I. Hand hygiene—single most important and effective means of preventing the spread of infection and antibiotic-resistant microorganisms.
A. Gloves reduce but do not eliminate risk of contamination
B. Washing agents
   1. Plain or antimicrobial soap
   2. Alcohol-based hand agent—preferred because it has greater ability to kill microbes
C. Hand hygiene protocol
   1. Before and after patient contact
   2. Before donning gloves and after removing gloves
   3. Before performing procedures
   4. After removing personal protective equipment
   5. After touching contaminated equipment
   6. Before going to break
   7. Before leaving the lab at the end of your shift
II. Personal protective equipment (PPE)—tasks and PPE requirements per facility protocols
A. Protect skin, mucous membranes, and clothing from contact with infectious agents
B. PPE includes
   1. Fluid-resistant gowns
      a. Function: Keep blood/body fluid from soaking through clothing
      b. When to use
         i. Performing vascular procedures
         ii. Handling of blood/body fluids if anticipating splashes, spray, spatter, or droplets of blood or other potentially infectious materials (OPIM)
   2. Aprons
      a. Function: Keep blood/body fluid from soaking through clothing
      b. When to use: handling of blood/body fluid

3. Masks—May be used with goggles per facility protocol
   a. Function: protect mucous membranes of mouth and nose
   b. When to use
      i. Risk of airborne particles
      ii. Procedures with risk of splashes, spray, spatter, or droplets of blood, or OPIM
4. Goggles—worn with mask per facility protocol
   a. Function: protect mucous membranes of eyes
   b. When to use: procedures with risk of splashes, spray, spatter, or droplets of blood or OPIM
5. Face shields—worn with goggles per facility protocol
   a. Function: protect mucous membranes of eyes, nose, and mouth
   b. When to use: procedures with risk of splashes, spray, spatter, or droplets of blood or OPIM
6. Respirators
   a. Function: protect against small droplets of respiratory fluid and airborne particles (i.e., tuberculosis [TB])
   b. When to use: care of patients with active TB
   c. Type: N95 respirators
      i. Tight fit with filters—fit test required
      ii. Filter out 95% of airborne particles
7. Shoe covers
   a. Function: protect shoes/feet
   b. When to use: procedures with risk of splashes, spray, spatter, or droplets of blood or OPIM
8. Gloves
   a. Function: protect hands against blood/body fluid exposure; does not protect against sharps
   b. When to use
      i. Handling of blood/body fluid
      ii. Performing vascular procedures
C. Order of donning PPE
   1. Gown
   2. Mask, respirator, or face shield and goggles—fit check
   3. Gloves

D. Order of removing PPE
1. Gloves
2. Face shield or goggles
3. Gown
4. Mask or respirator
III. Standard Precautions
A. 1996 CDC guidelines—minimum level of precautions
B. Combines the major features of universal precautions and body substance isolation for patient care in the hospital setting
1. Universal precautions apply to non-hospital settings
2. Universal precautions apply to blood, other body fluids if visibly bloody, such as semen and vaginal secretions, but not to feces, nasal secretions, sputum, sweat, tears, urine, saliva and vomit unless these others contain visible blood or are likely to contain blood
C. Based on the principle that transmissible infectious agents may be present in all blood, body fluids, secretions, excretions except for sweat, nonintact skin, and mucous membranes
D. Infection control (prevention) measures to prevent contact between skin or mucous membranes and blood, body fluids, tissue, and OPIM
1. Use barrier protection
2. Use work practice controls
3. Applies to *all* persons
E. Standard Precautions include:
1. Hand hygiene
2. Gloves
3. Gowns
4. Face protection—mask, goggles, face shield
5. Sharps disposal—no recapping; activate safety device, use punctures-resistant containers
6. Respiratory hygiene and cough etiquette
a. New Standard Precautions component 2003—response to severe acute respiratory syndrome (SARS)
b. Prevent transmission of respiratory infections
c. Apply to everyone—patients, families, workers
d. Guidelines
i. Post signs—cover mouth, nose when coughing/sneezing with tissue

ii. Dispose of tissue in trash
iii. Hand hygiene
iv. Supply tissues, alcohol-based hand agents
v. Mask and separate patients in waiting areas

Occupational Safety and Health Administration (OSHA)
I. Regulatory enforcement agency for employee health and safety
II. Authority over all industries, including hospitals and health care facilities
III. Gave 1992 Standard Precautions the authority or power of the law
IV. 2001 OSHA revised the Standards; clarified sharps safety issues

OSHA Bloodborne Pathogens Standard
I. Requires employers provide the following to employees:
A. Written bloodborne pathogen exposure control plan
B. Proper personal protective equipment (PPE)
C. Mandated policy that all blood, body fluids, and OPIM are treated as infectious
1. Body fluids
a. Blood, semen, vaginal secretions
b. Cerebrospinal, synovial, pleural, pericardial, peritoneal, and amniotic fluids
c. Saliva in dental procedures
d. Any fluid visibly contaminated with blood or difficult to determine such status
2. OPIM—tissues and such
D. Work practice and engineering controls to minimize or prevent exposure
E. Immunization against hepatitis B virus free of charge
F. Free medical follow-ups in the event of accidental exposure
G. Education and safety training at the time of hire and annually
H. Additional training, education, and containment policies for HIV and hepatitis B virus (HBV)
I. Policies for regulated waste to include labeling (biohazardous) requirements and disposal
J. Written schedule, procedure, type of disinfectant for cleaning
K. Records documenting exposures and training sessions

Isolation Control Measures
I. Isolation
    A. Separation of an infection source from susceptible hosts
    B. Breaks the chain of infection
    C. Isolation control measures
        1. Protect the patient from infectious agents
            a. Environment
            b. Carried by staff or visitors
        2. Protect staff, visitors, other patients from infectious patients
II. Types of isolation
    A. Protective environment (protective isolation or reverse isolation)—HEPA filters, positive air flow
        1. Immunocompromised patients
            a. Chemotherapy patients
            b. Transplant patients
        2. PPE required per facility protocol
            a. Gloves
            b. Mask
            c. Gowns
    B. Isolation precautions: two-tiered system
        1. Tier 1
            a. Use for all patients without regard to diagnosis or infectious state
            b. Purpose to prevent transmission of pathogens
            c. Use Standard Precautions
        2. Tier 2
            a. Targets patients known or suspected to be infected with highly transmissible pathogen
            b. Applies to epidemiologically important pathogens
                i. MRSA
                ii. VRE
            c. Use expanded precautions— Standard Precautions plus
                i. Airborne precautions—diseases spread by droplet nuclei
                    A) PPE: N95 respirator—certified by NIOSH
                    B) Diseases: measles, varicella, TB
                ii. Droplet precautions—diseases spread by large infectious droplets (see Box 4-1 on p. 45 in textbook)
                    A) PPE: Mask within 3 feet of patient
                    B) Diseases: certain pneumonias, meningitis, influenza, etc.
                iii. Contact precautions—diseases spread by direct patient contact or items in patient's environment (see Box 4-2 on p. 46 of textbook)
                    A) PPE: Gown, gloves

            B) Only necessary phlebotomy items enter room
            C) Nothing comes out unless in biohazard bag (i.e., tubes)
            D) Diseases: GI, respiratory, skin or wound infections, RSV, etc.

Bloodborne Pathogens
I. Bloodborne pathogens (BBPs)
    A. Infectious agents in the blood, certain body fluids, tissues
    B. Most common BBPs
        1. Hepatitis
            a. HBV—hepatitis B virus
            b. HCV—hepatitis C virus
            c. HDV—hepatitis D virus
        2. HIV
        3. Human T-lymphotropic virus (HTLV) I and II
        4. Syphilis
        5. Malaria
        6. Babesiosis
        7. Colorado tick fever
II. Bloodborne pathogens exposure risks in phlebotomy
    A. Percutaneous injury via needlestick or puncture
        1. 30% to 40% risk of acquiring HBV
        2. 0.3% risk of acquiring HIV
        3. 1.8% risk of acquiring HCV
        4. Other infectious agents—rare, isolated occurrences
    B. Mucous membranes—splashes
        1. 0.1% risk of acquiring HIV
        2. Not well documented for HBV and HCV but presumed less than percutaneous exposure
    C. Nonintact skin—splashes, contaminated gloves or hands
        1. Less than 0.1% risk of acquiring HIV
        2. Not well documented for HBV and HCV but risk is present
    D. Intact skin exposure
        1. No known risk of HBV transmission
        2. No known risk of HIV transmission
    E. Human bite—risk negligible but possible
    F. Contact with contaminated equipment or lab instruments—same as nonintact skin
    G. Droplet transmission—removal of stoppers, centrifuge accidents, splashes
        1. Risk dependent on type of exposure— mucous membrane, intact or nonintact skin
        2. See related risks previously addressed

II. Viral survival outside body—viability
  A. Hepatitis B
    1. Stable in dried blood and blood products
    2. Viable at 25° C for at least 7 days
  B. Hepatitis C
    1. Viable up to 4 days outside body
    2. Many feel viability only 16 hours at R.T.
  C. Hepatitis D
    1. Requires HBV for survival
  D. HIV
    1. Stable 1 to 3 days after drying
    2. Longer viability if frozen or lyophilized (freeze-dried)
  E. Syphilis
    1. Viable for a few hours outside of body
    2. 3 days in stored blood for transfusions
III. Cleaning up a spill
  A. Wipe up excess
  B. Flood with OSHA-approved disinfectant
    1. 10% household bleach
    2. EPA-registered hospital grade disinfectant chemical germicides (tuberculocidal)
    3. EPA registered as effective against HIV
  C. Let sit for 20 minutes and wipe up
  D. Large spills—powder or gel kits

CERTIFICATION PREPARATION QUESTIONS

1. Proper hand-washing technique requires scrubbing of palms, backs of hands, between and under nails for a minimum of:
  a. 1 minute
  b. 10 seconds
  c. 20 seconds
  d. 2 minutes

2. CDC guidelines for health care facilities and professionals include the use of Standard Precautions, which serve to:
  a. Protect the privacy of patients and their families
  b. Determine who should be hospitalized and for how long
  c. Reduce the risk of transmission of blood-borne and other pathogens
  d. Keep health care costs down for hospitalizations and medical procedures

3. Which of the following is an example of Standard Precautions?
  a. Wearing gloves as sole PPE during specimen processing
  b. Wearing gloves as sole PPE during a venipuncture procedure
  c. Laundering your PPE lab smock/jacket each night at home
  d. Use of a surgical mask during venipuncture on a TB patient

4. OSHA requires the potential exposure to blood, body fluids, or OPIM be assessed by:
  a. Employees on a case-by-case basis
  b. Employees during their annual review
  c. Employers for each job classification and task
  d. Employers on a case-by-case basis

5. OSHA regulation requires that all health care personnel in job classifications where there is exposure to blood and body fluids be offered the opportunity to receive a vaccination free of charge or sign a declination form for which of the following infectious agents:
  a. HAV
  b. HBV
  c. HCV
  d. HIV

6. You were in a hurry and failed to notice that the patient was in contact isolation until the nurse brings it to your attention. You should:
  a. Stop the procedure and immediately report to the employee health nurse for a medical review
  b. Follow isolation protocol from that point on, complete the procedure, change clothes, and report the incident
  c. Stop the procedure, leave and don a mask, and return to complete the venipuncture procedure
  d. No problem, you had on your lab coat; complete the procedure, wash hands, and move to the next patient

7. Health care–associated infections are:
  a. Contracted by health care workers on the job
  b. Always airborne through aerosols
  c. Contracted by patients in the health care setting
  d. Appear only in the elderly

8. Standard Precautions combine the major features of:
   a. Universal precautions and body substance isolation
   b. Body substance isolation and Bloodborne Pathogen Standard
   c. Bloodborne Pathogen Standard and universal precautions
   d. Body substance isolation and protective environment

9. The three *main* components of the chain of infection requiring continuous linkage include all of the following, *except*:
   a. Portal of entry
   b. Source
   c. Susceptible host
   d. Mode of transmission

10. Choose the correct order for putting on PPE:
    a. Mask, gloves, gown
    b. Gown, mask, gloves
    c. Gloves, mask, gown
    d. Gown, gloves, mask

11. An example of a health care–associated infection (nosocomial infection) is:
    a. A patient admitted to the hospital with pneumonia
    b. An employee who becomes colonized with MRSA
    c. A patient whose surgical wound becomes infected
    d. An employee who contracts HBV from a needlestick

12. The single most important and most effective means of preventing the spread of infection and organisms that are antibiotic resistant to patients and other health care workers is:
    a. Proper hand washing
    b. Using proper cough/sneeze etiquette
    c. Wearing gloves
    d. Getting vaccinated

13. The greatest bloodborne pathogen risk to laboratory employees is:
    a. HBV infection
    b. HIV infection
    c. Syphilis
    d. Tuberculosis

14. The use of which handwashing agent(s) is best at killing microbes?
    a. Soap and water
    b. Antimicrobial soap and water
    c. Plain water
    d. Alcohol-based hand solution

15. Which of the following potential exposures presents the *least* risk to the phlebotomist:
    a. Cut on hand from a broken tube of blood while cleaning up
    b. Blood leaks through the glove onto badly chapped hands
    c. Blood sprays onto exposed intact skin during venipuncture
    d. Rub eyes without washing hands while processing specimens

16. Which of the following viruses may be stable in dried blood and blood products at 25° C for at least 7 days?
    a. HAV
    b. HIV
    c. HBV
    d. HCV

17. A patient is admitted to the hospital with a diagnosis of influenza. The patient is admitted under tier 2 isolation precautions that include the use of which of the following precautions:
    a. Airborne
    b. Expanded
    c. Isolation
    d. Protective environment

18. The correct order for removing PPE:
    a. Mask, gloves, gown
    b. Gown, gloves, mask
    c. Gloves, gown, mask
    d. Gloves, mask, gown

19. Airborne precautions are to be used for patients who are suspected of having:
    a. Tuberculosis
    b. *Clostridium difficile*
    c. HIV
    d. Streptococcal (Group A) pharyngitis

20. Infections spread throughout a population with an invasion and growth of microorganisms when the following pathway is complete:
    a. Cellular communication

   b. Lytic cycle
   c. Chain of infection
   d. Means of transmission

21. Preventing the spread of infection to patients, health care workers, and visitors requires breaking the chain of infection through use of all of the following, *except*:
   a. PPE
   b. Hand hygiene
   c. Standard Precautions
   d. HIPAA

22. Immunocompromised patients are at risk for infection and would be identified as a(n) _____ within the chain of infection:
   a. Reservoir
   b. Fomite
   c. Infectious agent
   d. Susceptible host

23. The term that describes the ability of bloodborne pathogens to survive for a limited time outside of the host organism on surfaces such as clothing, countertops, equipment, etc., is referred to as:
   a. Virulence
   b. Viability
   c. Stamina
   d. Potency

24. The phlebotomist is about to enter the room of a patient in airborne isolation. Which of the following PPE will be needed?
   a. Gloves, gown
   b. Gloves, faceshield
   c. Gloves, faceshield, goggles
   d. Gloves, N95 respirator

25. A patient with an unidentified enteric infection is admitted to the hospital and placed in which of the following isolations?
   a. Airborne
   b. Contact
   c. Droplet
   d. Standard Precautions

26. Minimum PPE for routine venipuncture requires the use of gloves for the purpose of protecting the:
   a. Patient from the risk of HCAIs from the phlebotomist
   b. Phlebotomist from patient blood exposure

   c. Phlebotomist from risk of a needlestick
   d. Patient from chemicals in the hand washing agents

27. Bloodborne pathogens include all of the following diseases, *except*:
   a. Syphilis
   b. HTLV I
   c. Malaria
   d. TB

28. All of the following body fluids require Standard Precautions, *except*:
   a. Sweat
   b. Spinal fluid
   c. Urine
   d. Peritoneal fluid

29. The Bloodborne Pathogen Standard set by OSHA includes all of the following, *except*:
   a. Written bloodborne pathogen exposure control plan
   b. Respiratory hygiene and cough etiquette protocol
   c. Free HBV immunization for employees
   d. Written schedule and procedure for decontaminating surfaces

30. While performing an outpatient dermal puncture, the phlebotomist's gloves contaminate the outside of the microtainer tube with blood. After capping the specimen, the phlebotomist should:
   a. Disinfect the outside of the microtainer tube with an alcohol pad
   b. Rinse the outside of the microtainer tube with water
   c. Disinfect the outside of the microtainer tube with 10% bleach
   d. Put the microtainer tube in a biohazard bag

31. Bloodborne Pathogen Standards policies are designed for the protection of health care workers and include free immunizations for:
   a. HIV
   b. HBV
   c. HCV
   d. b and c

32. A patient is placed in a protective environment or reverse isolation for the purpose of:
   a. Protecting an immunocompromised patient from infectious agents

b. Protecting other patients and visitors in the hospital from possible contamination

c. Protecting the patient from inflicting personal injury during their hospital stay

d. Protecting health care workers from patients with highly infectious diseases

33. The mandate requiring employers to provide PPE to their employees comes from:
    a. Standard Precautions policy
    b. OSHA Bloodborne Pathogen Standard
    c. NIOSH standards
    d. Centers for Disease Control and Prevention

34. N95 respirators must be certified by which agency:
    a. OSHA
    b. CDC
    c. TJC
    d. NIOSH

35. HIV is viable outside of the host organism for:
    a. 1 to 3 days
    b. 7 days
    c. 16 hours
    d. Not viable outside of the host

36. The phlebotomist begins to have a runny nose and tickling cough and suspects early signs of possible influenza but isn't sure. The phlebotomist should employ all of the following precautions, *except*:
    a. Turn head away from patient to cough into the air
    b. Wear a surgical mask when in contact with patients
    c. Keep alcohol-based hand washing agent on phlebotomy tray
    d. Inform supervisor for possible reassignment of duty

37. A person who is a carrier of a disease-causing microorganism but exhibits no signs of illness is said to be a:
    a. Susceptible host
    b. Reservoir
    c. Agent
    d. Portal of entry

38. Which of the following would *not* put a patient at increased risk of infection?
    a. Nuclear cardiac scan

b. Chemotherapy
c. Appendectomy
d. Oral antibiotic therapy

39. Fomites include all of the following, *except*:
    a. Telephone
    b. Mosquito
    c. Door knob
    d. Countertop

40. Another name for nosocomial infection is:
    a. Transient infection
    b. Health care–associated infection
    c. Indigenous infection
    d. Exogenous infection

ANSWERS AND RATIONALES

1. **Answer: C**
   Rationale: Proper hand washing technique requires a vigorous scrub for about 15 to 20 seconds.
   Text Reference: p. 47

2. **Answer: C**
   Rationale: Standard Precautions employ the use of infection prevention practices designed to protect health care workers from infection.
   Text Reference: p. 44

3. **Answer: B**
   Rationale: Standard Precautions require at a minimum the use of gloves during routine venipuncture. Specimen processing is a task where splashes and spills can be anticipated and thus require the use of a fluid-resistant lab coat, goggles and face shield, or table-top safety shield in addition to gloves. A smock or jacket that is not impermeable to blood and body fluids does not provide adequate protection when performing procedures where there is the likelihood of contamination of clothing or skin with blood or body fluids. If the intended function of the smock or jacket is to act as PPE, then it is the employer's responsibility to launder, repair, replace, and dispose of it at the workplace. Performing venipunctures on patients who have TB requires the use of an N95 respirator, not a surgical mask.
   Text Reference: p. 40

4. **Answer: C**
Rationale: OSHA requires employers to make occupational exposure determinations and assess each job classification and task for risk. Employers are also required to provide employee training on the appropriate methods that would allow them to recognize other potential risks in the workplace that might expose them to blood, body fluids, and OPIM. In addition, training must include discussion of the limitations of PPE.
Text Reference: p. 44

5. **Answer: B**
Rationale: Employers must offer and provide the hepatitis B vaccine to employees free of charge. In the event of a bloodborne pathogen exposure, employees must provide counseling, testing, and medical treatment to their employees. Employees who decline the initial offer are able to reverse their decision and receive the vaccine free of charge.
Text Reference: p. 44

6. **Answer: B**
Rationale: Contact precautions are used to prevent spread of organisms to another patient from an infected patient through direct touching of the patient or indirect touching of surfaces or objects that may have been in contact with the patient. Required practices include hand hygiene and putting on gloves and a gown before entering the room. All equipment is to be disposed of in the patient's room, PPE removed, and hand hygiene performed before exiting the room. Blood tubes are to be placed in a biohazard bag before exit as well. In this instance, if the phlebotomist does not have a biohazard bag available, one should be sent for. The phlebotomist's tray is now contaminated and needs to be bagged and facility protocol followed for decontamination. The phlebotomist's clothes are now contaminated and need replacing per facility protocol.
Text Reference: p. 45

7. **Answer: C**
Rationale: Infections contracted by *patients* during their hospital stay are termed health care–associated infections. HCAIs are acquired through failure of hospital personnel to follow infection control practices (i.e., hand hygiene). They may also be acquired through direct contact with other patients in the facility.
Text Reference: p. 34

8. **Answer: A**
Rationale: Standard Precautions combine the major features of universal precautions (UP) and body substance isolation (BSI) and are based on the principle that all blood, body fluids, secretions, excretions except sweat, nonintact skin, and mucous membranes may contain transmissible infectious agents. Standard Precautions include a group of infection prevention practices that apply to all patients, regardless of suspected or confirmed infection status, in any setting in which health care is delivered. These include: hand hygiene; use of gloves, gown, mask, eye protection, or face shield, depending on the anticipated exposure; and safe injection practices. Also, equipment or items in the patient environment likely to have been contaminated with infectious body fluids must be handled in a manner so as to prevent transmission of infectious agents.
(From Siegel JD, Rhinehart E, Jackson M, Chiarello L, and the Healthcare Infection Control Practices Advisory Committee, 2007 Guideline for Isolation Precautions: Preventing Transmission of Infectious Agents in Healthcare Settings *http://www.cdc.gov/ ncidod/dhqp/pdf/isolation2007.pdf.*)
Text Reference: p. 44 and Content Overview (earlier in this chapter)

9. **Answer: A**
Rationale: The chain of infection requires that there be continuous linkage between a source, a means of transmission, and a susceptible host. Other links include a portal of entry whereby the infectious agent gains entry into the host and a portal of exit whereby the infectious agents leave the host.
Text Reference: p. 34

10. **Answer: B**
Rationale: In putting on PPE: 1. gown; 2. mask, goggles, or face shield; 3. gloves.
Text Reference: pp. 41-42

11. **Answer: C**
Rationale: Health care–associated infections (or nosocomial infections) are infections contracted by patients during a hospital stay. HCAIs may be due to direct contact with other patients, but are most often caused by failure of hospital personnel to follow infection control practices. A patient with pneumonia already had the infection before hospital admission. HCAIs are not conditions associated with employees.
Text Reference: p. 34

12. **Answer: A**
Rationale: The single most important and effective means of preventing the spread of infection and antibiotic-resistant microorganisms to patients and other health care workers is using proper hand hygiene.
Text Reference: p. 36

13. **Answer: A**
Rationale: The most frequently occurring lab-acquired infection is the HBV infection (hepatitis) due to accidental needlestick. The risk is 40% for HBV, 0.3% for HIV, and 1.8% for HCV.
Text Reference: p. 46 and Content Overview (earlier in this chapter)

14. **Answer: D**
Rationale: The hand washing agent that kills more microbes than other agents is an alcohol-based agent. While other hand hygiene agents do include plain water, regular soap and water, and antimicrobial soap and water, alcohol-based agents are best.
Text Reference: p. 36

15. **Answer: C**
Rationale: Exposure of blood, body fluids, or OPIM on intact skin presents the lowest risk of transmission of HIV, HBV, and HCV or the pathogenic organisms.
Text Reference: p. 46 and Content Overview (earlier in this chapter)

16. **Answer: C**
Rationale: The hepatitis B virus is viable in dried blood and blood products for at least 7 days. Hepatitis C virus is said to be stable for up to 4 days but some feel viability is only

16 hours at room temperature. HIV is viable outside of the body for 1 to 3 days.
Text Reference: p. 46

17. **Answer: B**
Rationale: Tier 2 isolation uses expanded precautions for all patients diagnosed with or suspected of being infected with a highly transmissible pathogen. Tier 1 isolation precautions refers to Standard Precautions, which are used for all patients in the hospital, regardless of diagnosis or infection status to prevent the transmission of infectious agents through blood or body fluids, etc. Patients diagnosed with or suspected of having a disease transmitted by airborne droplet nuclei are placed in airborne precautions.
Text Reference: p. 45

18. **Answer: C**
Rationale: Removing personal protective apparel is the opposite of putting on PPE: remove the gloves, mask, goggles or face shield, and then the gown. The order of removal is important to prevent contamination of your skin and clothing.
Text Reference: p. 42

19. **Answer: A**
Rationale: Airborne precautions are to be used for patients with a disease that is transmitted by airborne droplet nuclei such as TB. *Clostridium difficile* is an enteric pathogen requiring contact precautions. Streptococcal Group A pharyngitis is a droplet precaution illness. HIV is a blood-borne pathogen requiring Standard Precautions.
Text Reference: pp. 45-46

20. **Answer: C**
Rationale: The chain of infection requires that a source, a means of transmission, and a susceptible host be in continuous linkage for the spread of infection to occur.
Text Reference: p. 34

21. **Answer: D**
Rationale: Breaking the chain of infection to prevent the spread of disease to patients, visitors, and health care workers requires that PPE be used, hands be washed before and after patient, blood, body fluid, and OPIM

contact, and that Standard Precautions be followed.
Text Reference: pp. 36-40

22. **Answer: D**
Rationale: Within the chain of infection, immunocompromised patients would be identified as susceptible hosts. A fomite is a contaminated inanimate object. The infectious agent is the microorganism. The reservoir is a person who is a carrier of the infectious agent but is not sick.
Text Reference: pp. 34-35

23. **Answer: B**
Rationale: The ability of organisms to survive outside of the host organism is referred to as viability. Virulence refers the ability of an organism to cause disease (i.e., its degree of pathogenicity).
Text Reference: p. 46

24. **Answer: D**
Rationale: Standard Precautions requires at a minimum the use of gloves when performing routine venipuncture. Expanded precautions for a patient in airborne isolation require the use of gloves and an N95 respirator. The use of an N95 respirator versus a surgical face mask is mandated according to disease-specific recommendations as listed in the Respiratory Protection II.E.4, and Appendix A of the HICPAC/CDC Isolation Guideline.
Text Reference: pp. 40, 45

25. **Answer: B**
Rationale: Enteric infections with low infection dose or prolonged environmental survival are placed in contact precautions. Unknown enteric infections require isolation until the identification of the organism has been determined.
Text Reference: p. 46

26. **Answer: B**
Rationale: OSHA requires the use of gloves during routine venipuncture to protect the health care worker from exposure to the patient's blood. Gloves do not protect against a needlestick. The gloves used are not sterile in this instance and could become a source of contamination to the patient if the health care worker touches surfaces that could be contaminated. The phlebotomist

must be careful to only touch the items used in the venipuncture procedure and not items that could serve as fomites.
Text Reference: p. 40

27. **Answer: D**
Rationale: Bloodborne pathogens include HBV, HCV, HDV, HIV, HTLV I, HTLV II, syphilis, malaria, babesiosis, Colorado tick fever, Creutzfeldt-Jakob disease, etc. Tuberculosis is not considered a bloodborne pathogen. It is spread via droplet nuclei.
Text Reference: pp. 45-46

28. **Answer: A**
Rationale: Standard Precautions states that all human blood and certain body fluids are potentially infectious and pose the greatest risk to the exposed health care professional if acquired. Body fluids may include blood, semen, vaginal secretions, cerebrospinal, synovial, pleural, pericardial, peritoneal, and amniotic fluids, saliva in dental procedures, any body fluid that is visibly contaminated with blood, and all body fluids in situations where it is difficult or impossible to differentiate among those fluids. Universal precautions applies to non-hospital settings and applies other body fluids if visibly bloody including semen and the vaginal secretions, but not to the feces, nasal secretions, sputum, sweat, tears, urine, saliva and vomit unless these others contain visible blood or are likely contain blood. See CDC guidelines.
Text Reference: p. 44 and Content Overview (earlier in this chapter)

29. **Answer: B**
Rationale: Respiratory hygiene and cough etiquette protocol is a part of Standard Precautions, not the Bloodborne Pathogen Standard. The others are a part of the BBP Standard.
Text Reference: pp. 40, 44

30. **Answer: C**
Rationale: Decontamination of work surfaces, equipment, phlebotomy trays, and blood collection tubes that have been contaminated with blood should be performed using 10% bleach or other hospital-approved disinfectant.
Text Reference: p. 47

31. **Answer: B**
    Rationale: To date, the only immunization available to protect against the three primary bloodborne pathogens is the HBV vaccination. There are no vaccinations available for HCV or HIV.
    Text Reference: p. 44

32. **Answer: A**
    Rationale: Immunocompromised patients may be placed in their own isolation unit to minimize the risk of acquiring environmentally caused infections and prevent infection from others. Patients requiring reverse isolation include chemotherapy and radiation therapy patients who may have severely reduced WBC counts, burn patients, AIDS patients, transplant patients, etc.
    Text Reference: p. 44

33. **Answer: B**
    Rationale: The OSHA BBP Standard requires employers to provide the proper PPE to employees at no charge, train employees in the use of PPE, and requires employees to wear PPE as mandated by job classification and task.
    Text Reference: p. 44

34. **Answer: D**
    Rationale: OSHA sets the filtration efficiency capability for respirators, which must then be certified by NIOSH.
    Text Reference: p. 40

35. **Answer: A**
    Rationale: HIV is reported to be viable outside of the host organism for 1 to 3 days; there is a longer viability period if lyophilized or frozen. HBV is viable for about 7 days and HCV is viable for 4 days, with some reports saying 16 hours.
    Text Reference: pp. 46-47 and Content Overview (earlier in this chapter)

36. **Answer: A**
    Rationale: At the first sign of illness, the phlebotomist needs to take extreme precautions so as not to infect patients, visitors, and other health care workers. Depending on the signs and symptoms, proper respiratory and cough etiquette and hand hygiene may be sufficient. Asking the supervisor for possible reassignment without patient contact, such as specimen processing, restocking inventory, tallies, etc., are all viable options.
    Text Reference: pp. 40, 44

37. **Answer: B**
    Rationale: A reservoir is a person who carries an infectious agent but is not sick. The susceptible host is the person whose immune system is compromised by illness, surgery, or other disease and thus at risk for HCAIs. The agent is the microorganism capable of causing disease or illness. The portal of entry is the route that the microorganism gains entry into the susceptible host.
    Text Reference: pp. 34-35

38. **Answer: A**
    Rationale: Patients who are sick, have had surgery, or are undergoing chemotherapy or antibiotic therapy are at greater risk for acquiring further infections and diseases. The immune system becomes compromised and does not respond to infectious agents as effectively in these conditions as it would in a normal healthy person.
    Text Reference: pp. 44-45 and Content Overview (earlier in this chapter)

39. **Answer: B**
    Rationale: Fomites are contaminated objects and include inanimate objects. A mosquito is a vector that carries a disease but is not harmed by it.
    Text Reference: pp. 34, 36

40. **Answer: B**
    Rationale: Health care–associated infections or nosocomial infections acquired through failure of hospital personnel to follow infection control practices (i.e., hand hygiene). They may also be acquired through direct contact with other patients in the facility.
    Text Reference: p. 34

INTRODUCTION

The practice of medicine requires many specialized words whose meanings may at first seem impenetrably mysterious. In fact, most medical terms are formed from Latin or Greek and use prefixes, roots, combining vowels, and suffixes. Understanding the way in which words are constructed and memorizing the meanings of some of the most common word parts will allow you to decipher many terms encountered in the workplace. Abbreviations are also very common and should become familiar to you.

CONTENT OVERVIEW

Parts of a Word

I. Root or main part (see Table 5-3 on pp. 54-55 in textbook)
   A. Core of the word
   B. Essential meaning of the term: cardio = heart; hepato = liver
II. Prefix (see Table 5-1 on pp. 53-54 in textbook)
   A. Part at the beginning
   B. Modifies the meaning of term: epi- = above; sub- = below
III. Suffix (see Table 5-2 on p. 54)
   A. Part at the end, follows word root
   B. Modifies or adds meaning to word root: -osis = condition; -pathy = disease
IV. Combining vowel
   A. Important connector—usually an "o"
      1. Root and the suffix: neur/o/pathy
      2. Two word roots: pneum/o/thorax
   B. Added to make pronunciation easier
   C. Has no meaning of its own
   D. Rules of use
      1. Use if suffix does *not* begin with a vowel: gastr/o/stomy
      2. Normally *not* used if suffix starts with a vowel: hepat/ic
      3. Used when combining two word roots even if vowels are present: oste/o/arthritis
      4. *Not* used to connect prefix and word root: epi/derm/al

V. Combining form
   A. Word root plus combining vowel separated by slash: gastr/o
VI. Defining medical terms
   A. Start by defining the suffix
   B. Move to the prefix or if no prefix, first word root
   C. Lastly, the word root
   D. Example: gastro/enter/itis
      1. -itis means inflammation
      2. Gastr/o means stomach
      3. Enter- means intestines
      4. Total word analysis meaning—inflammation of the stomach and intestines
VII. Plurals (see Table 5-4 on p. 55 in textbook)
   A. Word ending in -a: retain the a and add an e
      1. Example: axilla → axillae
   B. Word ending in -en: drop -en and add -ina
      1. Example: lumen → lumina
   C. Word ending in -is: drop -is and add -es
      1. Example: naris → nares
   D. Word ending in -ix or -ex: drop -ix or -ex and add -ices
      1. Example: cervix → cervices
      2. Example: apex → apices
   E. Word ending in -nx: drop the x and add -ges
      1. Example: pharynx → pharynges
   F. Word ending in -on: drop the -on and add a
      1. Example: spermatozoon → spermatozoa
   G. Word ending in -um: drop -um and add -a
      1. Example: ovum → ova
   H. Word ending in -us: drop -us and add -i
      1. Example: nucleus → nuclei
      2. Exception to the rule: sinus → sinuses; virus → viruses
   I. Word ending in -ux: drop -ux and add -uces
      1. Example: hallux → halluces
   J. Word ending in -ax: drop the x and add -ces
      1. Example: -ax → aces

K. Word ending in -y: drop the y and add -ies
   1. Example: deformity → deformities
L. Word ending in -ma: retain the ma and add ta
   1. Example: carcinoma → carcinomata

Abbreviations

I.   Way of shortening words or phrases
II. Symbols are objects or signs that represent words or phrases
III. Only one widely used meaning within the medical field for each abbreviation
IV. Must use designated abbreviation precisely— uppercase only, lower case only, mix of both (see Table 5-5 on pp. 55-57 in textbook)
   A. CC means chief complaint
   B. cc means cubic centimeter, which equals mL
   C. C means Centigrade
   D. Ca or CA means cancer
   E. Ca means calcium
   F. MD = doctor
   G. HIV = human immunodeficiency virus
   H. Rx = prescription

CERTIFICATION PREPARATION QUESTIONS

1. The word part of en/ceph/al/itis that is the suffix:
   a. En
   b. Cephal
   c. Alitis
   d. Itis

2. The following word part is a prefix:
   a. Arterio
   b. Hypo
   c. Osis
   d. Hemo

3. The word root *gastr-* refers to:
   a. Gallbladder
   b. Liver
   c. Stomach
   d. Intestines

4. The plural form of ovum is:
   a. Ovums
   b. Ova
   c. Ovia
   d. Ovina

5. The term that refers to RBCs is:
   a. Erythrocytes
   b. Leukocytes
   c. Thrombocytes
   d. Erythemia

6. Inflammation of a vein is referred to as:
   a. Thrombosis
   b. Arteritis
   c. Phlebitis
   d. Phlebotomy

7. The medical abbreviation NPO means:
   a. Nephrology postoperative
   b. Nonprofit organization
   c. New personnel orientation
   d. Nothing by mouth

8. The prefix *inter-* means:
   a. Above
   b. Within
   c. Between
   d. Below

9. The suffix *-osis* means:
   a. Condition
   b. Disease
   c. Originating from
   d. Shape or form

10. The word roots *pneu* and *pnea* refer to:
    a. Veins
    b. Lungs
    c. GI tract
    d. Breath

11. A patient suffering from heart disease is said to have:
    a. Carditis
    b. Cardiopathy
    c. Atherosclerosis
    d. Cardiogenic

12. The term *angioplasty* means:
    a. Removal of an artery
    b. Fixation of a vessel
    c. Cutting a vein
    d. Reshaping or forming a vessel

13. The abbreviation *BID, bid* means:
    a. Twice a day
    b. Every two days

c. Couple of times a day
d. Twice a night

14. The term *hepatitis* means:
    a. Fixation of the liver
    b. Inflammation of the liver
    c. Inflammation of the blood
    d. Liver disease

15. The abbreviation *UTI* means:
    a. Upper thorax infection
    b. Until further identification
    c. Urinary tract infection
    d. Under the intestines

16. The following word parts represent prefixes:
    a. Peri, micro, nano
    b. Oma, statis, tomy
    c. Genous, post, tetra
    d. Pulmon, ren, bili

17. The prefix in the term *leukocyte* means:
    a. Cyst
    b. White
    c. Cell
    d. Pale

18. The suffix in the term *hemostasis* means:
    a. Slow
    b. Control
    c. Condition
    d. Blood

19. The word root for the term *pulmonectomy* is:
    a. Pulmo
    b. Pulmon
    c. Pulmone
    d. Pulmono

20. Which of the following terms means paralysis of all four extremities:
    a. Peraplegia
    b. Quadristasis
    c. Quadriplegia
    d. Tetraparesis

21. Which of the following terms means a condition in which the bones are dying?
    a. Osteopathy
    b. Necrosteoitis
    c. Osteonecrosis
    d. Osteosis

22. Which of the following metric prefixes represents millionth?
    a. Centi
    b. Milli
    c. Micro
    d. Nano

23. The following suffix means blood condition:
    a. Pathy
    b. Osis
    c. Penia
    d. Emia

24. Which of the following word parts contains a combining form?
    a. Micro
    b. Reno
    c. Oma
    d. Pro

25. The plural form of lumen is:
    a. Lumens
    b. Lumina
    c. Luminata
    d. Luminae

26. Which of the following terms means slow heartbeat?
    a. Bardycardia
    b. Tachycardia
    c. Hypocardia
    d. Cardiopenia

27. Which of the following suffixes means opening?
    a. Tomy
    b. Stomy
    c. Ectomy
    d. Genic

28. Which of the following word pairs is correct:
    a. Pharynx, pharynxes
    b. Fornix, fornices
    c. Ova, ovas
    d. Nuclei, nuclae

29. The word root(s) in *megacardiopathy* is/are:
    a. Mega, cardio
    b. Cardio, patho
    c. Cardio
    d. Diopath

30. The word analysis for the term *toxogenic* means:
    a. Originating from poisons
    b. Condition of poisons
    c. Form of poisons
    d. Disease from poisons

31. Which of the following prefixes means half?
    a. Bi
    b. Hemi
    c. Para
    d. Di

32. All of the following prefixes reference a size, *except:*
    a. Poly
    b. Micro
    c. Macro
    d. Mega

33. All of the following prefixes refer to time, *except:*
    a. Pre
    b. Ante
    c. Pro
    d. Post

34. All of the following prefixes refer to position or location, *except:*
    a. Ambi
    b. Exo
    c. Intra
    d. Inter

35. All of the following pairs are opposites, *except:*
    a. Micro, mega
    b. Ecto, endo
    c. Brady, tachy
    d. Pre, ante

36. Which of the following abbreviations means chief complaint?
    a. cc
    b. CC
    c. CA
    d. C

37. Thrombocytosis means:
    a. Increased number of platelets
    b. Normal hemostasis
    c. Decreased clotting time
    d. Formation of blood clots

38. All of the following prefixes refer to a color, *except:*
    a. Albi
    b. Lute
    c. Nigr
    d. Bili

39. The following term means a decrease of red blood cells:
    a. Leukocytosis
    b. Thrombocytopenia
    c. Erythrocytopenia
    d. Erythrocytosis

40. The following term means slow breathing:
    a. Eupnea
    b. Hyperpnea
    c. Micropnea
    d. Bradypnea

ANSWERS AND RATIONALES

1. **Answer: D**
   Rationale: The suffix is *-itis. En* is a prefix and *cephal* is a word root (i.e., the form of the word after all affixes have been removed). It is the foundation for the meaning of the word. *-alitis* is an incorrect form of the suffix.
   Text Reference: p. 53

2. **Answer: B**
   Rationale: Hypo- is the prefix that is at the beginning of a medical word. *Arterio* is a word root meaning artery; *hemo-* is a word root meaning blood, and *-osis* is a suffix meaning abnormal condition.
   Text Reference: p. 53

3. **Answer: C**
   Rationale: Gastr- means stomach. The medical term for: gallbladder is *cholecyst.* The word root for intestines is *enter/o.* The word root for liver is *hepat/o.*
   Text Reference: p. 54

4. **Answer: B**
   Rationale: To change singular words ending in *um* change to plural form: drop the *um* and add *a*
   Text Reference: p. 55

5. **Answer: A**
Rationale: *Erythr-* means red, *-cyte* means cell, thus erythrocyte means red blood cell or RBCs. *Leuko-* is a word root meaning white, and *thrombo-* is a word root meaning clot. The term *erythemia* refers to redness of the skin as a result of congestion of blood in the capillaries.
Text Reference: p. 53

6. **Answer: C**
Rationale: *-itis* means inflammation, *phlebo* means vein, thus phlebitis means inflammation of a vein. *Arteritis* refers to inflammation of the arterial walls; *thrombosis* refers to blood clot in a vessel; *phlebotomy* refers to cutting into a vein.
Text Reference: p. 53

7. **Answer: D**
Rationale: NPO means nothing by mouth.
Text Reference: p. 56

8. **Answer: C**
Rationale: *Inter-* means between; *hyper-* is above or excessive; and *intra-* means within, and *hypo-* means below.
Text Reference: p. 53

9. **Answer: A**
Rationale: *-osis* means condition; *-pathy* means disease; *-gen, -genic, -genous* means originating from; *-plasty* means shape or form.
Text Reference: p. 54

10. **Answer: D**
Rationale: *Pneu* and *pnea* both refer to the breath.
Text Reference: pp. 54

11. **Answer: B**
Rationale: The meaning for the suffix *-pathy* is disease, *cardi* means heart; thus cardiopathy means disease of the heart. Carditis is inflammation of the heart; cardiogenic means originating in the heart.
Text Reference: p. 54

12. **Answer: D**
Rationale: The suffix *-plasty* means to shape or form; the word root *angi/o* means

vessel, thus angioplasty means reshaping or forming a vessel.
Text Reference: p. 54

13. **Answer: A**
Rationale: *BID* or *bid* is the abbreviation for twice a day. *BIN* means twice a night.
Text Reference: p. 55

14. **Answer: B**
Rationale: The suffix *-itis* means inflammation; the word root *hepat-* means liver, thus hepatitis is inflammation of the liver.
Text Reference: p. 54

15. **Answer: C**
Rationale: The abbreviation *UTI* stands for urinary tract infection.
Text Reference: p. 57

16. **Answer: A**
Rationale: *peri-, micro-, nano-* are all prefixes; *-oma, -stasis, -tomy* are all suffixes; *-genous* is a suffix but *post-, tetra-* are prefixes; *pulmon-, ren-,* and *bili-* are all word roots.
Text Reference: pp. 53-55

17. **Answer: B**
Rationale: The prefix *leuko-* is a color prefix meaning white. The word root is *cyte*.
Text Reference: p. 54

18. **Answer: B**
Rationale: The suffix *-stasis* means stopping or control, the word root *heme* means blood, thus hemostasis means stopping the flow of blood.
Text Reference: p. 54

19. **Answer: B**
Rationale: The word root in the term *pulmonectomy* is *pulmon*. The combining form would be *pulmon/o*.
Text Reference: p. 55

20. **Answer: C**
Rationale: The prefix *quad-* means four; the suffix *-plegia* means paralysis, thus quadriplegia means paralysis of all four limbs.
Text Reference: p. 54

21. **Answer: C**
Rationale: The suffix *-osis* means condition; the word root *oste-* means bone; the word root *necro-* means death, thus osteonecrosis means that bones are dying.
Text Reference: p. 54

22. **Answer: C**
Rationale: The metric prefix *micro-* means millionth; *centi* means hundredth; *milli-* means thousandth; *nano-* means billionth.
Text Reference: p. 54

23. **Answer: D**
Rationale: The suffix *-emia* means blood condition. The other terms are general condition terms in that *-pathy* means disease; *-osis* means condition. The suffix *-penia* refers to a deficiency.
Text Reference: p. 54

24. **Answer: B**
Rationale: A combining form is usually the letter "o." The word root *ren-* means kidney and is presented in the combining form as *ren/o*. There are two prefixes that end in "o": *micro-* and *pro-*. There is one suffix that begins with "o": *-oma*.
Text Reference: p. 54

25. **Answer: B**
Rationale: The rule for making a medical term ending in *-en* plural requires that the *-en* be dropped and *-ina* added. Thus, lumen becomes lumina.
Text Reference: p. 55

26. **Answer: A**
Rationale: The suffix *-ia* means pertaining to; the prefix *brady-* means slow; the word root *cardi/o* means heart. Thus, the term bradycardia means pertaining to slow heartbeat.
Text Reference: pp. 53-54

27. **Answer: B**
Rationale: The suffix *-stomy* means opening; *-tomy* means to cut; *-ectomy* means surgical removal; and *-genic* means originating from.
Text Reference: p. 54

28. **Answer: B**
Rationale: To change a singular medical term ending in *ix* to plural, simply drop the *ix* and add *-ices*. Pharynx becomes plural by dropping *-nx* and adding *-nges* for pharynges. Ova is already plural. The singular form of ova is ovum. Nuclei is already plural. The singular form of nuclei is nucleus.
Text Reference: p. 55 and Content Overview (earlier in this chapter)

29. **Answer: C**
Rationale: The word root in *megacardiopathy* is *cardio-*; *mega-* is a prefix; *-pathy* is a suffix.
Text Reference: pp. 53-54

30. **Answer: A**
Rationale: The suffix *-genic* means originating from; the word root *tox-* or *toxico-* means poison. Thus, the word analysis for toxogenic means originating from poison.
Text Reference: p. 55

31. **Answer: B**
Rationale: The prefix *hemi-* means half; *bi-* and *di-* mean two; and *para-* means beside.
Text Reference: pp. 53-54

32. **Answer: A**
Rationale: Micro-, macro-, and *mega* refer to size—small, large, and large—respectively. The prefix *poly-* refers to a quantity (i.e., many).
Text Reference: p. 53

33. **Answer: C**
Rationale: The prefixes referring to time are *pre-*, which means before; *ante-*, which means before; *post-*, which means after. The prefix *pro-* means for or in front of.
Text Reference: pp. 53-54

34. **Answer: A**
Rationale: The following prefixes refer to position or location: *exo-* means outside; *intra-* means within; *inter-* means between. The prefix *ambi-* means both.
Text Reference: p. 53

35. **Answer: D**
Rationale: The following pairs are opposites: *micro-/mega-* meaning small/big; *ecto-/endo-* meaning outside/inside; *brady-/tachy-* meaning slow/fast. The prefix *pre-/ante-* both mean before.
Text Reference: pp 53-54

36. **Answer: B**

     Rationale: The designation of uppercase and lowercase letters is critical in the interpretation of an abbreviation, especially when the same letter or letters are used for different terms. The abbreviation CC means chief complaint; cc means cubic centimeter; CA means cancer; and C means Celsius. Remember, uppercase or lowercase letters make a difference in meaning.

     Text Reference: p. 55

37. **Answer: A**

     Rationale: Thrombocytosis means an increase in the number of platelets in the blood. The suffix *-osis* means condition; *thrombo-* means clot; *cyt-* means cell. For this particular term, an analysis of the word parts gives a clue to definition but not an exact meaning.

     Text Reference: pp. 54-55

38. **Answer: D**

     Rationale: The following prefixes refer to color: *albi-* means white; *lute-* means yellow;

nigr- means black. The following term is a word root: *bili-* meaning liver.

Text Reference: p. 54

39. **Answer: C**

     Rationale: The suffix *-penia* means deficiency or decrease; the prefix *erythro-* means red; and the word root *cyt/o-* means cell. Thus, erythrocytopenia means a decrease of red blood cells. The suffix *-osis* means condition, the prefix *leuko-* means white; and the word root *thrombo-* means clot.

     Text Reference: pp. 54-55

40. **Answer: D**

     Rationale: The prefix *brady-* means slow; the word root *pnea-* means breath. Thus, bradypnea means slow breathing. The prefix *eu-* means good or normal; *hyper-* means increased; *micro-* means small.

     Text Reference: pp. 53-54

HUMAN ANATOMY AND PHYSIOLOGY

Pamela Primrose

INTRODUCTION

An understanding of human anatomy and physiology allows the phlebotomist to interact more knowledgeably with both patients and other health care professionals. The tissues, organs, and body systems work together to create and maintain homeostasis, the integrated control of body function that is characteristic of health. Each body system is prone to particular types of diseases and is subject to particular tests that aid in diagnosing those diseases. As a phlebotomist, many of the patients you collect samples from will be undergoing diagnosis or treatment for diseases or other disorders. Others may require blood collection for reasons not related to illness, such as pregnancy or blood donation.

CONTENT OVERVIEW

Levels of Organization

I. Cells
   A. Smallest living units in the body
   B. Function: carry out metabolic functions via organelles
   C. Examples of organelles (see p. 64 in textbook)
      1. Nucleus—houses DNA/genes to direct protein production
      2. Mitochondria—powerhouse of cell, ATP
      3. Plasma membrane—regulates materials coming in and out of cell
II. Tissues
   A. Cells of similar structure and function
   B. Four basic types of tissue
      1. Epithelial tissue
         a. Function: cover or line some organs and body cavities
         b. Examples:
            i. Skin
            ii. Mouth
      2. Muscle tissue
         a. Function/examples:
            i. Skeletal or striated voluntary—moves skeleton
            ii. Cardiac or striated involuntary—pumps blood
            iii. Smooth—nonstriated involuntary—regulates passage of materials through vessels, gut, etc.
      3. Nerve tissue
         a. Function: intracellular communication
         b. Examples:
            i. Neurons—excitable cells
            ii. Neuroglial cells—nourish and support neurons
            iii. Myelin sheath—insulates nerves to facilitate transmission of impulses
      4. Connective tissue
         a. Function: bind and support other three types of tissue
         b. Examples:
            i. Bone
            ii. Blood
            iii. Adipose
III. Organs
   A. Two or more kinds of tissue
   B. Function: carry out specialized and complex function
   C. Examples:
      1. Heart
      2. Lungs
      3. Kidneys
IV. Body systems
   A. Groups of organs
   B. Function: work together to form complex body functions
   C. Examples:
      1. Cardiovascular
      2. Pulmonary

Anatomic Terminology

I. Anatomic position:
   A. Body is erect
   B. Facing forward
   C. Arms at the sides
   D. Palms facing forward
II. Directional terms
   A. Ventral and anterior—front
   B. Dorsal and posterior—back
   C. Lateral—side

D. Medial—midline
E. Distal—away from point of origin/ attachment
F. Proximal—nearest point of attachment
G. Inferior—below
H. Superior—above
I. Prone—lying on back
J. Supine—lying on abdomen
K. Flexion—bend joint
L. Extension—straighten joint
M. Abduction—away
N. Adduction—closer

III. Body planes
A. Frontal plane (coronal plane)—front/back
B. Sagittal plane (lateral plane)—left/right
C. Transverse plane (axial plane)—top/bottom

IV. Body cavities
A. Ventral cavities
1. Thoracic cavity
a. Heart
b. Lungs
c. Mediastinum—middle section of chest cavity
i. Heart, aorta, thymus
ii. Portion of trachea, esophagus, lymph nodes, nerves
2. Abdominopelvic cavity
a. Abdominal
i. Stomach
ii. Intestines
iii. Liver, gallbladder
iv. Pancreas
v. Kidneys
b. Pelvic
i. Bladder
ii. Rectum
iii. Ovaries, testes
B. Dorsal cavities
1. Cranial cavity
a. Brain
2. Spinal cavity
a. Spinal cord

Skeletal System
I. Function
A. Support body
B. Provide movement
C. Protect internal organs
D. Store minerals—calcium/phosphorus
E. Hematopoiesis—blood cell formation
II. Components
A. Bones—connective tissue makes up skeleton (206 bones)

B. Ligaments—bone to bone
C. Tendons—muscle to bone
D. Cartilage—dense connective tissue in joints, ribs, etc.
III. Features of bones
A. Function and examples of bone cells
1. Osteocytes—mature bone cells—structure
2. Osteoblasts—make bone
3. Osteoclasts—break down bone to release stored minerals
B. Classified by their shapes—long, short, flat, sesamoid, irregular
IV. Features of joints
A. Function
1. Connect bones
B. Example of joint types
1. Immovable (synarthrosis)
a. Cranium
b. Facial (some)
2. Partially movable (amphiarthrosis)
a. Vertebrae
3. Free moving (diarthrosis)
a. Shoulder
b. Elbow
c. Knee
C. Components of freely moving joints
1. Ligaments (see above)
2. Synovial cavity—fluid filled
3. Articular cartilage—lines weight bearing surfaces
V. Bone and joint disorders (see Box 6-1 on p. 72 in textbook)
A. Fractures—simple
B. Metabolic diseases—osteoporosis
C. Infections—osteomyelitis
D. Neoplastic diseases—osteoma
E. Developmental abnormalities—scoliosis
VI. Common lab tests for bone and joint disorders (see Table 6-1 on p. 72 in textbook)
A. Alkaline phosphatase
B. Rheumatoid factor (RF)
C. Synovial fluid analysis

Muscular System
I. Function of muscular system
A. Types and function of muscle previously discussed in Tissue
B. Attachments—previously discussed in components Skeletal System
C. Occur in antagonistic pairs
1. Biceps flexes, triceps extends

II. Components
  A. Muscle types previously discussed—muscle structure beyond scope of knowledge
III. Disorders of muscular system (see Box 6-2 on p. 73 in textbook)
  A. Trauma—tendonitis
  B. Genetic disease—muscular dystrophy
  C. Metabolic disease—mitochondrial
  D. Autoimmune disease—myasthenia gravis
  E. Motor neuron disease—Lou Gehrig's disease (ALS)
IV. Common lab tests for muscle disorders (see Table 6-2 on p. 73 in textbook)
  A. CK isoenzymes—CK–MM, CK–MB
  B. Creatine kinase
  C. Myoglobin

Integumentary System
I. Function
  A. Protection—barrier against microbes, chemicals
  B. Thermoregulation of body temperature— evaporation of sweat
  C. Sensation—sensory receptors
II. Components
  A. Skin
  B. Hair
  C. Nails
  D. Glands
  E. Nerves
III. Features of the integumentary system
  A. Epidermis—outer layer
    1. Melanocytes—pigmentation
  B. Dermis—inner layer
    1. Glands—sweat/sudoriferous, oil/sebaceous
    2. Hair follicles
    3. Nerves
    4. Sensory receptors
    5. Capillary bed
  C. Subcutaneous
    1. Connective tissue—adipose
    2. Larger blood vessels
    3. Nerves
IV. Disorders of the integumentary system (see Box 6-3 on p. 74 in textbook)
  A. Infection—fungal infection
  B. Neoplastic disease—melanoma
  C. Inflammation—acne
V. Common lab tests for integumentary disorders (see Table 6-3 on p. 74 in textbook)
  A. C & S
  B. Skin biopsy

Nervous System
I. Function
  A. Controls, regulates, and communicates internal and external stimuli
    1. Maintains homeostasis
    2. Works with the endocrine system
II. Divisions of nervous system
  A. Central nervous system
    1. Function
      a. Receives sensory input from entire peripheral system
      b. Integrates and processes input for understanding of response needed
        i. Directs movement of muscles
        ii. Directs actions of organs and glands
    2. Components
      a. Brain
        i. Cerebrum
          A) Thought
          B) Emotion
          C) Memory
        ii. Cerebellum
          A) Fine-tuning motor commands
        iii. Thalamus
          A) Relay station for incoming sensory information
        iv. Brain stem
          A) Basic life process
            1) Respiration
            2) Heart beat
            3) Blood pressure
      b. Spinal cord
        i. Transmission of neural impulses between brain and body
      c. Cerebrospinal fluid
        i. Nourish, remove wastes, and cushion brain
        ii. Circulates around brain, spinal cord, ventricles
      d. Meninges—three membranes surrounding brain/spinal cord
        i. Pia mater
        ii. Arachnoid
        iii. Dura mater
  B. Peripheral nervous system (PNS)
    1. Function
      a. Carry information to central nervous system
    2. Divisions of PNS
      a. Sensory nervous system
        i. Function: sends information to CNS from:
          A) Internal organs
          B) External stimuli

b. Motor nervous system
  i. Function: sends information from CNS to:
    A) Organs
    B) Muscles
    C) Glands
  ii. Divisions/function of motor nervous system
    A) Somatic nervous system: voluntary control of skeletal muscles
    B) Autonomic nervous system: involuntary control of cardiac and smooth muscle
III. Disorders of the nervous system (see Box 6-4 on p. 77 in textbook)
  A. Trauma—concussion
  B. Stroke—embolic, hemorrhagic
  C. Infection—meningitis
  D. Neoplastic disease—neuroma
  E. Degenerative disease—Alzheimer's
  F. Autoimmune disease—Multiple sclerosis
  G. Developmental disorders—cerebral palsy
  H. Psychiatric illness—schizophrenia
IV. Common lab tests for neurologic disorders (see Table 6-4 on p. 77 in textbook)
  A. CSF analysis
  B. Protein
  C. Glucose

Digestive System
I. Function
  A. Digestion of food
    1. Mechanical—chew, stomach churning
    2. Chemical—enzymes from saliva, stomach, intestines
      a. Carbohydrases—carbohydrates
      b. Proteases—proteins
      c. Lipases—fats
      d. Bile—fats
  B. Absorption of nutrients—through villi in small intestines via peristalsis
  C. Elimination of waste—defecation
II. Components
  A. Mouth—tongue/teeth—chemical/mechanical digestion
  B. Esophagus—passageway to stomach
  C. Stomach—chemical/mechanical digestion
  D. Small/large intestines—absorption
  E. Rectum—holds feces until passed
  F. Anus—opening to expel feces
  G. Accessory digestive organs
    1. Liver—makes bile (and has other functions)

  2. Gallbladder—stores bile, secretes as needed
  3. Pancreas—secretes enzymes amylase, lipase (others that are not part of digestion)
III. Disorders of the digestive system (see Box 6-5 on p. 79 in textbook)
  A. Infection—ulcer, HAV
  B. Inflammation—colitis, cholecystitis
  C. Chemical damage—cirrhosis
  D. Autoimmune disease—Crohn's disease
IV. Common lab tests for digestive disorders (see Table 6-5 on p. 79 in textbook)
  A. Amylase
  B. Ammonia
  C. Occult blood

Urinary System
I. Function
  A. Remove metabolic wastes
  B. Maintain acid-base balance
  C. Regulate body hydration
  D. Produce hormones
    1. Renin—controls blood pressure
    2. Erythropoietin—regulates production of RBCs
  E. Process
    1. Filtration
    2. Secretion
    3. Reabsorption
II. Components
  A. Kidneys
    1. Nephron: functional unit of the kidneys that forms urine
  B. Ureters—drain urine from kidneys to bladder
  C. Bladder—temporary reservoir for urine
  D. Urethra—passageway for urine to be excreted
III. Disorders of the urinary system (see Box 6-6 on p. 82 in textbook)
  A. Infection—UTI
  B. Chemical—renal calculi
IV. Common lab tests for urinary disorders (see Table 6-6 on p. 82 in textbook)
  A. BUN
  B. Creatinine
  C. C & S

Respiratory System
I. Function
  A. Relies on circulatory system
    1. Transport gases to tissues from lungs
    2. Transport gases to lungs from tissues

B. Obtain oxygen for use by cells
   1. *External respiration*—exchange of gases in lungs
      a. Between alveoli and capillaries
   2. Oxygen binds to hemoglobin in RBCs and is carried to all cells
C. Expel carbon dioxide waste generated by metabolism
   1. *Internal respiration*—exchange of oxygen and carbon dioxide at cellular level
      a. Between systemic capillaries and tissues
   2. Carbon dioxide diffuses out of cells, carried by bicarbonate ion and back to lungs for release
II. Components
   A. Upper airways
      1. Nasal passages
      2. Throat
   B. Lower airways
      1. Trachea—airway to lungs
      2. Larynx—voice box
      3. Lungs
         a. Bronchi—branches off trachea into lungs
         b. Bronchioles—smaller branches leading to alveoli
         c. Alveoli—site of exchange of gases, tiny air sacs
III. Disorders of the respiratory system (see Box 6-7 on p. 83 in textbook)
   A. Infection—pneumonia
   B. Inflammation—bronchitis
   C. Obstruction—asthma
   D. Insufficient ventilation—spinal cord injury
   E. Developmental disorder—infant respiratory distress syndrome
   F. Neoplastic disease—lung cancer
IV. Common lab tests for respiratory system (see Table 6-7 on p. 83 in textbook)
   A. ABGs
   B. Electrolytes
   C. Throat swabs

Endocrine System
I. Function
   A. Work with nervous system
   B. Maintain homeostasis
   C. Regulate other endocrine glands via feedback loops
   D. Release powerful chemical substances directly into bloodstream to act on target organs or tissues

II. Components
   A. Hormones
      1. Function
         a. Released into circulation by endocrine glands
         b. Exert effect on target cells by binding to receptor sites
      2. Types of hormones
         a. Steroid
            i. Testosterone
            ii. Progesterone
         b. Amine
            i. Thyroxine
            ii. Epinephrine
         c. Peptide—protein
            i. Insulin
            ii. Growth hormone
   B. Endocrine glands
      1. Pituitary gland
         a. Function
            i. Master gland
            ii. Controls other glands via feedback loops
         b. Location: base of hypothalamus
         c. Hormones
            i. Anterior lobe
               A) TSH
               B) FSH
               C) Growth hormone
            ii. Posterior lobe
               A) ADH
               B) Oxytocin
      2. Thyroid gland
         a. Function
            i. Regulate basal metabolic rate
         b. Location: front of neck below larynx
         c. Hormones
            i. Thyroxine (T_4)
            ii. Triiodothyronine (T_3)
      3. Parathyroid gland
         a. Function
            i. Regulates amount of calcium and phosphorus in blood
         b. Location: behind thyroid
         c. Hormone
            i. Parathormone
      4. Thymus gland
         a. Function
            i. Role in early development of immune system
            ii. Adult role unknown
         b. Location: behind sternum

c. Hormone
  i. Thymosin
5. Pancreas
  a. Function
    i. Regulates blood glucose level
      A) Hyperglycemia: may indicate diabetes mellitus
      B) Hyperglycemia: elevated blood glucose level
      C) Hypoglycemia: low blood glucose level
    ii. Nonhormonal function—produces digestive enzymes
  b. Location: behind the stomach
  c. Hormones
    i. Insulin
    ii. Glucagon
6. Adrenal glands
  a. Function
    i. Medulla: role in coping with physical and emotional stress—fight or flight
    ii. Cortex: role in body metabolism
  b. Location: above each kidney
  c. Hormones
    i. Adrenal medulla
      A) Epinephrine
      B) Norepinephrine
    ii. Adrenal cortex
      A) Corticosterone
      B) Aldosterone
7. Gonads are the ovaries and testes
  a. Function
    i. Steroid hormone production
    ii. Gametogenesis
  b. Location
    i. Ovaries: pelvic cavity
    ii. Testes: external to abdominopelvic cavity
  c. Hormones
    i. Testes
      A) Testosterone
    ii. Ovaries
      A) Estrogens
      B) Progesterone
III. Disorders of the endocrine system (see Box 6-8 on p. 85 in textbook)
  A. Hyposecretion
    1. Insulin: diabetes mellitus
    2. Thyroxine: hypothyroidism
  B. Hypersecretion
    1. Growth hormone: acromegaly or gigantism
    2. Insulin (due to tumor): hyperinsulinism

IV. Common lab tests for endocrine system (see Table 6-8 on p. 86 in textbook)
  A. Thyroid panel
  B. FSH
  C. FBS
  D. Calcium

Reproductive Systems
I. Function
  A. Male reproductive system
    1. Spermatogenesis
    2. Ejaculation of sperm
  B. Female reproductive system
    1. Oogenesis
    2. Fertilization of ovum
    3. Host and nourish embryo
II. Components
  A. Male reproductive system
    1. Scrotum—climate control and protection of testes
    2. Testes—sperm and testosterone production
    3. Epididymis—stores sperm
    4. Vas deferens—functions in ejaculation
    5. Urethra—pass urine; passageway for sperm
    6. Penis—copulation to pass sperm into female reproductive tract
    7. Glands—fluid plus sperm makes semen
      a. Prostate—25% to 30% of sperm fluid
      b. Seminal vesicles—60% of sperm fluid
      c. Bulbourethral gland—lubricate urethra, neutralize urine acidity
  B. Female reproductive system
    1. Ovaries—eggs; ovulation; estrogen production
    2. Fallopian tubes—site of fertilization
    3. Uterus—reproduction: site of implantation, nourishment, and growth
    4. Cervix—provides uterine support
    5. Vagina—copulation and receptacle for sperm
III. Disorders of the reproductive system (see Box 6-9 on p. 87 in textbook)
  A. Male reproductive system
    1. STDs: examples—gonorrhea, HIV
    2. Prostate cancer
  B. Female reproductive system
    1. STDs: examples—syphilis, genital herpes

2. Endometriosis
3. Fibroids
4. Cancer
IV. Common lab tests for reproductive system
   (see Table 6-9 on p. 87 in textbook)
   A. Semen analysis
   B. PSA
   C. Pap smear
   D. HCG

CERTIFICATION PREPARATION QUESTIONS

1. The levels of organization in the body from simplest to complex are:
   a. Cell, organ, tissue, system
   b. Cell, tissue, system, organ
   c. Cell, tissue, organ, system
   d. Cell, system, tissue, organ

2. The function of the system level of organization is to:
   a. Carry out common tasks
   b. Form discrete units of function
   c. Organize to form complex tissues
   d. Communicate and coordinate body parts

3. When the body acts to maintain a dynamic steady state, it is referred to as:
   a. Hemostasis
   b. Homeostasis
   c. Chemostasis
   d. Biostatic

4. Striated involuntary muscles are:
   a. Epithelial muscle
   b. Smooth muscle
   c. Skeletal muscle
   d. Cardiac muscle

5. Nerve tissue consists of:
   a. Striated tissue
   b. Osteoblasts
   c. Neurons
   d. Dura mater

6. The thorax is located _____ to the pelvis.
   a. Anterior
   b. Inferior
   c. Deep
   d. Superior

7. An organ located in the dorsal cavity is the:
   a. Stomach
   b. Liver
   c. Lungs
   d. Spinal cord

8. The plane that divides the body into top and bottom:
   a. Sagittal
   b. Coronal
   c. Transverse
   d. Frontal

9. The liver is located within the:
   a. Mediastinum
   b. Thoracic cavity
   c. Abdominal cavity
   d. Dorsal cavity

10. Classification of bones includes all of the following, *except*:
    a. Sesamoid
    b. Irregular
    c. Round
    d. Short

11. Functions of the skeletal system include all of the following, *except*:
    a. Store minerals
    b. Support body
    c. Hematopoiesis
    d. Thermoregulation

12. The articular cartilage, ligaments, and synovial fluid are all parts of which type of joint:
    a. Freely movable
    b. Immovable
    c. Fixed
    d. Partially movable

13. A disorder of the skeletal system is:
    a. Tendonitis
    b. Poliomyelitis
    c. Cerebral palsy
    d. Sarcoma

14. The following lab test is used for bone and joint disorders:
    a. Calcium
    b. Troponin
    c. Potassium
    d. Sodium

15. Muscles attach to the skeletal system by use of:
    a. Ligaments
    b. Joints
    c. Tendons
    d. Cartilage

16. Muscles usually occur in:
    a. Synergistic quads
    b. Antagonistic pairs
    c. Opposable triceps
    d. Freely movable agonists

17. Which of the following is a disorder of the muscular system?
    a. Tendonitis
    b. Neurosarcoma
    c. Cerebral palsy
    d. Parkinson disease

18. A muscular skeletal test includes:
    a. BUN
    b. Amylase
    c. Creatine kinase
    d. Magnesium

19. The layer of the integumentary system that is rich with capillaries is the:
    a. Dermis
    b. Epidermis
    c. Subcutaneous
    d. Epithelial

20. Functions of the integumentary system include all of the following, *except*:
    a. Protection
    b. Thermoregulation
    c. Sensation
    d. Integration

21. Glands of the integumentary system include:
    a. Pineal
    b. Sebaceous
    c. Thymus
    d. Meninges

22. A substance produced by the integumentary system to protect cellular DNA:
    a. Melatonin
    b. Melanin
    c. Carotene
    d. Keratin

23. A disorder of the integumentary system:
    a. Ringworm
    b. Cushing disease
    c. Endometriosis
    d. Cystitis

24. The brain and spinal cord are parts of the _____ system.
    a. Peripheral nervous
    b. Central nervous
    c. Somatic nervous
    d. Autonomic nervous

25. The brain and the spinal cord are protected by three layers of membranes called:
    a. Vertebrae
    b. Schwann cells
    c. Neuroglial cells
    d. Meninges

26. The part of the brain responsible for basic life functions:
    a. Cerebrum
    b. Cerebellum
    c. Brain stem
    d. Occipital lobe

27. A disorder of the nervous system includes:
    a. Multiple sclerosis
    b. Tendonitis
    c. Fibromyalgia
    d. Mitochondrial disorders

28. The following is a component of the digestive system:
    a. Alveoli
    b. Liver
    c. Adrenal cortex
    d. Nephron

29. Digestion of food begins with mastication or chewing, which is referred to as:
    a. Secretion
    b. Mechanical digestion
    c. Peristalsis
    d. Chyme

30. Section of the GI tract where absorption of digested molecules of food occurs:
    a. Cecum
    b. Small intestine
    c. Sigmoid
    d. Colon

31. All of the following are common lab tests for the digestive system, *except*:
    a. Occult blood
    b. Ammonia
    c. Bilirubin
    d. Microalbumin

32. Bile is produced by which organ?
    a. Liver
    b. Pancreas
    c. Islets of Langerhans
    d. Gallbladder

33. A disorder of the digestive system:
    a. Hepatitis
    b. Osteoporosis
    c. Asthma
    d. Graves' disease

34. Components of the urinary system include all of the following, *except*:
    a. Ureters
    b. Nephron
    c. Dendrites
    d. Glomerulus

35. The function of the urinary bladder is:
    a. Filtration
    b. Secretion
    c. Reabsorption
    d. Storage

36. Which of the following is a test for urologic disorders?
    a. Creatine kinase
    b. Blood urea nitrogen
    c. Myoglobin
    d. Human chorionic gonadotropin

37. A patient suffering from cystitis has inflammation of the:
    a. Kidneys
    b. Renal calyces
    c. Urinary bladder
    d. Ureters

38. Structures associated with the respiratory system include:
    a. Alveoli
    b. Pressure receptors
    c. Bowman capsule
    d. Convoluted tubules

39. The function of the respiratory system includes all of the following, *except*:
    a. Internal respiration
    b. External respiration
    c. Exhalation of carbon dioxide
    d. Efferent transportation

40. The site of internal respiration is at the _____ level.
    a. Cellular
    b. Alveoli and capillary
    c. Bronchiole
    d. Nares

41. A disorder of the respiratory system:
    a. URI
    b. UTI
    c. ALS
    d. RA

42. Regulation of body functions to maintain homeostasis is a function of the _____ system.
    a. Nervous
    b. Digestive
    c. Muscular
    d. Endocrine

43. The master gland of the endocrine system refers to which gland?
    a. Thymus
    b. Thyroid
    c. Pituitary
    d. Adrenal

44. This gland regulates carbohydrate metabolism through secretion of insulin and glucagon, which serve to maintain normal blood glucose levels.
    a. Pituitary
    b. Liver
    c. Pancreas
    d. Thyroid

45. Hyperglycemia is a symptom of which endocrine disorder?
    a. Diabetes insipidus
    b. Hyperinsulinemia
    c. Diabetes mellitus
    d. Nephritis

46. Endocrine disorder tests include:
    a. FSH

b. RSV
c. HCV
d. CSF

47. Which of the following structures is a part of the male reproductive system?
    a. Bulbourethral gland
    b. Ureters
    c. Collecting duct
    d. Ventricles

48. A function of the reproductive system includes production of:
    a. Hormones
    b. Enzymes
    c. TRH
    d. Reagin

49. Fertilization of the embryo occurs in the:
    a. Ovaries
    b. Fallopian tubes
    c. Fimbriae
    d. Uterus

50. A disorder associated with the reproductive system is:
    a. Shingles
    b. Cystitis
    c. Giardiasis
    d. Syphilis

ANSWERS AND RATIONALES

1. **Answer: C**
   Rationale: The organization in the body from simplest to complex is cell, tissue, organ, and then body system.
   Text Reference: p. 63

2. **Answer: A**
   Rationale: Cells join together to form tissues that then interact to form discrete units of function called organs. When different organs interact to carry out common tasks they are referred to as an organ system.
   Text Reference: p. 63

3. **Answer: B**
   Rationale: Homeostasis is the process at each level of organization in the body that functions to maintain a dynamic steady state or metabolic equilibrium. Hemostasis refers to

stopping the flow of blood. Chemostasis is the continuous cultivation of cells. Biostatic refers to the inhibition of the growth of an organism.
   Text Reference: p. 63

4. **Answer: D**
   Rationale: Cardiac muscle or heart muscle is striated in appearance and involuntarily controlled by the autonomic nervous system. Smooth muscle is nonstriated involuntary muscle found in the tunica media layer of blood, lymph vessels, GI tract, bladder, and uterus. Skeletal muscle is striated voluntary muscle that is attached to the skeleton.
   Text Reference: p. 65

5. **Answer: C**
   Rationale: Nerve tissue is comprised of neurons and neuroglial cells. Osteoblasts are cells that make bone; striated tissue is a type of muscle tissue; dura mater is the outer covering of the brain.
   Text Reference: pp. 65-66, 70, 77

6. **Answer: D**
   Rationale: Superior means above. The thorax is above the pelvis. Anterior means to the front and inferior means below the surface of the body.
   Text Reference: p. 68

7. **Answer: D**
   Rationale: The organs of the central nervous system include the brain and spinal cord, which are located in the dorsal cavity. The liver, lungs, and stomach are located in the ventral cavity. In addition, the stomach and liver are located in the abdominal cavity; the lungs are located in the thoracic cavity.
   Text Reference: p. 68

8. **Answer: C**
   Rationale: The transverse plane divides the body into top and bottom. The sagittal plane divides the body into left and right. The coronal or frontal plane divides the body into front and back.
   Text Reference: pp. 68-69

9. **Answer: C**
   Rationale: The liver is located within the upper abdominal cavity. The lungs are located in the thoracic cavity. The dorsal

cavity contains the cranial and spinal cavities, which house the brain and spinal cord, respectively. The mediastinum is the space between the lungs that contains the heart, aorta, thymus gland, portion of the trachea, esophagus, lymph nodes, and important nerves.
Text Reference: pp. 68-69 and Content Overview (earlier in this chapter)

10. **Answer: C**
Rationale: Bones are classified by their shapes and include long, short, flat, sesamoid, and irregular bones.
Text Reference: p. 70

11. **Answer: D**
Rationale: The functions of the skeletal system include support, movement, and protection, storage of minerals, and hematopoiesis. Thermoregulation is a function of the integumentary system.
Text Reference: pp. 69, 73

12. **Answer: A**
Rationale: A free moving joint such as the elbow, shoulder, knee, etc., consists of ligaments, a fluid-filled synovial cavity, and articular cartilage.
Text Reference: p. 71

13. **Answer: D**
Rationale: Sarcoma is a malignant neoplastic disorder of the skeletal system. Tendonitis is a trauma disorder and poliomyelitis is a motor neuron disease, both of the muscular system. Cerebral palsy is a developmental disorder of the nervous system.
Text Reference: pp. 72-73

14. **Answer: A**
Rationale: Calcium is a mineral that is stored in the bone along with phosphorus. Troponin is used to assess myocardial infarction. Potassium and sodium are electrolytes used to assess acid-base imbalances that would result in respiratory disorders.
Text Reference: pp. 72, 83

15. **Answer: C**
Rationale: Tendons are a type of fibrous connective tissue that attaches muscles

to bones. Ligaments are tough, fibrous connective tissues that hold two bones together. Cartilage is a tough, fibrous, elastic tissue found in the joints, outer ear, larynx, etc.
Text Reference: pp. 70-71

16. **Answer: B**
Rationale: Muscles usually occur in antagonistic pairs with opposable actions, whereby one muscle contracts as another relaxes.
Text Reference: p. 71

17. **Answer: A**
Rationale: Tendonitis is a muscular disorder. Neurosarcoma, cerebral palsy, and Parkinson disease are all nervous system disorders.
Text Reference: pp. 73, 77

18. **Answer: C**
Rationale: Creatine kinase is a test of the muscular system to assess muscle damage. BUN is blood urea nitrogen and is used to assess kidney disease; amylase is an enzyme of the digestive system and testing is performed to assess the presence of pancreatitis. Magnesium is a mineral of the skeletal system and is used to assess mineral imbalance.
Text Reference: pp. 72-73, 82

19. **Answer: A**
Rationale: The dermis is the layer of skin that is rich in capillaries along with oil and sweat glands, nerves, and sensory cells. This is the targeted site for microcollection procedures. The epidermis is the outermost layer of skin, whereas the subcutaneous layer is the innermost layer and consists of fat and collagen.
Text Reference: p. 73

20. **Answer: D**
Rationale: The integumentary functions include protection against invasion of microbes and chemicals; thermoregulation through sweating and constriction; sensation through specialized cells that allow the brain to perceive hot, cold, pain, etc. Integration is a part of the nervous system function.
Text Reference: p. 73

21. **Answer: B**
    Rationale: Sebaceous glands are oil glands located in the dermal layer of the skin in the integumentary system. The pineal and thymus glands are parts of the endocrine system. Meninges refers to the three membranes of the central nervous system.
    Text Reference: pp. 73, 77, 80

22. **Answer: B**
    Rationale: Melanin is a pigment produced by melanocytes in the epidermal layer of the skin in the presence of UV light to protect the DNA of the skin. It also gives rise to the pigmentation of skin colors of the various races. Melatonin is a hormone produced by the pineal gland. Carotene is a provitamin A, and keratin is a protein in skin and nails.
    Text Reference: p. 73 and Content Overview (earlier in this chapter)

23. **Answer: A**
    Rationale: Ringworm is an infection of the integumentary system. Cushing disease is an endocrine disorder that arises from hypersecretion of cortisol and ACTH. Endometriosis is a reproductive disorder in women due to the extrauterine presence of endometrial cells. Cystitis is a bladder infection.
    Text Reference: pp. 74, 80, 85, 87

24. **Answer: B**
    Rationale: The brain and spinal cord are parts of the central nervous system. The peripheral nervous system refers to all neurons outside of the CNS. The somatic system refers to the voluntary innervations of muscles, and the autonomic nervous system refers to the involuntary innervations of cardiac and smooth muscle.
    Text Reference: pp. 73, 77

25. **Answer: D**
    Rationale: Meninges are the three layers of membranes that encase and protect the brain and the spinal cord: dura mater, arachnoid, and the pia mater. Vertebrae are the bones of the spinal column; Schwann cells produce the myelin sheath; and neuroglial cells provide nourishment and support to the neurons of the CNS.
    Text Reference: p. 77

26. **Answer: C**
    Rationale: The brain stem controls basic life processes including respiration, heartbeat, and blood pressure. The cerebrum controls thoughts, emotions, memory; the cerebellum fine tunes motor commands; and the occipital lobe is the visual processing center.
    Text Reference: p. 76 and Content Overview (earlier in this chapter)

27. **Answer: A**
    Rationale: Multiple sclerosis is an autoimmune disorder of the nervous system due to demyelination of the CNS neurons. Tendonitis, fibromyalgia, and mitochondrial disorders are all disorders of the muscular system.
    Text Reference: pp. 73, 77

28. **Answer: B**
    Rationale: The liver is an accessory organ that functions within the digestive system. Alveoli are part of the respiratory system and function in the exchange of gases during external respiration. The adrenal cortex is the outer portion of the adrenal gland. The nephron is the functional unit of the urinary system.
    Text Reference: pp. 77, 81, 84

29. **Answer: B**
    Rationale: Mechanical digestion (chewing, churning action of stomach) and chemical digestion (enzymes in saliva; enzymes, chemicals in stomach and small intestines) break food down into small molecules, which are then absorbed by the intestines. Peristalsis is the wavelike motion of smooth muscle of the GI tract moving food into and through the GI tract. As food moves into the stomach and undergoes further mechanical and chemical digestion, it turns into chyme, which is a thick, soupy mixture that then moves through the GI system. Digestive enzymes and chemicals are hormonally controlled and released through secretion when food is present.
    Text Reference: pp. 77-78

30. **Answer: B**
    Rationale: Absorption of digested food molecules occurs in the small intestine where numerous fingerlike projections called villi are surrounded by a rich capillary bed

that aids in rapid and efficient absorption of nutrients. The cecum, colon, and sigmoid are all parts of the large intestine.
Text Reference: pp. 78-79

31. **Answer: D**
Rationale: Occult blood, ammonia, and bilirubin are all lab tests for digestive disorders. Microalbumin is a renal test.
Text Reference: pp. 79, 82

32. **Answer: A**
Rationale: The liver produces bile that is stored in the gallbladder, which releases it into the small intestine to aid in the digestion of fats. The pancreas produces insulin and glucagon, which function in carbohydrate metabolism. The islets of Langerhans are a group of specialized tissue that make and secrete hormones such as insulin, glucagon, somatostatin, etc.
Text Reference: pp. 79, 85

33. **Answer: A**
Rationale: Hepatitis is an inflammation of the liver, which is an accessory organ to the digestive system. Osteoporosis is a skeletal disorder, which can be partially prevented through dietary inclusion of calcium. Asthma is a respiratory disorder that new studies indicate may be linked to diet in addition to other causes. Graves' disease is a thyroid disorder resulting from hypersecretion of thyroid hormones.
Text Reference: pp. 72, 79, 83, 85

34. **Answer: C**
Rationale: The ureters, nephron, and glomerulus are all structures of the urinary system. Dendrites are the branched projections of the neuron in the nervous system.
Text Reference: pp. 67, 81

35. **Answer: D**
Rationale: The urinary bladder functions as a temporary reservoir or storage unit for urine until it is expelled from the body through micturition. The kidneys function to clear blood of waste products through filtration, secretion, and reabsorption.
Text Reference: p. 80 and Content Overview (earlier in this chapter)

36. **Answer: B**
Rationale: Blood urea nitrogen (BUN) is a test of the urinary system. Creatine kinase and myoglobin are muscular system tests. HCG is a substance produced as a result of fertilization of the ovum and is a reproductive system test used to assess pregnancy. HCG testing can be performed on urine, but it is not a test of the urinary system.
Text Reference: p. 82

37. **Answer: C**
Rationale: Cystitis is inflammation of the bladder. *Cyst/o* means bladder, the suffix *-itis* means inflammation. The kidneys contain renal calyces, which are branches of the renal pelvis surrounding the renal medulla. The ureters connect the kidneys to the bladder and function to allow the urine filtrate to drain into the bladder.
Text Reference: pp. 82, Box 6-6

38. **Answer: A**
Rationale: Alveoli are the final branching structures in the lungs that serve as the site for gas exchange between the atmosphere and the blood. Pressure receptors are structures in the dermal layer of skin; the Bowman capsule houses the glomerulus in the nephron unit of the urinary system; and convoluted tubules are structures with the nephron unit.
Text Reference: pp. 74, 80-82

39. **Answer: D**
Rationale: The functions of the respiratory system are internal respiration for the exchange of oxygen and carbon dioxide at the cellular level; external respiration for the exchange of gases in the lungs; and for the expulsion of carbon dioxide generated from metabolic processes.
Text Reference: p. 80

40. **Answer: A**
Rationale: Trachea branches into the bronchi leading to the bronchioles that then terminate in the alveoli where the capillaries wrap around providing a network for the exchange of gases between the alveoli and blood. Nares refer to the nose. Internal respiration occurs at the cellular level as

oxygen is released from RBCs and carbon dioxide diffuses out of the tissue into the blood.
Text Reference: pp. 81-82

41. **Answer: A**
Rationale: The abbreviation URI stands for upper respiratory infection; UTI is urinary tract infection; ALS is amyotrophic lateral sclerosis; and RA is a test for rheumatoid arthritis.
Text Reference: pp. 72-73, 82-83

42. **Answer: D**
Rationale: The function of the endocrine system is to regulate body functions to maintain homeostasis. The digestive system is for absorption and elimination of waste; the muscular system is for movement of the skeleton, pumping of blood, and regulation of passage of materials through vessels depending on the type of muscular tissue; the nervous system controls, regulates, and communicates as a system by receiving, processing, and responding to nerve impulses.
Text Reference: p. 83

43. **Answer: C**
Rationale: The pituitary gland is referred to as the master gland because it regulates many other endocrine glands through feedback loops.
Text Reference: p. 82

44. **Answer: C**
Rationale: The pancreas produces insulin and glucagon that regulate the level of the sugar glucose in the blood. The pituitary is the master gland of the endocrine system and produces a number of hormones that regulate other glands. The thyroid gland secretes T_3, T_4, and calcitonin and functions to regulate the body's metabolism and calcium levels. The liver secretes bile.
Text Reference: p. 85

45. **Answer: C**
Rationale: Diabetes mellitus results from hyposecretion of insulin causing a rise in blood glucose. Hyperinsulinemia can cause low blood glucose levels due to insulin overdose or tumor. Diabetes insipidus is the result of hyposecretion of ADH. Nephritis is inflammation of the kidney.
Text Reference: pp. 80, 85

46. **Answer: A**
Rationale: FSH is follicle-stimulating hormone produced by the pituitary gland. RSV is a test for viral pneumonia; HCV is hepatitis C virus and is a test for disorders of the digestive system; and CSF is cerebral spinal fluid, a test of the nervous system.
Text Reference: pp. 77, 79, 86

47. **Answer: A**
Rationale: The bulbourethral gland is a part of the male reproductive system. The ureters and the collecting duct are parts of the urinary system. The ventricles are located in the brain.
Text Reference: pp. 77, 80, 86

48. **Answer: A**
Rationale: The reproductive system produces the hormones estrogen in the ovaries and testosterone in the testes.
Text Reference: p. 86

49. **Answer: B**
Rationale: Fertilization of the egg occurs in the fallopian tube, which continues on to the uterus where implantation occurs.
Text Reference: p. 86

50. **Answer: D**
Rationale: Syphilis is a sexually transmitted disease associated with the reproductive system. Cystitis refers to a bladder infection; giardiasis is a parasitic infection of the digestive system; and shingles is a nervous system disorder that is a latent infection of varicella-zoster.
Text Reference: pp. 77, 79, 82, 87

CIRCULATORY, LYMPHATIC, AND IMMUNE SYSTEMS

Pamela Primrose

INTRODUCTION

The circulatory system transports blood containing oxygen and nutrients throughout the body and picks up metabolic waste products for disposal. Beginning at the heart, blood passes from arteries to capillaries to veins, and then back to the heart. The structure of each type of blood vessel is adapted to its function within the system. In addition to its role in nutrient and waste transport, blood transports hormones and enzymes, along with clotting factors that minimize blood leakage in the event of injury. Hemostasis ensures that a rupture in a blood vessel is repaired quickly. A separate but linked circulatory system, the lymphatic system, redistributes intercellular fluid and provides an important route of transport for cells of the immune system. The immune system fights foreign invaders through a combination of cellular and chemical defenses.

CONTENT OVERVIEW

Circulatory System

I. Function
   A. Pulmonary circulation
      1. Carries blood between heart and lungs
      2. Gas exchange in external respiration
   B. Systemic circulation
      1. Carries blood between heart and rest of body tissues
      2. Gas exchange in internal respiration
II. Components
   A. Heart
      1. Structure
         a. Muscular double pump
         b. Pericardium—double-layered sac surrounding heart
            i. Support
            ii. Lubrication
         c. Three layers
            i. Epicardium: outer layer of epithelial cells
            ii. Myocardium: middle layer of cardiac tissue
            iii. Endocardium: inner layer of modified epithelium
         d. Four chambers
            i. Left/right atria: upper chambers
            ii. Left/right ventricles: lower chambers
         e. Valves
            i. Right atrioventricular (AV) or tricuspid valve
               A) Separates right atrium from right ventricle
            ii. Pulmonary semilunar valve
               A) Separates right ventricle from pulmonary arteries
            iii. Left atrioventricular or bicuspid or mitral valve
               A) Separates left atrium from left ventricle
            iv. Aortic semilunar valve
               A) Separates left ventricle from aorta
            v. Septum
               A) Separates right and left sides of heart
               B) Keeps blood from crossing over
III. Circulation through the heart
   A. Pulmonary circulation
      1. Deoxygenated blood enters heart
      2. Pulmonary arteries—transport deoxygenated blood to lungs
      3. Pulmonary veins—transport oxygenated blood to heart
   B. Systemic circulation
      1. Aorta pumps oxygenated blood to tissues
      2. Capillaries—site of gas exchange between blood and tissues
      3. Veins return blood to heart to repeat circulatory system process
   C. Summary of blood flow:
      Inferior/superior venae cavae → Rt atrium → AV/tricuspid valve → Rt ventricle → Pulmonary semilunar valve → Rt/Lft pulmonary arteries → Lungs → Rt/Lft pulmonary veins → Lft atrium → Mitral valve → Lft ventricle → Aortic semilunar valve → Aorta → Arteries → Arterioles → Capillaries → Venules → Veins

IV. Blood vessels
  A. Anatomy of vessels
    1. Arteries and veins
      a. Tunica media—middle smooth muscle
      b. Tunica media—middle smooth muscle
      c. Tunica intima—inner single layer endothelial cells
    2. Capillaries
      a. Single layer of endothelial cells
  C. Arteries
    1. Function—carry blood to tissues
    2. Structure and location
      a. Thick muscular wall
        i. Expand as blood enters
        ii. Contract to maintain flow and pressure in diastole
      b. Deeper in tissue—feel for pulse
      c. Branch into smaller arterioles, which branch into capillaries
  D. Capillaries
    1. Function—site of exchange of gases, nutrients, wastes between blood and tissues
    2. Structure and location
      a. Single layer to maximize diffusion
      b. Complex network connecting arterioles and venules
      c. Present in all tissues
    3. Lead to venules, the smallest veins, which flow into veins
  E. Veins
    1. Function—carry blood back to heart
    2. Structure and location
      a. Thinner walls, less muscle
      b. Minimal fluctuation in blood pressure
      c. Valves—prevent backflow of blood
      d. Closer to surface of skin
V. Contraction of the heart and blood pressure
  A. Heartbeat cycle
    1. Contraction—systole
      a. Atria contract simultaneously slightly before ventricles contract
        i. Blood moves to ventricles
      b. Ventricles contract simultaneously
        i. Blood moves to lungs and aorta
    2. Relaxation—diastole
      a. Both atria and ventricles fill again
  B. Blood pressure
    1. Ratio of ventricular systole to diastole i.e., 110/80 mm Hg
    2. Varies in different points in circulatory system

3. Always measured from brachial artery
  a. Sphygmomanometer: measures force of blood on arterial wall
VI. Disorders of the heart and blood vessels (see Table 7-1 on p. 99 in textbook)
  A. Arteries
    1. Aneurysm
    2. Arteriosclerosis
  B. Veins
    1. Varicose veins
    2. Hemorrhoids
  C. Heart
    1. Coronary artery disease
    2. Myocardial infarction
      a. Atherosclerosis
      b. Blood clot
      c. Arteriospasm
        i. Stress
        ii. Drugs (i.e., cocaine)
        iii. Exposure to extreme cold
        iv. Cigarette smoking
VII. Tests used to diagnose an MI (see Box 7-1 on p. 99 in textbook)
  A. Troponin T and troponin 1
  B. Myoglobin

Veins for Phlebotomy Procedures
I. Peripheral blood
  A. Antecubital veins
  B. Hand/wrist veins
  C. Foot/ankle veins
  D. Fingertip
  E. Heel pad
  F. Earlobe
II. Circulatory anatomy of the antecubital fossa
  A. Location—below elbow joint
  B. Use in phlebotomy
    1. Accessible
    2. Prominent veins—resemble "M" or "H"
      a. Cephalic vein—thumb side
      b. Median cubital vein—center
      c. Basilic vein—inner
    3. Other structures
      a. Brachial artery—across front crease of elbow
      b. External cutaneous nerve—close to cephalic
      c. Internal cutaneous nerve—close to basilica
  C. Potential complications during venipuncture
    1. Puncturing artery

2. Hitting nerve
   a. Maybe no deeper than veins
   b. May pass over veins

Blood Facts
I. Blood
   A. Components
      1. Plasma
         a. Fluid portion—clear pale yellow; may be slightly hazy due to fibrinogen
         b. 55% of volume of blood
         c. 90% water
         d. 10% dissolved substances (examples)
            i. Albumin
               A) Protein—60% of plasma protein
               B) Functions to maintain osmotic pressure
               C) Transports molecules
                  1) Unconjugated bilirubin
                  2) Calcium
                  3) Hormones (thyroid hormones and some fat-soluble hormones)
                  4) Cortisol (15% of total; more if cortisol levels are elevated)
                  5) Drugs—warfarin, phenylbutazone, etc.
            ii. Immunoglobulins or antibodies
               A) Immune system
               B) Fight invasion of pathogens, etc.
            iii. Fibrinogen and other clotting factors
            iv. Complement
               A) Immune system proteins
               B) Destroy target cell by puncturing membranes
            v. Electrolytes
               A) Major ions of plasma—examples
                  1) Na^+
                  2) K^+
                  3) Cl^-
                  4) HCO_3^-
                  5) Ca^{2+}
         e. Formed in vitro through use of anticoagulant
            i. Examples of use
               A) Hematology—EDTA
               B) Coagulation—sodium citrate
               C) STAT chemistry—lithium heparin

2. Serum
   a. Plasma without clotting factors—clear pale yellow fluid removed from clot; may be hazy from lipids
   b. Formed when blood clots
      i. Examples of use
         A) Chemistry—SST
         B) Immunology—red top
   c. Fibrinogen → fibrin
      i. Uses up clotting factors
      ii. Traps cellular elements
      iii. Separate serum from cells via centrifugation
3. Formed elements
   a. Formed in bone marrow from stem cells
   b. 45% of blood volume
   c. RBCs: 99% (5 million/microliter)
      i. Function
         A) Carry hemoglobin—red color
         B) Iron-containing oxygen transports protein
         C) Carry CO_2
      ii. Released from bone marrow as reticulocyte
      iii. Mature into erythrocyte day or so later
      iv. Lifespan 120 days → break down
         A) Iron—recycled
         B) Amino acids—recycled
         C) Bilirubin—transported to liver as waste
      v. Old RBCs removed from blood
         A) Liver
         B) Bone marrow
         C) Spleen
   d. WBCs: <1%
      i. Function
         A) Fight infection
         B) Aid in immune process
         C) Produced in bone marrow
         D) Mature in bone marrow and thymus
         E) Reside in bone marrow, thymus, other lymphoid tissue
         F) Lifespan varies
      ii. Types of cellular elements in circulation
         A) Granulocytes
            1) Neutrophils: (PMN, segs) 40% to 60%
               a) Phagocytes—attack and digest bacteria
               b) Lifespan 3 to 4 days

2) Eosinophils: 1% to 3% (eosin dye—red)
  a) Phagocytic—parasites and antibody-labeled foreign molecules
  b) Lifespan 18 hours in circulation; approximately 6 days in tissue
3) Basophils: <1% (basic dye—deep purple)
  a) Capable of ingesting foreign particles
  b) Produce heparin and histamine
  c) Lifespan several days in circulation; as mast cell in tissue several weeks to months

B) Mononuclear
  1) Monocytes: 3% to 8%
    a) Largest phagocytic cell—roving sentries
    b) Activate B cells (lymph) to make antibody
    c) Diapedesis into peripheral tissues from circulatory system → macrophage
    d) Lifespan is said to be several months
  2) Lymphocytes: 20% to 40%
    a) Most reside in lymph nodes
    b) Circulate—circulatory and lymphatic system
    c) Increase—viral infections
    d) Lifespan said to be about 4 years for 80% of lymphs and some almost 20 years
    e) Types
      i) B cells: differentiate into plasma cells to make antibodies or become memory cells
      ii) T cells: cellular immunity

      iii) Natural killer (NK) cells: destroy foreign cells, infected cells
C. Thrombocytes: <1% (platelets)
  1) Membrane-bound packets of cytoplasm
  2) Function: coagulation
  3) Lifespan: 9 to 12 days

II. Hemostasis
  A. Process of blood vessel repair to stop the flow of blood
  B. Series of steps
    1. Muscular contraction
      a. Vascular phase—30 minutes vasoconstriction
    2. Clot formation
      a. Platelet phase: primary hemostasis
        i. Platelet adhesion
        ii. Platelet aggregation
      b. Coagulation phase: secondary hemostasis
        i. Cascade of enzymes and factors → fibrin clot
        ii. Begins within 30 seconds to several minutes of injury
    3. Removal of clot
      a. Fibrinolysis phase
        i. Breakdown of fibrin by plasmin
        ii. Occurs when tissue repair commences
        iii. Tests to assess rate of fibrinolysis
          A) FDP—fibrin degradation products
          B) FSP—fibrin split products
        iv. Exogenous substances to dissolve clots in strokes, MIs, pulmonary embolism, etc.
          A) Synthetic t-PA (tissue plasminogen activator)
          B) Urokinase
          C) Streptokinase

III. Blood disorders—examples (see Table 7-2 on p. 106 in textbook)
  A. RBCs and hemoglobin
    1. Anemia
    2. Sickle cell anemia
  B. WBCs
    1. Leukemia
    2. Mononucleosis
  C. Hemostasis, platelets, and clotting
    1. Hemophilia
    2. Thrombosis

IV. Common laboratory tests for blood disorders (see Table 7-2 on p. 106 in textbook)
  A. CBC—anemia, leukemia
  B. Sickle-cell solubility—sickle cell disease
  C. Monospot—infectious mononucleosis
  D. PT—monitor Coumadin
  E. PTT—monitor heparin

Lymphatic System Facts

I. Lymphatic system
  A. Components
    1. Lymphatic vessels
      a. Closed at distal ends
      b. Valves keep fluid moving in one direction
      c. Empty into venous system distal to superior vena cava
    2. Lymph organs
      a. Lymph nodes—populated by lymphocytes
        i. Locations throughout body—cervical, axillary, inguinal, etc.
        ii. Screen lymph fluid—for presence of infectious or foreign agents
        iii. Example: tonsils
    3. Associated organs
      a. Spleen—removes old RBCs; examines blood by T, B cells
      b. Thymus—maturation of T cells
    4. Lymph fluid
      a. Derived from interstitial fluid—combination of plasma and cellular fluid
      b. Contains proteins or molecules from infectious agents
        i. Examined by WBCs in lymph nodes for immune response
      c. Transports fat, keeping it out of capillary circulation in intestines
    5. Lymphocytes
      a. T cells: cellular immunity
      b. B cells: make antibody
  B. Lymphatic system disorders
    1. Lymphedema—accumulation of interstitial fluid in tissues
    2. Lymphoma—tumor of lymph gland
      a. Example: Hodgkin disease

Immune System Facts

I. Immune system
  A. Nonspecific immunity
    1. Defense against infectious agents
    2. Independent of specific chemical markers
    3. Types
      a. Physical barriers
      b. Complement system
      c. Phagocytes—monos and neutrophils
      d. Inflammation
        i. Increases blood flow—redness, heat
        ii. Capillary permeability—swelling
        iii. Activation of macrophages
        iv. Increases temperature
        v. Clotting reaction—walls off infection
        vi. Activates specific immunity
      e. Fever
  B. Specific immunity
    1. Cellular immunity
      a. Molecular recognition of markers
        i. Antigens
      b. Involves T cells
    2. Humoral immunity
      a. B cells → plasma cells → memory cells
        i. Antibodies
        ii. Specific to antigen
  C. Immune system disorders
    1. Autoimmunity—attack own tissues
    2. Allergy—inappropriate immune response
    3. Severe-combined immune deficiency (SCIDS)—genetic lack of T and B cells
    4. AIDS

CERTIFICATION PREPARATION QUESTIONS

1. The function of the circulatory system includes transportation of all of the following, *except*:
   a. Blood throughout body
   b. Hormones, enzymes, nutrients, clotting factors
   c. Wastes for removal
   d. Lymph fluid

2. Pulmonary circulation carries blood between the:
   a. Heart and body tissues
   b. Heart and the lungs
   c. Heart and visceral organs
   d. Heart and venae cavae

3. The flow of oxygenated blood through the circulatory vessel system as it leaves the heart is as follows:
   a. Aorta → veins → capillaries → venules → arteries → venae cavae
   b. Venae cavae → arteries → capillaries → arterioles → veins → aorta

   c. Aorta → arteries → arterioles → capillaries
     → venules → veins → venae cavae
   d. Arterioles → arteries → venules →
     capillaries → veins → venae cavae

4. The exchange of dissolved gases, nutrients, and waste products in the blood occurs in the:
   a. Capillary beds
   b. Venous network
   c. Arterial beds
   d. Lymphatic organs

5. The heart is surrounded by a thin membranous sac referred to as the:
   a. Epicardium
   b. Pericardium
   c. Myocardium
   d. Endocardium

6. The coronary arteries that supply blood to the heart are embedded in which layer?
   a. Epicardium
   b. Myocardium
   c. Endocardium
   d. Pericardium

7. The heart consists of how many chambers?
   a. Two
   b. Three
   c. Four
   d. Five

8. Another name for the tricuspid valve is:
   a. Left atrioventricular valve
   b. Right atrioventricular valve
   c. Pulmonary semilunar valve
   d. Mitral valve

9. The left atrioventricular valve is also referred to as the:
   a. Mitral valve
   b. Bicuspid valve
   c. Aortic semilunar valve
   d. A and B

10. Before entering the heart, deoxygenated blood from the systemic circulation collects in the:
   a. Left atrium
   b. Venae cavae
   c. Right ventricle
   d. Aorta

11. Oxygenated blood exits the heart through the:
   a. Pulmonary veins
   b. Left atrium
   c. Aortic semilunar valve
   d. Right ventricle

12. A cardiac cycle is described as being the:
   a. Flow of blood through the pulmonary circuit
   b. Flow of blood through the systemic circuit
   c. One complete contraction and relaxation of each heart chamber
   d. "Lubb-dupp" sound of the heartbeat

13. Systole is a measure of the:
   a. Relaxation phase of the heart
   b. Movement of blood through the systemic circuit
   c. Contraction phase of the heart
   d. Venous pressure

14. The difference between arteries and veins is that:
   a. Veins contain a thicker muscular wall and are closer to the surface of tissue
   b. Arteries have a thicker muscular wall and are deeper than veins in tissue
   c. Veins have a thinner wall, valves, and are deeper than arteries in tissue
   d. Arteries have a thicker muscular wall, are close to the surface, and identified by a pulse

15. Blood pressure is a measure of the:
   a. Force of blood on arteriole walls
   b. Force of blood on arterial walls
   c. Force of blood on the walls of the heart chambers
   d. Force of blood on venous walls

16. Impaired blood flow leading to reduced level or lack of oxygen to a tissue is referred to as:
   a. Ischemia
   b. MI
   c. Heart attack
   d. CVA

17. The venous system functions to:
   a. Provide nutrients to tissues
   b. Carry oxygenated blood to tissues
   c. Divert blood from arteries into visceral organs
   d. Return blood back to the heart

18. A patient diagnosed with an MI is undergoing investigative testing to determine the cause of the heart attack. MIs may be due to any of the following conditions, *except*:
    a. Atherosclerosis
    b. Coronary arteriospasm
    c. Thrombus
    d. Phlebitis

19. A patient is admitted to the ER complaining of severe chest pain. All of the following laboratory tests may be ordered to assist in the diagnosis of a myocardial infarct, *except*:
    a. Troponin I
    b. Myoglobin
    c. CBC
    d. CK-MB

20. Veins suitable for possible venipuncture in the antecubital area include all of the following, *except*:
    a. Basilic vein
    b. Cephalic vein
    c. Median cubital vein
    d. Brachial veins

21. Formed or cellular elements of the blood include all of the following, *except*:
    a. Platelets
    b. WBCs
    c. RBCs
    d. Plasma

22. The plasma: cellular composition of whole blood is:
    a. 35% plasma: 65% cellular elements
    b. 55% plasma: 45% cellular elements
    c. 75% plasma: 25% cellular elements
    d. 90% plasma: 10% cellular elements

23. Plasma consists of:
    a. 90% water, 10% solutes
    b. 55% water, 45% solutes
    c. 10% water, 90% solutes
    d. 60% water, 40% solutes

24. The phlebotomist needs to collect a sample that will yield approximately 5 mL of plasma for the test that has been ordered. He will need to collect a minimum of _____ mL of blood.
    a. 15 mL
    b. 7 mL

    c. 10 mL
    d. 5 mL

25. Blood enters the left atrium through:
    a. Pulmonary vein
    b. Venae cavae
    c. Right ventricle
    d. Systemic circulation

26. Blood enters the left ventricle from the:
    a. Pulmonary vein
    b. Venae cavae
    c. Left atrium
    d. Systemic circulation

27. Characteristics of veins include all of the following, *except*:
    a. Have a thicker wall to move blood up to the heart
    b. Have valves to prevent backflow of blood
    c. Are closer to the skin surface than arteries
    d. Blood flows into veins from venules

28. A plasma protein that serves to help regulate blood volume by maintaining osmotic pressure and by transporting many different types of molecules is:
    a. Fibrinogen
    b. Complement
    c. Albumin
    d. Antibody

29. Serum is the liquid portion of blood that lacks:
    a. Electrolytes
    b. Clotting factors
    c. Colloidal particles
    d. Complement

30. The phlebotomist must draw blood for a STAT glucose, BUN, and electrolytes in ER and deliver it to the lab for testing as the I-STAT instrument is not functioning properly. Which type of sample is *most* appropriate?
    a. Serum
    b. Plasma
    c. Whole blood
    d. All of the above

31. Which cell loses its nucleus before release from the bone marrow?
    a. RBC
    b. WBC

   c. Platelet
   d. Stem cells

32. Mature RBCs are referred to as:
   a. Reticulocytes
   b. Leukocytes
   c. Thrombocytes
   d. Erythrocytes

33. A patient has been diagnosed with anemia and the physician wants to assess how well the bone marrow is producing RBCs. The physician requests which of the following tests to be drawn and tested?
   a. Hemoglobin
   b. Hematocrit
   c. Reticulocyte
   d. CBC

34. Normal RBC counts average about:
   a. 2 million/µL
   b. 5 million/µL
   c. 10 million/µL
   d. 15 million/µL

35. One of the primary functions of erythrocytes is to:
   a. Deliver oxygen to body tissues
   b. Phagocytize foreign substances
   c. Produce antibodies
   d. Participate in the coagulation cascade

36. Another term for WBC is:
   a. Erythrocyte
   b. Leukocyte
   c. Thrombocyte
   d. Histiocyte

37. The normal WBC reference range is:
   a. 2000 to 4000/µL
   b. 5000 to 10,000/µL
   c. 8000 to 12,000/µL
   d. 9000 to 14,000/µL

38. The primary function of WBCs is to:
   a. Deliver nutrients to body tissues
   b. Remove metabolic waste products
   c. Participate in the coagulation cascade
   d. Protect the body against infection

39. The WBC that is most prevalent in the blood is:
   a. Lymphocyte
   b. Neutrophil
   c. Monocyte
   d. Eosinophil

40. The WBC that is associated with antibody production is:
   a. Neutrophil
   b. Lymphocyte
   c. Monocyte
   d. Basophil

41. The cellular element that plays an important role in coagulation is:
   a. RBC
   b. WBC
   c. Platelet
   d. Fibrinogen

42. The lifespan of a platelet is:
   a. 3 to 4 days
   b. 9 to 12 days
   c. 10 to 15 days
   d. 110 to 120 days

43. The normal platelet reference range averages:
   a. 50,000/µL
   b. 100,000/µL
   c. 200,000/µL
   d. 500,000/µL

44. The process by which blood vessels are repaired after injury is referred to as:
   a. Homeostasis
   b. Chemostasis
   c. Cytostasis
   d. Hemostasis

45. A patient is recovering from deep vein thrombosis and the doctor wishes to assess the rate of fibrinolysis. The physician orders which of the following tests?
   a. FDP
   b. D-dimer
   c. FSP
   d. All of the above

46. Two slightly hazy, pale yellow liquid specimens have been received into the lab in transfer tubes from the physician's office for a glucose and a PT test. The labels are handwritten and contain the patient's name, date, date of birth, and time of draw—no test has been designated on the labels. How do you determine which specimen to use for the PT test?
   a. Haziest specimen is the PT plasma specimen so use it
   b. Both tubes are plasma—send one to coagulation and one to chemistry

c. Call the physician's office to clarify
d. Cannot make a determination, patient needs to be redrawn

47. A hereditary blood disorder that results in a decreased production of hemoglobin and anemia is:
a. Thalassemia
b. Sickle-cell anemia
c. Polycythemia
d. Iron-deficiency anemia

48. A 14-year-old patient is experiencing signs and symptoms of malaise, fever, sore throat, swollen lymph nodes. The physician suspects a blood disorder caused by Epstein-Barr virus and orders a test to assess if the patient has:
a. HIV
b. Bacterial infection
c. DIC
d. Mononucleosis

49. The phlebotomist receives a STAT order for a series of coagulation tests for a newborn who had undergone a circumcision earlier in the day and is experiencing prolonged bleeding as a result of the procedure. The doctor suspects the newborn may have:
a. Hemophilia
b. Bacterial infection
c. Thrombosis
d. Polycythemia vera

50. Which of the following exhibits a pulsation on palpation?
a. Arteriole
b. Venule
c. Vein
d. Artery

51. Leukopenia refers to:
a. Elevated WBC count
b. Decreased neutrophil count
c. Increased RBC count
d. Decreased WBC count

52. All of the following are functions of the lymphatic system, *except*:
a. Assist in the systemic circulation of blood
b. Return tissue fluid to circulatory system
c. Screen lymphatic fluid for signs of infection
d. Provide a passageway for lymphocytes patrolling tissues

53. Lymph fluid is derived from:
a. Serum
b. Interstitial fluid
c. Plasma
d. Peritoneal fluid

54. Lymph organs include all of the following, *except*:
a. Tonsils
b. Spleen
c. Liver
d. Thymus

55. A condition where there is an accumulation of interstitial fluid in the tissues due to a blocked lymphatic vessel:
a. Lymphoma
b. Inflammation
c. Lymphedema
d. Thrombosis

ANSWERS AND RATIONALES

1. **Answer: D**
Rationale: The circulatory system transports blood, which contains oxygen, nutrients, enzymes, hormones, clotting factors, etc., throughout the body. It also picks up metabolic wastes for removal from the body by various mechanisms. Lymph fluid is carried by the lymphatic system.
Text Reference: p. 94

2. **Answer: B**
Rationale: Pulmonary circulation carries deoxygenated blood coming into the heart from the inferior and superior venae cavae through the pulmonary arteries to the lungs for oxygenation and then back to the heart through the pulmonary veins for distribution to the rest of the body.
Text Reference: p. 94

3. **Answer: C**
Rationale: The flow of blood moves from the heart through the aorta, to the arteries, to the arterioles, to the capillaries, to the venules, and to the veins that merge into the superior and inferior venae cavae, which then return deoxygenated blood back into the heart for reoxygenation.
Text Reference: pp. 95-97

4. **Answer: A**

   Rationale: The walls of capillary vessels consist of a single-cell layer that allows for the exchange of dissolved gases, nutrients, waste products, etc., to occur between the blood and the fluid bathing the tissues.

   Text Reference: p. 95

5. **Answer: B**

   Rationale: The pericardium is the sac surrounding the heart that provides support and lubricates the heart. The epicardium is the outer layer of the heart, the myocardium is the cardiac muscle, and the endocardium is the innermost layer of the heart.

   Text Reference: p. 95

6. **Answer: A**

   Rationale: The epicardium is the outer layer of the heart and consists of epithelial cells and underlying fibrous connective tissue in which the coronary arteries that provide blood flow to the heart itself are embedded.

   Text Reference: p. 95

7. **Answer: C**

   Rationale: The heart consists of four chambers: two atria and two ventricles.

   Text Reference: p. 95

8. **Answer: B**

   Rationale: The tricuspid valve, consisting of three flaps, is also referred to as the right atrioventricular or AV valve and separates the right atrium and the right ventricle. The left atrioventricular valve consists of two flaps and is also known as the mitral or bicuspid valve and separates the left atrium from the left ventricle.

   Text Reference: p. 95

9. **Answer: D**

   Rationale: The left atrioventricular valve is also called the mitral valve or the bicuspid valve consisting of two flaps that separate the left atrium from the left ventricle. The aortic semilunar valve separates the left ventricle from the aorta.

   Text Reference: p. 95

10. **Answer: B**

    Rationale: Deoxygenated blood from the systemic circulation returns to the heart via the venous system and collects in the superior and inferior venae cavae, which then empty into the right atrium. Blood then moves through the tricuspid valve into the right ventricle and is pumped through the pulmonary semilunar valve into the pulmonary arteries to be transported to the lungs for oxygenation. Blood returns to the left atrium via the pulmonary veins moving into the left ventricle through the mitral valve as the heart contracts. Contraction of the left ventricle forces blood through the aortic semilunar valve into the aorta for distribution of oxygenated blood to the systemic circulatory system.

    Text Reference: pp. 95-97

11. **Answer: C**

    Rationale: Contraction of the left ventricle forces oxygenated blood to move out of the ventricle and into the aorta for distribution to body tissues via the major arteries and arterioles to the capillary beds where the exchange of nutrients, gases, metabolic waste products, etc., occurs. Blood returns to the heart via the venous system.

    Text Reference: p. 97

12. **Answer: C**

    Rationale: Each heartbeat cycle is composed of a complete contraction and relaxation of each heart chamber. Flow of blood through the pulmonary circuit involves the reoxygenation of blood as it flows from the heart to the lungs. The flow of blood through the systemic circuit refers to oxygenated blood being carried from the heart to the rest of the body tissues. The "lubb-dupp" sound of the heartbeat is the sound of the valves closing. The "lubb" is heard when the two AV valves close at the start of ventricular systole and the "dupp" is heard when the two semilunar valves close at the start of ventricular diastole.

    Text Reference: p. 97

13. **Answer: C**

    Rationale: Systole is the term used for the contraction phase of the heart because the contraction develops pressure forcing blood through the system. The relaxation phase of the cardiac cycle allows the chamber to fill again.

    Text Reference: p. 97

14. **Answer: B**
Rationale: Arteries have a thick muscular wall to withstand the high blood pressure that is generated by ventricular contraction. The arteries expand as the blood is pumped into them and contract during diastole to maintain blood flow and pressure. Arteries are located deeper in the tissue than veins and can be located by feeling for a pulse.
Text Reference: p. 97

15. **Answer: B**
Rationale: Blood pressure is the measure of the force of blood on the arterial walls and is measured by a sphygmomanometer.
Text Reference: p. 97

16. **Answer: A**
Rationale: Another term for impaired blood flow leading to reduced or lack of oxygen in tissue is ischemia. Hypoxia is an inadequate supply of oxygen to cells and tissues as a result of impaired respiratory process, altitude, anemia, cerebral events (i.e., cardiopulmonary arrest, traumatic birth, fetal placental or cord disorders). Anoxia means absence of oxygen. The medical abbreviations MI and CVA refer to myocardial infarct and cerebral vascular accident, respectively.
Text Reference: p. 97

17. **Answer: D**
Rationale: Venules and veins function to return blood back to the heart for reoxygenation. Arteries carry oxygenated blood away from the heart to the tissues. The aorta branches off into major arteries that carry blood to the various organs (i.e., renal artery, hepatic artery).
Text Reference: p. 97

18. **Answer: D**
Rationale: Myocardial infarctions or heart attacks can result from CAD or atherosclerosis, thrombus, or spasm of the coronary artery. Phlebitis is inflammation of a vein.
Text Reference: p. 97 and Content Overview (earlier in this chapter)

19. **Answer: C**
Rationale: Serum markers in myocardial infarction include Troponin I, myoglobin, and CK-MB. Troponin and CK-MB are specific to cardiac muscle. Troponin I and CK-MB begin to rise about 3 to 6 hours after the onset of the MI. Myoglobin, while not specific for cardiac muscle, can help to rule out MI and rises before CK-MB. CBC is a complete blood count and assesses the number of RBCs, WBCs, platelets, types of WBCs, and RBC morphology, etc.
Text Reference: p. 99

20. **Answer: D**
Rationale: Veins in the antecubital area include the basilic, cephalic, and median cubital vein. The brachial veins are venae comitantes that accompany the brachial artery and are located deep in the tissue.
Text Reference: p. 101

21. **Answer: D**
Rationale: Formed or cellular elements in the blood include platelets, WBCs, and RBCs. Plasma is the fluid portion of blood.
Text Reference: p. 101

22. **Answer: B**
Rationale: The composition of whole blood is 55% plasma and 45% cellular or formed elements.
Text Reference: p. 101

23. **Answer: A**
Rationale: Normal plasma constitutes 55% of the volume of blood and consists of 90% water and 10% dissolved substances that include proteins, amino acids, electrolytes, gases, sugars, hormones, lipids, vitamins, and waste products (i.e., urea).
Text Reference: pp. 101-102

24. **Answer: C**
Rationale: The phlebotomist will need to collect a minimum of 10 mL of blood to yield approximately 5 mL of plasma, because plasma comprises 55% of the blood volume and cellular elements account for the other 45%. Thus, $0.55 \times 10\,mL = 5.5\,mL$ of plasma.
Text Reference: p. 101

25. **Answer: A**
Rationale: Blood leaves the lungs and re-enters the heart into the left atrium via the pulmonary vein.
Text Reference: pp. 95-97

26. **Answer: C**
Rationale: Blood enters the left ventricle through contraction of the left atrium.
Text Reference: pp. 95-97

27. **Answer: A**
Rationale: Veins are closer to the surface of the skin, have valves to prevent the backflow of blood, and the flow of blood moves from venules to veins. Arteries must be able to withstand the high blood pressure of blood that results from ventricular contractions that move oxygenated blood throughout the body.
Text Reference: p. 99

28. **Answer: C**
Rationale: Albumin comprises about 60% of the plasma proteins and is produced by the liver. It plays an important role in plasma osmotic pressure, providing about 80% of the osmotic pressure and serves as a carrier protein for unconjugated bilirubin, calcium, thyroid and some fat soluble hormones, cortisol, and some drugs. It also serves as a marker of chronic liver disease and nutritional status. Other factors must also be considered when evaluating high or low concentration levels of albumin.
Text Reference: p. 102 and Content Overview (earlier in this chapter)

29. **Answer: B**
Rationale: Plasma that lacks clotting factors is referred to as serum. When a blood sample is collected in a Vacutainer tube or syringe that does not contain an anticoagulant, the coagulation cascade will result in a clot as fibrinogen is converted to fibrin, which traps all of the cellular elements. Centrifugation of a clotted sample will yield serum.
Text Reference: p. 102

30. **Answer: B**
Rationale: STAT testing requires quick turn-around times, thus a plasma specimen would be the best choice in this instance because the sample can be spun and loaded onto the instrument in a matter of minutes. A serum sample would require a minimum of 30 minutes to clot before spinning, thereby delaying the delivery of test results to the physician. Whole blood can be used in the

I-STAT instrument but is not operational at this point in time.
Text Reference: p. 102

31. **Answer: A**
Rationale: RBCs initially contain a nucleus, but as the cell matures the nucleus is expelled and the cell is then referred to as a reticulocyte. Nucleated RBCs are not normally seen in the peripheral blood of healthy individuals.
Text Reference: p. 102

32. **Answer: D**
Rationale: An erythrocyte is a mature RBC. A reticulocyte is the maturation stage of a RBC just before the erythrocyte stage. Leukocytes are WBCs and thrombocytes are platelets.
Text Reference: p. 102

33. **Answer: C**
Rationale: The reticulocyte count is a test that assesses the bone marrow's production of RBCs. Hemoglobin and hematocrits are useful in assessing anemia, blood loss, polycythemia, etc. A CBC is a complete blood count that assesses the number of formed cellular elements of the blood and differentiates the types of WBCs.
Text Reference: p. 102

34. **Answer: B**
Rationale: Normal reference ranges for RBCs are 4.7 to 6.1 million/µL (microliter) for men and 4.2 to 5.4 million/µL for women. The best answer from the choices is 5 million/µL.
Text Reference: p. 102

35. **Answer: A**
Rationale: RBCs carry approximately 280 million hemoglobin molecules, which are the iron-containing oxygen transport proteins in RBCs. Oxygen binds to the hemoglobin molecules in the lungs and is then transported to all body tissues. RBCs pick up CO_2 in the tissues for delivery back to the lungs where it is released.
Text Reference: p. 102

36. **Answer: B**
Rationale: Leukocyte is another term for WBC. An erythrocyte is a RBC, a thrombocyte is a platelet, and a histiocyte is a macrophage found in connective tissue.
Text Reference: p. 102

37. Answer: B
Rationale: The normal reference range for WBC counts is typically listed at 4800 to 10,800/μL. The answer approximating that range is 5000 to 10,000/μL. Reference ranges typically vary somewhat according to geographic areas but for the most part are very similar.
Text Reference: p. 102

38. Answer: D
Rationale: The primary function of WBCs is to protect the body against infection. Different types of WBCs (i.e., neutrophils, lymphocytes, monocytes, eosinophils, and basophils) perform specific functions in cell-mediated and humoral immunity processes that function to remove bacteria, viruses, parasites, and other invasive substances from the body in an effort to limit, prevent, and recover from illness.
Text Reference: p. 102

39. Answer: B
Rationale: Neutrophils comprise 40% to 60% of all leukocytes present in the blood; lymphocytes comprise 20% to 40%; monocytes comprise 3% to 8%; and eosinophils comprise 1% to 3%.
Text Reference: p. 103

40. Answer: B
Rationale: Lymphocytes, in particular B-lymphocytes that have transformed into plasma cells, play an important role in the humoral immune response by producing antibodies against foreign antigens, acting as antigen presenting cells, and making memory cells against the antigens in the event of a future exposure.
Text Reference: p. 103

41. Answer: C
Rationale: Platelets play a critical role in the coagulation process by sticking to the endothelial cells during adhesion in the coagulation process.
Text Reference: p. 104

42. Answer: B
Rationale: Platelets remain in the circulatory system for approximately 9 to 12 days.
Text Reference: p. 104

43. Answer: C
Rationale: Normal reference ranges for platelet counts typically range from 150,000 to 450,000 platelets/μL, with an average of 200,000 platelets/μL.
Text Reference: p. 104

44. Answer: D
Rationale: Hemostasis literally means stopping the flow of blood. When blood vessels are injured, the process of repairing them to stop the flow of blood requires platelets and other coagulation factors. Homeostasis is referred to as dynamic equilibrium of metabolic processes, whereby the body processes work to maintain internal equilibrium by constant adjustment of the body's physiological processes. Chemostasis refers to the cultivation of cells (microorganisms) in a chemostat. Cytostasis refers to prevention of the growth and multiplication of cells.
Text Reference: p. 104

45. Answer: D
Rationale: FDP—fibrin degradation products, D-Dimer, and FSP—fibrin split products can all be used to assess the rate of fibrinolysis.
Text Reference: p. 105

46. Answer: D
Rationale: Visual inspection of serum or plasma specimens reveal similarities in terms of color, which is pale yellow; clarity, which may be clear for both or slightly hazy for plasma due to the presence of fibrinogen. However, the presence of lipids in the blood may impart a haziness to serum as well. The PT test requires a plasma specimen from a sodium citrate tube. The glucose test can be a serum sample or a plasma sample from a lithium heparin tube, for example. Thus, in this instance there is no way to determine which specimen is plasma from a blue or green stoppered tube or which is serum. The patient must be redrawn.
Text Reference: pp. 101-102

47. Answer: A
Rationale: Thalassemia is an inherited blood disorder that results in the decreased production of either α- or β-globin protein chains depending on the genetic mutation.

The result is mild to severe anemia. Sickle-cell anemia is an inherited disorder that results in the formation of sickle-shaped cells during periods of oxidative stress. Polycythemia is a condition of increased RBCs. Iron-deficiency anemia results from decreased absorption of iron and can be due to a number of factors, such as decreased dietary intake, increased demand due to pregnancy, increased blood loss, etc.
Text Reference: p. 106

48. **Answer: D**
Rationale: Mononucleosis is due to an infection of the B-lymphocytes by the Epstein-Barr virus, resulting in atypical or reactive T-cells that are visible on a peripheral blood smear. Symptoms include general malaise, loss of appetite, fever, sore throat, and lymphadenopathy (i.e., swollen lymph nodes).
Text Reference: p. 106

49. **Answer: A**
Rationale: Hemophilias are a group of inherited coagulation disorders marked by a decrease in the production of certain clotting factors and an increase in clotting time. The most common hemophilia is due to a factor VIII deficiency.
Text Reference: p. 106

50. **Answer: D**
Rationale: Arteries pulsate as a result of pressure waves that move through the arteries as the ventricles contract, forcing blood into the aorta and stretching it. The stretching produces a wave of distention, referred to as pulse waves, that gradually become faster as blood moves toward the peripheral vessels. It is used to denote the frequency rate of the heartbeat per minute.
Text Reference: p. 97

51. **Answer: D**
Rationale: Leuko- means white, -penia means decrease, thus leukopenia means decreased WBC count.
Text Reference: pp. 102-103

52. **Answer: A**
Rationale: Functions of the lymphatic system include returning tissue fluid to the circulatory system, screening lymph fluid for signs of infection, and providing a passageway for lymphocytes.
Text Reference: p. 106

53. **Answer: B**
Rationale: Lymphatic fluid is derived from fluid between the cells called interstitial fluid. It is a combination of plasma forced out of capillaries and cellular fluid exiting cells through osmosis.
Text Reference: p. 107

54. **Answer: C**
Rationale: Organs of the lymphatic system include the tonsils, spleen, and thymus. The tonsils are large lymph nodes where resident T and B lymphocytes screen lymph fluid for signs of infection. The spleen removes old RBCs, and resident T and B lymphocytes examine blood for signs of infection. The thymus is involved in the maturation of T lymphocytes. The liver is an accessory organ in the digestive system.
Text Reference: p. 108

55. **Answer: C**
Rationale: Lymphedema is an accumulation of interstitial fluid in tissues as a result of a blocked lymphatic vessel. A lymphoma is a tumor of lymph tissue that is usually malignant. Inflammation is the response of body tissue to injury or irritation and is evidenced by pain, swelling, redness, and heat. Thrombosis is the condition of a blood clot in a vessel.
Text Reference: p. 108

VENIPUNCTURE EQUIPMENT

Pamela Primrose

INTRODUCTION

Equipment for routine venipuncture includes material needed for the safe and efficient location of a vein and collection of a blood sample, plus equipment to ensure the safety and comfort of both the patient and the user. Most venipuncture procedures are performed with a double-ended multisample needle that delivers blood into an evacuated tube with a color-coded stopper. The stopper indicates the additives used in the tube. Learning what each color signifies, and in what order different-colored tubes should be drawn, is essential for a phlebotomist.

CONTENT OVERVIEW

Phlebotomy Equipment

I. Purpose
   A. Collection of blood specimens
      1. Needles
      2. Color-coded tubes
      3. PPE
   B. Protection of sample integrity
      1. Light-sensitive substances
      2. Temperature-sensitive substances
II. Responsibility of phlebotomist
   A. Maintain clean, well-stocked tray
   B. Collect appropriate blood specimen safely and efficiently
      1. Correct patient
      2. Correct tube
      3. Correct volume
   C. Maintain integrity of specimen
   D. Deliver to correct department

Organizing and Transporting Equipment

I. Portable tray
   A. Clean
   B. Well stocked
   C. Organized
II. Inpatient
   A. Tray carry to patient's—room
      1. Place on solid surface—table
      2. Never on bed
   B. Cart—leave in corridor

III. Outpatient
   A. Special phlebotomy chair
   B. Bed or reclining chair
   C. Drawing station

Locating Veins

I. Tourniquet
   A. Impedes venous blood flow
   B. Results in distention or dilation of vein
   C. Types
      1. Latex
      2. Nonlatex
      3. Velcro closure
      4. Blood pressure cuff
         a. Pressure
            i. Above diastole
            ii. Below systole
         b. Training required
         c. Permission required
   D. Vein finders
      1. Transilluminators
         a. Uses red and white LEDS—absorbed by veins
         b. Shines through patient's skin → veins visible
         c. Example: venoscope transilluminator
      2. Infrared light
         a. Infrared light images vessels
         b. Example: AccuVein
         c. Example: VeinViewer
      3. Doppler ultrasound
         a. Blood is moving
         b. Ultrasonic waves reflected from blood vessels
         c. Examples: portable vein finder from Georgia Tech

Cleaning the Puncture Site

I. Antiseptic
   A. Purpose
      1. Clean living tissue
      2. Prevents sepsis
      3. Acts as bacteriostatic before venipuncture
   B. Types
      1. 70% isopropyl alcohol—most common
         a. Bacteriostatic—inhibits, doesn't kill
         b. 30- to 60-second contact

    c. Prepackaged prep pads

    d. Cotton balls and bottle of isopropyl alcohol

  2. Povidone-iodine (Betadine)

    a. Interferes with chemistry tests

    b. Not used routinely

    c. Patient allergies to iodine—use alternate antiseptic

    d. Wash off after use

  3. Chlorhexidine gluconate

    a. Not used on infants under 2 months of age

    b. For patients allergic to iodine

    c. Wash off after use due to harshness of chemicals

  4. Benzalkonium chloride (Zephiran chloride)

    a. For patients allergic to iodine

    b. Wash off after use due to harshness of chemicals

II. Disinfectant

  A. Cleans surfaces other than living tissue

  B. Destroys, neutralizes, or inhibits growth of pathogenic microorganisms

Protecting the Puncture Site

I. Stop bleeding—gauze pad applied with pressure

II. Post-bleeding wound care options

  A. Adhesive bandage

  B. Surgical tape over gauze

Needles

I. Purpose

  A. Penetrate vein for collection of blood

    1. Sterile

    2. Disposable

    3. One use

II. Features of needles

  A. Double-ended: penetrates skin and pierces rubber stopper on tube

  B. Point

    1. Sharp

    2. Inspect for burrs, other defects

    3. Smooth entry

  C. Bevel

    1. Angled cut on the tip of the needle shaft giving it a V-shaped tip

    2. Ease shaft into skin

  D. Shaft

    1. Length—¾ to 1½ inches

    2. Gauge—diameter of needle lumen

      a. Smaller the gauge, the larger the diameter

      b. Larger the number, the smaller the lumen

      c. Example: 21 gauge > 22 gauge > 23 gauze

      d. Needle lengths: 1½ inches; 1 inch; ¾ inch

        i. Depends on depth of vein

        ii. Type of procedure: hand vein, foot, antecubital fossa, etc.

      e. Choice of gauge *not* matter of preference but type of collection; patient condition; size of vein

        i. Blood donors—16 gauge

        ii. Routine adult collection—20 to 21 gauge

          A) Blood delivered quickly

          B) More damaging to tissue

          C) May collapse vein

        iii. Obese patient—size and depth of vein

          A) Deep veins need 1½ inch length

          B) Gauge depends on size of vein

        iv. Small, fragile veins—23 gauge

          A) Blood delivered more slowly

          B) Less tissue damage

          C) RBCs may hemolyze as they pass through lumen

    3. Lumen

      a. Hollow tube within shaft

      b. Measured by gauge

  E. Hub

    1. Point of attachment of needle to Vacutainer holder or syringe

III. Multisample needles

  A. Most common double-ended needle

  B. Retractable rubber sleeve on one end

    1. Used when collecting multiple tubes

    2. Keeps blood from leaking into adapter

IV. Safety syringes and safety syringe needles

  A. Patients with fragile or small veins

  B. Veins that may collapse

  C. Allows for controlled gentle vacuum

  D. Hypodermic needle with safety device

    1. 22 to 23 gauge—smaller may cause hemolysis

    2. 1 inch

  E. Advantage—blood appears in hub once vein entered

  F. Transfer blood into tubes

    1. Blood transfer device

    2. One-handed technique

V. Winged infusion sets or butterflies

  A. Used on small veins

    1. Hand

    2. Elderly

    3. Pediatric

B. Allows for greater flexibility
   1. Placing needle
   2. Manipulating needle
C. Size
   1. 23 gauge (25 gauge not recommended)
   2. ¾ to ½ inch long
D. Safety device attached
E. Used with evacuated collection tube holder or syringe

Needle Safety

I. CDC report
   A. Approximately 1000 needlestick injuries per day
      1. Nurses
      2. Phlebotomists
      3. Others
II. OSHA's 1999 Needle Safety and Prevention Act
   A. Increase "engineering controls" per needle safety of Bloodborne Pathogens Standard
   B. Federal legislation
      1. Enforces use of safety devices
   C. Many states have legislation
      1. Address safety devices
   D. Allows employers to choose the best method that works for their employees
III. Standard strategies
   A. Internally self-blunting needles—before removal from vein
   B. Retractable needles
      1. Blunt cannula inside needle tip
      2. Advanced beyond tip before removal from arm
   C. Retractable technologies
      1. Needle retracts
         a. Syringe
         b. Tube holder
         c. Other device
   D. Single-handed activation
   E. Recapping is *not* acceptable per OSHA's standards and guidelines.

Needle Adapters

I. Adapter usage
   A. Referred to as tube holder
   B. One-time use—discard with needle attached
      1. Contamination from leakage
      2. Contamination from aerosolization when switching tubes

C. Tube advancement mark
   1. Ensures proper connection between needle and tube
   2. Indicates how far tube can be advanced without losing vacuum

Evacuated Collection Tubes

I. Types of tubes and additives
   A. Color-coded
      1. Glass, no additive
      2. Plastic
         a. Shatter-resistant
         b. Safer in transport
         c. Safe in high speed centrifugation
   B. Additives (see Tube Additives section)
      1. Clot (platelet) activators—reduce clotting time
      2. Anticoagulants—chemicals prevent clotting
         a. Manufacturer recommends full draw
         b. Underfilling or overfilling disrupts blood:anticoagulant ratio
            i. Underfilling: over-anticoagulated
               a) Alters test results
               b) EDTA
                  1) RBCs shrink
                  2) MCHC, Hct values incorrect
                  3) Sedimentation rates erroneous
            ii. Overfilling: too little anticoagulant
               a) Microclot formation
               b) Test results erroneous
   C. Stopper types
      1. Thick rubber stopper
      2. Rubber stopper with plastic top
         a. BC Vacutainer Hemogard
         b. Minimizes aerosol spray on stopper removal
   D. Size and volume
      1. Sizes of tubes vary
         a. Length
         b. Internal diameter
      2. Volume: 1.8-15 mL
         a. Tube vacuum determines volume
            i. CLSI guidelines: ±10% of stated draw volume through shelflife
            ii. Draw volume decreases over time
               a) Plastic tubes (polyethylene terephthalate) permeable
               b) Tubes requiring full draw: check for volume acceptability
         b. Sodium citrate tubes—inner narrow tube allowing draw of 1.8 mL

3. Larger tube greater vacuum pull; vice versa
4. Needle gauge selection
   a. Based on tube size
   b. Small vein, smaller needle, smaller tube size
      i. Reduces risk of hemolysis
      ii. Two small tubes versus one large tube
      iii. Partial draw tubes
5. Determining tube size
   a. Volume of sample required for test (see Chapter 7)
   b. Expense of tube size—smaller more costly
   c. Instrumentation requires specific size
6. Expiration dates
   a. Discard expired tubes
   b. Decreased vacuum—short draw
   c. Degraded additives
   d. Problems using old tubes
      i. Improper test results
      ii. Redraw patient

Types of Blood Specimens

I. Blood samples used for analysis
   A. Whole blood
      1. Anticoagulated blood
      2. Departments
         a. Hematology—cell counts
         b. Blood bank—blood typing
         c. Chemistry—hormones, metals
   B. Serum
      1. Fluid remaining after specimen clots
         a. Does not contain fibrinogen
         b. Missing some clotting factors used up in process
         c. Cannot be used for coagulation studies
      2. Clotting time: 30 to 60 minutes
      3. Centrifugation separates serum from cells
      4. Departments
         a. Chemistry
         b. Immunology
   C. Plasma
      1. Fluid portion from anticoagulated specimen
         a. Contains fibrinogen
         b. Contains other clotting factors
      2. Whole blood plus anticoagulant
      3. Centrifugation separates plasma from cells
      4. Departments
         a. Chemistry
            i. STAT testing
            ii. No waiting for specimen to clot
         b. Coagulation studies

Tube Additives

I. Additive type, stopper color, characteristics, and test affected
   A. In all tubes except glass red top
   B. Require gentle inversion 5 to 8 times to mix
   C. Types
      1. Types of anticoagulants and modes of action (see following table)
         a. Correct ratio blood to anticoagulant required
         b. Choice of anticoagulant: dependent on test

Anticoagulants and Modes of Action				
Function	**Additive**	**Tube**	**Characteristics**	**Tests Affected**
Bind calcium to inhibit coagulation cascade	EDTA: Sodium or potassium ethylenediamine-tetraacetic acid Chelates calcium	Lavender Royal blue Pink Tan (plastic) Pearl	• CBC • Toxicology • Blood bank • Lead • Viral loads • Preserves blood cell integrity • Prevents platelet clumping • Compatible with blood staining	• Calcium (Ca^{++}) • Coagulation tests: PT, PTT • Sodium (Na^+) • Potassium (K^+)
	Sodium citrate binds calcium ions forming soluble complex	Light blue	• Coagulation	• Ca^{++}

Anticoagulants and Modes of Action—cont'd

Function	Additive	Tube	Characteristics	Tests Affected
	Potassium oxalate—forms insoluble complex with calcium	Gray	• Glucose testing • Combined with antiglycolytic agents (inhibits glycolysis) • Sodium fluoride: preserves glucose 3 hr • Iodoacetate—preserves glucose 24 hr	• Coagulation tests: PT, PTT • K^+ • Cellular morphology (i.e., RBCs) • Some enzymes
	Sodium polyethanol sulfonate (SPS)	Yellow	• Blood cultures • Inhibits immune system: complement and phagocytosis • Neutralizes antibiotics in patient's blood	N/A
Inhibit conversion of prothrombin to thrombin—temporary effect, forms clots within 24 hr	Heparin—sodium, lithium, ammonium	Green; light green Royal Blue Tan (glass)	Preferred for plasma chemistry tests, ABGs	• PT, PTT, etc. • Na^+ • Li^+

COLOR-CODED TOPS: STOPPERS, ADDITIVES, SPECIMENS, EXAMPLES, DEPARTMENTS (see following table) Note: Chart presents examples of tubes/stoppers and is not all inclusive for BD or Greiner Bio-One. BD Vacutainer® blood collection tubes may be glass and/or plastic depending upon stopper color. Greiner Bio-One Vacuette® blood collection tubes are PET plastic only.

Tube	Additive	Specimen	Test Examples	Department
Red (Glass Tube)	None or silicone coated	Serum	Metabolic panel, RPR, type and screen	Chemistry, immunology, blood bank
Red (Plastic Tube)	Clot activator Silicone coated	Serum	Glucose, CRP	Chemistry, immunology
Light Blue-Clear Light Blue Requires full draw Nine parts blood to one part sodium citrate; 4.5 mL blood to 0.5 mL citrate	Sodium citrate CTAD-Citrate theophylline, adenosine, dipyridamole (for selected platelet function assays)	Plasma	PT, PTT	Coagulation
Lavender	EDTA: K_2 EDTA; sprayed on; CLSI preferred K_3 EDTA: liquid Na_2 EDTA: powder	Whole blood	CBC	Hematology

(Continued)

Tube	Additive	Specimen	Test Examples	Department
Pearl or PPT (plasma preparation tube)	Gel with EDTA	Plasma	Viral loads; molecular diagnostic tests	Molecular diagnostics
Gold, SST, Red/ Gray, Tiger Top	Clot activators, thixotropic gel	Serum	Glucose; metabolic panel, TSH	Chemistry
Gray	Antiglycolytic agent: Sodium fluoride Anticoagulants: Sodium oxalate or Na_2 EDTA	Plasma	Lactic acid, GTT, FBS, blood alcohol	Chemistry
Black	Sodium citrate—4 parts blood to 1 part citrate; full draw	Whole blood	Sedimentation rate	Hematology
Green	Heparin: Na Heparin; Li^+ Heparin; NH_4 Heparin	Plasma	STAT chemistry tests, ammonia, electrolytes, ABGs	Chemistry
Light green (PST—plasma separator tube); green/gray	Li^+ Heparin; thixotropic gel	Plasma	STAT potassium	Chemistry
Orange; yellow/ gray—for patients on anticoagulation therapy or STATS	Thrombin—5 minute clotting time	Serum	STAT chemistry tests	Chemistry
Royal blue— chemically clean; stopper formulation to prevent erroneous results	Heparin, EDTA, or none	Plasma or serum	Toxicology, trace metals such as manganese, copper; nutritional analytes	Toxicology
Tan—Formulated to contain < 0.1 μg/mL (ppm) lead	K_2 EDTA (plastic)	Plasma	Lead	Toxicology/ chemistry
Yellow—sterile	SPS—inhibits complement and phagocytosis	Whole blood	Blood culture	Microbiology
Yellow—nonsterile	Acid citrate dextrose (ACD) Dextrose nourishes, preserves RBCs; citrate acts as anticoagulant	Whole blood	Human leukocyte antigen (HLA) for paternity, tissue typing; DNA	Molecular diagnostics
Pink—Label/stopper meet AABB standards	K_2 EDTA	Plasma, whole blood	Antibody screen, compatibility	Blood bank, immunohematology

CLOT ACTIVATORS AND OTHER ADDITIVES (see following table) Note: Types of additives used are specific to the manufacturer of the tubes (i.e., BD, Greiner Bio-One).

Additive	Stopper Color	Characteristics	Test Interferences
Clot Activators: a. Thrombin	Orange, yellow/gray Gold, SST, tiger top	– Converts fibrineogen to fibrin STAT chemistry tests: clots in 5 minutes – Used to prevent stroke if patient on anticoagulants	Possibly tests requiring plasma/whole blood PT, PTT, thrombin time Blood bank tests
b. Inert substances: Glass; silica, siliceous earth, clay, Celite		– Surface for platelet activation – Invert 5-8 times to mix – Silica imparts white haze to interior of tube	
Thixotropic gel	Gold, SST, tiger top Light Green Pearl	– Inert, synthetic substance – Density between cells and serum or plasma – Centrifugation: moves between serum or plasma and cells – Prevents contamination of serum or plasma with cells – Easy separation	Blood bank tests Some drug screens, etc.
Silicone coating	Gold, SST, tiger top	Prevents RBCs from adhering to the interior wall of tube	
ACD (acid citrate dextrose)	Yellow nonsterile	Dextrose nourishes and preserves RBCs Citrate is an anticoagulant	

Order of Draw Standards: CLSI

I. CLSI recommendations
  A. Used when multiple tests drawn using multisample needle
    1. Prevents contamination of other tubes apart from technique (see Chapter 9)
      a. Anticoagulant
      b. Other materials
  B. Same for multitube draw and dispensing from syringe draw
    1. Some facilities use separate order of draw for syringes
      a. Dispense into anticoagulant tubes first—prevents microclot formation
  C. Revised to reflect increased use of plastic tubes with clot activators—interfere with coagulation tests
  D. CLSI Order of draw standards: most commonly used tubes (see following table)
  E. Variation of order of draw
    1. Institutional internal studies support variation
    2. Check and follow your institution's protocol

Needle Disposal and Containers

I. OSHA Bloodborne Pathogen Standards and OSHA's 1999 Needle Safety and Prevention Act requirements
  A. Dispose of needle/adapter as a unit
  B. Use sharps with engineered sharps injury protection i.e., safety needles, etc.
  C. Biohazard disposal container
    1. Closable or sealable
    2. Puncture resistant
    3. Leak proof
    4. Labeled with correct biohazard label

Tube	Note
Blood culture (SPS)	Drawn first to minimize contamination
Light blue	Use discard tube (nonadditive or citrate) only if drawing with butterfly to prime tubing with blood so vacuum is not exhausted with air—ensures full draw; adversely affected by other additives
Yellow (ACD)	
Red	Glass nonadditive may be drawn before citrate tube to prevent contamination by additives
Gold, SST, or red/gray	Carryover of clot activator into any tube other than blue is irrelevant—neutralized by anticoagulant; clot activator contamination of blue top → erroneous coagulation results
Green	With or without gel; less likely to interfere with EDTA tubes
Lavender	Binds calcium, other metals; erroneous test results: low Ca^{++}; high K^+; increases coagulation tests results
Gray	K^+ oxalate elevates K^+ levels; oxalate damages cell membranes—interferes with differentials; sodium fluoride elevates Na^+, inhibits many enzymes
Other additives	Check package insert and lab manual for protocol

CERTIFICATION PREPARATION QUESTIONS

1. To have extra tubes within arm's reach in case a tube needs to be replaced while the needle is still in the patient's arm, the phlebotomist should place the tray on the:
   a. Patient's bed
   b. Night stand
   c. Floor
   d. Window sill

2. Phlebotomy trays should be disinfected with bleach at least once per:
   a. Day
   b. Week
   c. Month
   d. Quarter

3. The phlebotomist is working in the outpatient department and has an order for a patient who routinely faints when his or her blood is drawn. The *best* practice to employ for this patient is to:
   a. Put the patient in the room with a reclining chair or bed
   b. Put the patient in a phlebotomy chair and lock the armrest
   c. Get a physician to draw the blood and assist in the process
   d. Distract the patient with small talk so he or she doesn't faint

4. Tourniquets should be disposed of:
   a. When there is visible contamination with blood or OPIMs
   b. The first of each month
   c. When worn out
   d. After each patient

5. Supplies that are used routinely in venipuncture include all of the following, *except*:
   a. Safety needles
   b. Evacuated tubes
   c. Disinfectant
   d. Tourniquet

6. The most commonly used antiseptic in routine venipuncture is:
   a. Povidone-iodine
   b. Benzalkonium chloride
   c. 70% isopropyl alcohol
   d. Chlorhexidine gluconate

7. The following antiseptic should *not* be used on infants under the age of two months:
   a. Povidone-iodine
   b. Chlorhexidine gluconate
   c. Benzalkonium chloride
   d. Betadine

8. A tourniquet is used in performing venipuncture to:
   a. Prevent venous blood flow out of the arm to enlarge the vein
   b. Make the skin taut for easier palpability and access to the vein
   c. Force hemoconcentration of analytes for more accurate assays
   d. Maximize pooling of arterial blood for enhanced visibility of veins

9. Use of a blood pressure cuff in lieu of a tourniquet requires all of the following parameters, *except*:
   a. Pressure above diastolic pressure
   b. Pressure below systolic pressure
   c. Referencing the patient's blood pressure from the chart
   d. Blood pressure training

10. The needle gauge describes the diameter of the needle's:
    a. Hub
    b. Shaft
    c. Lumen
    d. Bevel

11. A device that uses high-intensity red and white LEDs that penetrate deep into the patient's subcutaneous tissue to highlight veins is called a:
    a. Venoscope transilluminator
    b. AccuVein
    c. VeinViewer
    d. Vein stabilizer

12. The phlebotomist is preparing to draw blood on an elderly patient with small fragile veins and selects a needle gauge of:
    a. 16
    b. 20
    c. 21
    d. 23

13. The difference between a single-sample needle and a multisample needle is:
    a. Retractable sheath
    b. Length
    c. Gauge
    d. Luer lock

14. Advantages to using a syringe include all of the following, *except*:
    a. Controlled vacuum
    b. Vein less likely to collapse
    c. No need for evacuated tubes
    d. Blood appears in the hub on entry into the vein

15. The phlebotomist selects a winged infusion set with a syringe to draw blood from an infant. On completion of the draw, the phlebotomist begins to transfer blood into the appropriate tubes by:

a. Carefully inserting the needle tip of the butterfly into the tube
b. Removing the syringe from the hub adapter and attaching a blood transfer device
c. Attaching a needle onto the syringe and inserting it into a hand-held tube
d. Popping the tops off the tubes and dispensing required tube volume

16. The phlebotomist decides to use a winged infusion set and small-volume tubes on an accident victim who is bleeding internally and will be transferred to surgery as soon as the draw is completed. He carefully draws the coagulation tests, Chem 7, and a CBC, in that order, and delivers them to the lab for testing. There appears to be a problem with the coagulation results because:
    a. Order of draw was incorrect contaminating tubes with anticoagulants
    b. Internal bleeding causes hemoconcentration of coagulation factors
    c. Tube not completely full due to air space in the length of the tubing
    d. Butterflies should not be used for coagulation tests due to possible hemolysis

17. Engineering practices for needle safety recommended by OSHA include all of the following, *except*:
    a. Needle cutting device
    b. Retractable needles
    c. Self-blunting needles
    d. Safety shield devices

18. Use of a needle safety device that provides a high level of protection from needlestick injuries is one that is designed to:
    a. Be activated with one hand safely behind the needle
    b. Be deployed using two hands safely behind the needle
    c. Recap using one hand recapping device
    d. Allow needle insertion into a barrier gel

19. The tube advancement mark on the needle adapter functions to:
    a. Prevent loss of tube vacuum when assembling needle/tube apparatus
    b. Indicate how far to push tube onto the needle once inserted into the vein
    c. Ensure the needle is seated properly in the adapter

d. Guide hand placement on the adapter when inserting the tube

20. Additives are chemical substances added to tubes to:
   a. Prevent aerosolization of blood when removing the stopper
   b. Ensure continuation of cellular metabolism in vitro
   c. Promote or prevent certain changes in the blood sample
   d. Neutralize any blood-borne pathogen in the blood sample

21. On return to the lab after drawing an in-house patient, the phlebotomist discovers that she has used an expired lavender top tube. The right course of action is to:
   a. Redraw the patient if the test results are abnormal
   b. Discard the tube and redraw the patient using an unexpired tube
   c. Not worry about it because the tube was a full draw
   d. Pour the blood into an unexpired tube and mix thoroughly

22. The use of anticoagulants will yield which type of blood specimen?
   a. Whole blood and serum
   b. Plasma and serum
   c. Whole blood and plasma
   d. Plasma only

23. The type of specimen used for STAT chemistry testing in the laboratory is:
   a. Whole blood
   b. Serum
   c. Plasma
   d. Clotted blood

24. Which of the following additives function to promote coagulation?
   a. Anticoagulants
   b. Silica
   c. Thixotropic gel
   d. Silicone

25. Antiglycolytics include which of the following:
   a. Sodium fluoride
   b. SPS
   c. Sodium citrate
   d. EDTA

26. The phlebotomist has an order for a manganese testing and draws which tube:
   a. Lavender
   b. Light blue
   c. Light green
   d. Royal blue

27. A test for STAT electrolytes has been ordered, so the phlebotomist selects which tube to be drawn:
   a. Yellow
   b. Gold
   c. Lavender
   d. Green

28. Tube formulated to contain less than 0.1 µg/mL of lead:
   a. Yellow
   b. Pearl
   c. Royal blue
   d. Tan

29. The phlebotomist has a request from the blood bank to draw a nonadditive tube on a specific patient in addition to the pink top tube. The tube selected is:
   a. Red glass
   b. Red plastic
   c. Red/gray
   d. Lavender

30. Which of the following tubes does not contain EDTA?
   a. Gray
   b. Royal blue
   c. Pink
   d. Lavender

31. Which of the following tubes contain an anticoagulant that inhibits the conversion of prothrombin to thrombin?
   a. Lavender
   b. SPS
   c. Green
   d. Light blue

32. The appropriate tube for a STAT sodium level is:
   a. Sodium heparin
   b. Lithium heparin
   c. SST
   d. Red glass

33. Anticoagulant modes of action include all of the following, *except*:
    a. Bind calcium
    b. Inhibit conversion of prothrombin to thrombin
    c. Interfere with hepatic synthesis of coagulation proteins
    d. Forms an insoluble complex with calcium

34. Clot activators include all of the following, *except*:
    a. Thrombin
    b. Silicone
    c. Glass
    d. Silica

35. The additive that inhibits both complement and phagocytosis is:
    a. Sodium polyethanol sulfonate
    b. Potassium oxalate with iodoacetate
    c. Acid citrate dextrose
    d. Ammonium heparin

36. The phlebotomist has an order for routine CBC, metabolic panel, and a blood typing. The phlebotomist will select which of the following sets of tubes:
    a. Lavender, black, gold
    b. Blue, lavender, orange
    c. Tan, gold, lavender
    d. Gold, lavender, pink

37. Eventhough the blood bank can use a lavender top tube for compatibility testing, some labs prefer to use which of the following tubes?
    a. SST
    b. Green
    c. Pink
    d. Orange

38. The phlebotomist is in the midst of a difficult pre-op draw for a CBC, PT, PTT, and electrolytes. After placing the last tube in the tube holder, the phlebotomist picks up the previous two tubes to continue inversions and notices that the PT/PTT tube did not completely fill. The proper course of action is to:
    a. Finish collecting the last tube and then pop on another citrate tube
    b. Put the PT/PTT tube back on to see if it will completely fill

    c. Draw an appropriate discard tube first and then collect the PT, PTT
    d. Redraw the patient for the PT and PTT tests

39. The phlebotomist has an order for a CBC, ABO, Rh, antibody screen, hepatitis panel, kidney panel, RPR, CRP, RA, thyroid panel and PT. The *best* course of action in drawing the patient's blood is to:
    a. Draw one of each tube first and then go back and collect the remaining tubes
    b. Follow the correct order of draw and collect all tubes
    c. Draw one of each tube and prepare aliquots for each department
    d. Enter into the computer system the locations of tubes for departments that will share samples

40. The phlebotomist is preparing to go to several of the area nursing homes to collect routine blood draws for glucose and CBCs on several patients and will be gone for the morning. The following tube will be used to draw the glucose:
    a. Gold
    b. PST
    c. Gray
    d. SST

ANSWERS AND RATIONALES

1. **Answer: B**
   Rationale: The phlebotomist's tray should be placed on a solid surface, such as the patient's night stand or the overbed table, which is within close proximity of the patient for easy access. Trays should never be placed on the bed where they could be overturned or possibly cross-infect the patient because of contamination from other potentially infectious materials (OPIMs) from other patients' rooms. The floor contains contaminants and the window sill is generally too far out of reach.
   Text Reference: p. 115

2. **Answer: B**
   Rationale: Phlebotomy trays should be disinfected with bleach at the very least once per week unless visibly contaminated with

blood or OPIM, which then would require immediate decontamination.
Text Reference: p. 115

3. **Answer: A**
Rationale: If a patient is known to suffer from syncope each time their blood is drawn, the best practice is to simply put them in a room with a reclining chair or bed if available. If no bed is available then the next choice would be to make sure the armrest is locked securely, have smelling salts handy, and converse with the patient to distract his attention away from the venipuncture.
Text Reference: p. 116

4. **Answer: D**
Rationale: Studies have revealed the presence of pathogenic *Staphylococcus aureus, Streptococcus, Bacillus,* other microorganisms, blood stains, etc., on tourniquets that were used repeatedly on different patients. Thus, tourniquets are to be disposed of after each use to prevent cross-infection between patients. In-house patients may have a designated tourniquet that is kept in their room and used for the duration of their stay depending on hospital protocol.
Text Reference: p. 116

5. **Answer: C**
Rationale: Routine venipuncture supplies include safety needles, a variety of evacuated tubes, antiseptic, and a tourniquet. Disinfectants are chemicals that are used to decontaminate nonliving surfaces and are not used on patients.
Text Reference: p. 115

6. **Answer: C**
Rationale: 70% isopropyl alcohol is the most commonly used antiseptic for routine venipunctures. Povidone-iodine, benzalkonium chloride, and chlorhexidine gluconate are used for other invasive procedures, such as blood cultures and ABGs.
Text Reference: p. 117

7. **Answer: B**
Rationale: Chlorhexidine gluconate should not be used on infants under the age of 2

months. This antiseptic is chlorinated and similar in structure to hexachlorophene, which caused brain injury to infants in 1972. While said to be relatively safe, chlorhexidine gluconate is generally restricted to use on older infants.
Text Reference: p. 117

8. **Answer: A**
Rationale: The purpose of the tourniquet is to prevent the flow of venous blood out of the arm so that the veins become engorged for easier viewing and/or palpation.
Text Reference: p. 116

9. **Answer: C**
Rationale: Use of a blood pressure cuff in venipuncture requires training and supervisory permission. The pressure should be set less than the systolic but more than the diastolic pressures, typically in the range of 60 to 80 mm Hg. This requires that the patient's blood pressure be taken before the venipuncture procedure. The blood pressure cannot be referenced from the patient's chart because it typically fluctuates throughout the day along with a patient's condition. Medications may or may not have been administered that will have an impact on blood pressure readings.
Text Reference: p. 117

10. **Answer: C**
Rationale: The lumen is the hollow tube within the shaft. Its size (i.e., diameter) is described by the gauge. The hub is the point of attachment of the needle to the collecting device or syringe. The shaft is the section of the needle between the hub and the bevel. The bevel is the angular tip of the needle.
Text Reference: p. 117

11. **Answer: A**
Rationale: The Venoscope transilluminator uses red and white LEDs that transilluminate the subcutaneous tissue, whereby veins absorb the light and are rendered visible. AccuVein and VeinViewer use infrared light to visualize veins. A vein stabilizer is a device used to stabilize veins that are prone to rolling.
Text Reference: p. 117 and Content Overview (earlier in this chapter)

12. **Answer: D**
Rationale: For small fragile veins, a needle gauge of 23 is generally used. The typical gauge for routine adult venipuncture is 20 to 21 gauge. Blood donor collection uses 16-gauge needles.
Text Reference: p. 118

13. **Answer: A**
Rationale: A multisample needle contains a sheath that retracts over the needle tip as it penetrates the stopper of the tube. On changing tubes, the sheath reverts back to its original state covering the end of the needle so blood does not leak out and contaminate the Vacutainer holder and other tubes. Single-sample needles do not contain this sheath.
Text Reference: p. 118

14. **Answer: C**
Rationale: A syringe is very useful when drawing patients who have small or fragile veins. It allows for control over the vacuum pull on the vein by gradually and slowly pulling back on the plunger. This process is less likely to result in a collapsed vein. Blood appears in the hub on entry into the vein. Blood must be transferred into evacuated tubes at the end of the draw.
Text Reference: p. 118

15. **Answer: B**
Rationale: Use of a butterfly with a syringe to draw blood requires that the syringe be removed from the hub adapter and attached to a blood transfer device for safe delivery of the appropriate amounts of blood into each tube. Using the 23 or 25 gauge of the butterfly needle may cause hemolysis of the specimen and it goes through the small lumen a second time. Never hold a tube in the hand while inserting a syringe needle into it as accidental hand puncture may ensue. The one-handed technique should be employed if no blood transfer devices are available.
Text Reference: p. 119 and Content Overview (earlier in this chapter)

16. **Answer: C**
Rationale: A discard tube is required when using a butterfly to draw coagulation tests as a result of the air in the tubing, which partially exhausts the vacuum, resulting in

a short draw and thus incorrect blood to anticoagulant ratio. The order of the draw was correct, internal bleeding did not cause hemoconcentration of coagulation factors in the peripheral blood, and when properly used, a butterfly should yield an acceptable specimen for coagulation testing.
Text Reference: pp. 118-119 and Content Overview (earlier in this chapter)

17. **Answer: A**
Rationale: Recommended OSHA engineering practices include retractable needles that contain a blunt cannula inside the tip of the needle, retractable needles such as those on some syringes, self-blunting needles, etc. Recapping needles and cutting or bending needles is prohibited.
Text Reference: p. 119

18. **Answer: A**
Rationale: The Needlestick Safety and Prevention Act recognizes that there is not a single needle safety device that suits every institution. As such, employers may select with the help of employees, the type of device that meets their needs in reducing the number of needlestick injuries. Most require single-hand activation, which keeps the hand safely behind the needle.
Text Reference: p. 118 and Content Overview (earlier in this chapter)

19. **Answer: A**
Rationale: The tube advancement mark on the needle adapter indicates how far the tube can be pushed into the adapter without the loss of tube vacuum.
Text Reference: p. 119

20. **Answer: C**
Rationale: Additives are chemical substances that promote or prevent certain changes in the blood sample, such as enhancing the clotting process or preventing clotting.
Text Reference: p. 120

21. **Answer: B**
Rationale: Expired tubes can lead to erroneous test results because of decreased vacuums that may alter the blood to anticoagulant ratio and degradation of

additives that may affect sample integrity. Any sample that is drawn by mistake in an expired tube must be redrawn. Stock should be checked and rotated so that tubes are used before their expiration dates and not lurking in the back of storage cabinets.
Text Reference: p. 121

22. **Answer: C**
Rationale: Anticoagulants prevent the blood from clotting and would yield both a whole blood sample or on centrifugation, a plasma sample. Serum is the liquid portion of blood after a specimen clots.
Text Reference: p. 121

23. **Answer: C**
Rationale: Plasma is typically used for STAT chemistry testing because there is no waiting time for the specimen to clot. It is simply centrifuged on receipt in the lab and is then immediately placed on the instrument. Serum or clotted blood requires 30 minutes to fully clot before centrifugation and delays test results in STAT situations.
Whole blood is typically used in STAT bedside testing.
Text Reference: p. 121

24. **Answer: B**
Rationale: Silica or glass particles are commonly used in clot activator tubes to provide increased surface area for platelet activation that promotes the clotting process. Anticoagulants prevent blood from clotting. Thixotropic gel is an inert synthetic substance that functions to separate serum or plasma from cells on centrifugation. The silicone coating prevents the RBCs from adhering to the interior wall of the tube.
Text Reference: p. 121 and Content Overview (earlier in this chapter)

25. **Answer: A**
Rationale: Antiglycolytics are agents that preserve glucose and are used most often when there may be a delay between the time of the draw and separation of plasma from cells. Sodium fluoride preserves glucose for 3 days, whereas iodoacetate preserves glucose for 24 hours. SPS inhibits complement and phagocytosis. Sodium citrate is the anticoagulant in blue stopper

and black stopper tubes. EDTA is the anticoagulant in lavender stopper tubes.
Text Reference: p. 123

26. **Answer: D**
Rationale: Trace metals tests such as manganese tests are drawn in royal blue top tubes. The use of anticoagulant or no anticoagulant is dependent on the type of manganese test being performed (i.e., whole blood or serum) and the instrumentation used.
Text Reference: p. 122

27. **Answer: D**
Rationale: STAT testing requires a fast turnaround time, so the best choice would be the green top tube because it does not require clotting time and can be centrifuged immediately on receipt in the laboratory.
Text Reference: p. 123

28. **Answer: D**
Rationale: Lead analysis requires a tube that is virtually lead free. The tan top tubes are designed to contain less than 0.1 μg/mL of lead.
Text Reference: p. 123

29. **Answer: A**
Rationale: Of the tubes listed, the only one that contains no additives is the red glass. Red plastic and red/gray contain clot activators. Lavender top tubes contain EDTA.
Text Reference: p. 123

30. **Answer: A**
Rationale: Gray stopper tubes contain potassium oxalate plus an antiglycolytic agent. Royal blue stoppers are labeled to identify the type of additive: EDTA, heparin, or no additive. Pink and lavender stopper tubes contain EDTA.
Text Reference: pp. 122-123

31. **Answer: C**
Rationale: The mode of action of heparin in green top tubes is to inhibit the conversion of prothrombin to thrombin. EDTA in lavender, SPS in yellow, and sodium citrate in light blue prevent coagulation by interacting with calcium to make it unavailable for the coagulation process, thereby inhibiting specimen clotting.
Text Reference: pp. 122-123

32. **Answer: B**
Rationale: Lithium heparin would be the most appropriate choice for a STAT sodium. Although SST and red glass stopper tubes can be used for sodium assays, they require clotting time before centrifugation and thus are not the best choice for STAT testing. Sodium heparin contains sodium and would yield erroneously elevated sodium results.
Text Reference: pp. 122-123

33. **Answer: C**
Rationale: The modes of action include binding, chelating, or forming an insoluble complex with calcium: sodium citrate, EDTA, and potassium oxalate, respectively. Heparin inhibits the conversion of prothrombin to thrombin. The synthesis of coagulation proteins occurs in vivo not in vitro.
Text Reference: pp. 122-123 and Content Overview (earlier in this chapter)

34. **Answer: B**
Rationale: Thrombin, glass, and silica function to increase the rate at which a clot forms. Silicone is a coating on the interior walls of gold, SST, and orange/gray stopper tubes to prevent the RBCs from sticking.
Text Reference: p. 122 and Content Overview (earlier in this chapter)

35. **Answer: A**
Rationale: The additive that inhibits both complement and phagocytosis is SPS or sodium polyethanol sulfonate. Potassium oxalate with iodoacetate is an anticoagulant with an antiglycolytic agent. Acid citrate dextrose is the additive in nonsterile yellow stopper tubes that uses dextrose to nourish and preserve RBCs and citrate as the anticoagulant. Ammonium heparin is one of the heparin anticoagulants used in green stopper tubes.
Text Reference: pp. 122-123

36. **Answer: D**
Rationale: The metabolic panel is typically drawn in a gold stopper tube; CBC in a lavender topper tube; and blood typing in a lavender or pink. The only choice using all three tubes was D.
Text Reference: pp. 122-123

37. **Answer: C**
Rationale: Pink stopper tubes are similar to lavender but differ in that their closure and label are designed to meet the AABB standards.
Text Reference: p. 123

38. **Answer: C**
Rationale: The correct order of draw is PT/PTT, electrolytes, and then CBC. The last tube on the needle is the CBC and could cross-contaminate a blue top tube if subsequently placed on the needle. Since this is a difficult draw the best solution would be to draw out several milliliters of blood in a discard tube, such as a red glass or another blue top tube, followed by a new blue top tube. If a discard tube cannot be drawn, then the patient would need to be redrawn. The previous blue top may have a bad vacuum, hence the short draw, so using a new tube is the best choice.
Text Reference: pp. 122-123

39. **Answer: A**
Rationale: If the routine order of draw requires that a large number of a single-type tubes be drawn before others, it is advisable that the phlebotomist draw at least one of each required tube color before the remainder of the large group. The rationale is that if the patient is a difficult stick at least the majority of tests can be completed and aliquots made if the draw is short.
Text Reference: p. 124

40. **Answer: C**
Rationale: If separation of serum and cells for glucose testing will be delayed for several hours, it is best to collect the specimen in a gray top tube. These tubes contain antiglycolytic agents that will preserve glucose. Gray tops containing sodium fluoride are preserved for 3 days and gray tops containing iodoacetate are preserved for 24 hours.
Text Reference: p. 123

ROUTINE VENIPUNCTURE
Pamela Primrose

INTRODUCTION

Routine venipuncture is the most common procedure a phlebotomist performs. The single most important step in venipuncture is positive identification of the patient. For inpatients this is done by matching the information on the requisition with the information on the patient's identification band, or for outpatients, the information provided by the patient. Although most patients are suitable candidates for drawing blood with evacuated tubes, patients with fragile veins may be better candidates for syringe collection, with the blood being transferred to evacuated tubes after the draw.

CONTENT OVERVIEW

Requisitions
I. Origination
   A. Orders for blood testing
      1. Blood test must be authorized by physician
      2. In-house nursing staff may order per physician's instructions
         a. Followed up with physician's written orders later
         b. Depends on hospital protocol
II. Purpose
   A. Identify the patient correctly
   B. Specify specimens to be collected
   C. Give an indication of supplies needed before procedure
III. Types of requisitions
   A. Computer-generated
   B. Handwritten
IV. Information required:
   A. Patient demographics
      1. Name
      2. Date of birth (DOB)
      3. Sex
      4. Race
   B. ID number
      1. Inpatient—hospital ID number, DOB, room number, bed
      2. Outpatient—medical record number assigned
   C. Name or code of the ordering physician
   D. Tests requested along with ICD-9 code

E. Test status in order of priority
   1. STAT or medical emergency—first
      a. Results needed immediately
      b. Critical patients
         i. ER STATs first
         ii. In-house STATs second
         iii. Outpatient STATs third
      c. Alert lab when delivered
         i. May have color-coded label: orange or pink
      d. Examples
         i. ABGs
         ii. CBC or H & H
         iii. Cardiac tests
   2. Timed—second
      a. Specified time
      b. Timing critical to ensure accurate results
      c. Record actual time of draw
      d. Examples
         i. GTT
         ii. Therapeutic drug monitoring
   3. ASAP—third (may be second depending on situation or test)
      a. As soon as possible
      b. Results urgent but less than STAT
      c. Patient not critical
      d. Examples
         i. CBC or H & H
         ii. Glucose
   4. Fasting—fourth
      a. No food or beverage except water for 8 to 12 hours
      b. Verify fast
         i. Yes: proceed with specimen collection
         ii. No: contact physician to confirm collection or reschedule
      c. Examples
         i. Cholesterol
         ii. Triglycerides
         iii. Chemistry profile or metabolic panel
   5. Routine—last
      a. Standard procedure
      b. Diagnostic testing
      c. Monitor therapy or recovery
      d. No urgency—collect as received or batch

V. Miscellaneous information
  A. Bleeding complications
  B. Sites to avoid
VI. Special handling
  A. Usually not included on requisition
  B. General knowledge: (i.e., bilirubin protected from light)
  C. Nonroutine test knowledge: look-up in specimen collection manual
VII. Barcoding patients
  A. Ensures positive identification between patient and all procedures
    1. Blood specimens
    2. Other tests ordered
    3. X-rays
    4. Billing
    5. Other
  B. Linked to patient medical record
  C. Accurate, rapid, and reduces potential for error
VIII. Delivery of requisitions
  A. Sent to lab
  B. Pick up at nursing station
  C. Via computer order
  D. Fax
  E. Phone
    1. Hard copy to follow
    2. Computer order to follow (i.e., ER phone call)
  F. Outpatient brings along
IX. Receipt of requisitions
  A. Examine it for required information
  B. Check for duplicates
  C. Prioritize the requisitions—STAT, timed, etc. See Chapter Outline E. 1-5 previously discussed.
  D. Collect all equipment

Billing/Coding
I. Insurance codes—diagnostic codes
  A. ICD-9—international classification of diseases
    1. Used to code diagnoses
      a. Signs
      b. Symptoms
      c. Injuries
      d. Diseases
      c. Conditions
  B. CPT—current procedural terminology
    1. 5-digit code
    2. Used to describe services of physicians and other health care providers
      a. Medical
      b. Surgical

  c. Radiology
  d. Laboratory
  e. Anesthesiology
  f. Evaluation/management services
II. Billing
  A. CPT and ICD-9 codes must correlate for payment approval to occur
  B. Mismatched codes will be rejected for payment
  C. Software used to identify and reject claims for mismatched codes
  D. Medicare/Medicaid billing issues
    1. Centers for Medicare and Medicaid reimbursement
      a. Ensure the procedures are deemed medically necessary
      b. Identified tests requiring documentation of medical necessity
      c. System using ICD-9 codes to assess for tests' medical necessity
        i. Policies of local medical review boards (MRRBs)
        ii. Policies of national coverage determinations (NCDs)
        iii. Patient diagnosis determines medical necessity
    2. Advanced beneficiary notice (ABN)
      a. Used if tests deemed not a medical necessity or questionable
      b. Must be signed by patient *before* blood draw
        i. Cannot bill patient unless ABN signed and dated by patient
      c. Requires the following if reimbursement may be denied:
        i. Lab tests identified
        ii. Reason reimbursement likely to be denied
        iii. Ensures patient understands he/she may have to pay out of pocket
        iv. Allows beneficiary/patient to make an informed decision
      d. Patient can refuse to sign—then service not provided unless physician is willing to pay
      e. Must inform physician if patient refuses to sign

Routine Venipuncture Procedure
I. Knock on door before entry
  A. Alerts patient
  B. Respectful of privacy
  C. Gently wake sleeping patients

II.   Greet and identify self
III.   Identify correct patient
    A. Patient states full name and secondary identifier such as DOB, SS#, medical record number, which are then matched to the patient's ID band, etc., as indicated below per CLSI recommendations.
      1. Inpatient: match information to requisition and ID band
        a. ID band must be attached to patient
      2. Outpatient: match information to requisition and perform secondary checks per institutional protocol
        a. Check ID band if used
        b. Patient signs label to verify name if no ID band
        c. Photo ID
      3. Joint commission requirements: Use two acceptable identifiers such as patient's name, phone number, or other person-specific identifier.
        a. Patient's room number or physical location is not to be used as an identifier.
    B. Misidentification
      1. Incorrect diagnosis
      2. Incorrect treatment
      3. Death
      4. Grounds for dismissal
      5. Lawsuit
IV.   Explain what you need to do and obtain informed consent
    A. Doctor ordered test
    B. Do not discuss specifics—refer to physician
V.   Check pretest preparations
    A. Check for medication
      1. Blood thinning medications— Coumadin (warfarin), aspirin, etc.
        a. Requires longer compression time after draw
      2. Abstinence from medications
        a. Note on requisition any medications taken by patient
    B. Check fasting status if required
      1. Verify time of last meal or snack or beverage
VI.   Position and prepare the patient
    A. Seated
    B. Lying supine
    C. Arm straight out, elbow supported, palm up
    D. Request patient remove all foreign objects from mouth—gum, etc.
VII.   Wash hands and don gloves
VIII.   Assemble your equipment
    A. Routine venipuncture—good veins
    B. Syringe draw—small, fragile veins, collapsing veins; hand veins
    C. Butterfly draw—children, difficult or small fragile veins; hand veins
IX.   Apply the tourniquet
    A. 3 to 4 inches above puncture site
      1. Hand
        a. Place on proximal side of wrist at radius and ulna
      2. Wrist
        a. Place 3 to 4 inches above selected site
    B. On skin or sleeve if arm is hairy
      1. Watch for pinching of skin
    C. Do *not* leave on longer than 1 minute
      1. Hemoconcentration—alter test results
        a. Serum protein increased
        b. Potassium elevated
        c. Lactic acid increased
      2. Hemolysis—destruction of RBCs, increase in K^+
        a. Greater than 2 to 3 minutes
      3. Petechiae
        a. Indicate capillary wall or platelet defect
        b. May be prolonged bleeding at puncture site
X.   Select the site
    A. Antecubital fossa
      1. First choice: median cubital
        a. Well anchored
      2. Second choice: cephalic vein
        a. Tendency to move
      3. Third choice: basilic vein
        a. Least firmly anchored
        b. Near brachial artery and nerve
    B. Hand
    C. Wrist
    D. Foot/ankle—requires physician permission
XI.   Palpate the vein
    A. Depth
    B. Width
    C. Direction
    D. Spongy, bouncy, firm
      1. Arteries pulsate
      2. Tendons feel rigid
      3. Sclerosed veins are hard, cordlike
    E. Increase circulation for difficult veins
      1. Gentle massage
      2. Warm towel or other approved warming device
      3. No repeated fist clenching—elevated K^+ levels

F. Landmark veins not visible
  1. Freckle, mole, crease, hair
  2. Do not use pen to mark
  3. Avoid performing a blind-stick
    a. Vein is not visible or palpable
    b. Visibly mark the spot or anatomic area

XII. Remove tourniquet

XIII. Clean the site
  A. 70% isopropyl alcohol
  B. Concentric circles moving outward from site
  C. Air dry 30 to 60 seconds—do *not* blow or wipe
    1. Maximum bacteriostatic action
      a. 70% isopropyl alcohol dissolves cell membranes to kill organism
    2. Avoids hemolysis of RBCs
    3. Prevents stinging

XIV. Reapply the tourniquet

XV. Examine the needle
  A. Blunted/barbed point
  B. Obstructed lumen
  C. Bent shaft
  D. Do *not* touch needle on anything—get new needle if contaminated prior to insertion

XVI. Perform the venipuncture
  A. Anchor vein 1 to 2 inches below puncture site with thumb while fingers support the back side of the arm
  B. Warn patient of slight poke or pinch
  C. Insert needle at a 15° to 30° angle
  D. Bevel up
  E. Label down—can see blood flow
  F. Thread the needle into the vein to ensure bevel is completely in and seated
  G. Keep assembly angled downward
    1. Prevents backflow of blood into needle from tube
    2. Prevents contamination of needle with tube additive
    3. Prevents additive from entering patient's circulation

XVII. Fill the first tube
  A. Use flanges of adapter to stabilize needle as tube is pushed on
  B. Use small talk while filling tubes
    1. Distracts patient
    2. Helps relieve anxiety

XVIII. Remove the tourniquet
  A. Once blood flow is established
  B. Tourniquet on no longer than 1 minute
  C. Removed before needle removal
    1. Prevents hematoma

XIX. Advance and change the tubes
  A. Switch tubes when previous tube is full
    1. "Hissing" sound
      a. Needle out of vein—partially or totally
      b. Remove tourniquet and needle and start over
  B. Remove tube
    1. Forward pressure of thumb or finger against adapter
    2. Simultaneously pull tube off needle
    3. Balance push—pull to stabilize needle
  C. Invert tubes 5 to 8 times

XX. Prepare for needle removal
  A. Remove last tube first
  B. Prevents blood from dripping out of needle

XXI. Withdraw the needle
  A. Pull straight out
  B. Activate safety feature on needle

XXII. Apply pressure
  A. After needle is removed
  B. Arm straight out or slightly bent
    1. Do not bend arm upward over site
    2. Prevents hematoma
  C. Until bleeding stops
    1. Two minutes or longer for patients on anticoagulant therapy

XXIII. Dispose of the used needle/adapter unit in the needle collection container i.e., sharps container

XXIV. Label the tubes
  A. After collection
  B. Inpatient: at bedside
  C. Outpatient: in presence of patient
  D. *Never* prelabel tubes before the draw
  E. Use pen or permanent marker
  F. Required information
    1. Patient's name
    2. ID number
    3. Date
    4. Time of collection
    5. Phlebotomist's initials or employee number
    6. Optional—test

XXV. Attend to the patient
  A. Check site for bleeding
    1. Platelet plug formed and secure—bandage
    2. Continue pressure if still bleeding
  B. Apply bandage or tape
  C. Put everything back as found
    1. Bedrail up
    2. Patient covered

3. Overbed table within patient's reach
D. Dispose of contaminated materials in biohazard container
E. Remove gloves and wash hands
F. Thanks patient, smile
   1. Advise patient to leave bandage on at least 15 minutes
   2. Do not carry purse on forearm
   3. No heavy lifting with that arm for at least 1 hour
G. Report to nursing station if required
   1. Patient was fasting
   2. Patient medications withheld
XXVI. Deliver the specimen
A. Receive specimen(s) into lab via protocol
   1. Logbook
   2. Computer
B. Complete paperwork per laboratory protocol

Routine Venipuncture with a Syringe

I.   Perform steps I-XIV in the Routine Venipuncture procedure above
II.   Inspect the needle and prepare the syringe
  A. Inspect the needle for barbs, blunted tips, or bent shaft
  B. Pull plunger back to ensure moves easily
  C. Push plunger all the way back in to expel air
III.   Perform the venipuncture per step XVI in Routine Venipuncture
  A. Flash of blood in syringe hub
IV.   Fill the syringe
  A. Control vacuum by how fast plunger is pulled—slow is best
    1. 80% of hemolyzed samples are syringe draws
  B. Gently and slowly pull back on plunger
V.   Withdraw the needle and activate safety device per step XXI of Routine Venipuncture
VI   Apply pressure per step XXII of Routine Venipuncture
VII.   Transfer the blood to evacuated tubes
  A. Order of draw same as evacuated tube system
    1. Alternate order of draw as directed by institutional protocol
  B. Methods
    1. Needleless blood transfer device
    2. One-handed technique
    3. Never remove tube tops
    4. Never push on plunger
      a. Causes hemolysis
      b. Creates aerosol spray as needle removed

      c. Tube tops may pop off due to increased pressure
    5. Allow tube vacuum to pull blood into tube
    6. Position tube so blood flows down side of tube—prevents hemolysis
VIII.   Dispose of the needle, syringe, and transfer device in the needle collection container
IX.   Label the tubes per step XXIV of Routine Venipuncture
X.   Attend to the patient per step XXV of Routine Venipuncture
XI.   Deliver the specimen per step XXVI of Routine Venipuncture

---

CERTIFICATION PREPARATION QUESTIONS

1. Blood collection procedures begin with:
  a. Greeting the patient
  b. Requisition or order for blood test
  c. Patient's consent
  d. Knock on the door

2. Requests for blood draws are generated by the:
  a. Nurse
  b. Lab
  c. Physician
  d. Hospital

3. The *minimum* information required on a requisition includes all of the following, *except*:
  a. Patient demographics
  b. Special handling of lab tests
  c. ID number
  d. Name of physician

4. The phlebotomist receives a lab requisition and proceeds to use it for all of the following purposes, *except:*
  a. Ensure necessary equipment is on tray
  b. Determine specimens to be collected
  c. Assess patient diagnosis
  d. Verify patient identification

5. Verbal orders for lab tests must be followed up with a:
  a. Written order in hard copy or electronic format
  b. Verbal confirmation by the physician
  c. Phone call verifying the request
  d. Copy of results faxed to the physician's office

6. The phlebotomist is responsible for which of the following actions when lab requests are received electronically in the phlebotomy department:
   a. Prioritizing the requests
   b. Assigning accession numbers
   c. Informing the MLS/MT of incoming tests
   d. Logging in the requests

7. A system that allows for full integration of the hospital information system and the laboratory information system accurately connecting patients, requests for lab procedures, and blood specimens is:
   a. Accession numbers
   b. Barcodes
   c. Social security numbers
   d. Admission number

8. Which of the following tests must be drawn first?
   a. Fasting
   b. Timed
   c. STAT
   d. ASAP

9. A phlebotomist should knock on the patient's door before entering:
   a. When the door is closed
   b. During visiting hours
   c. When the physician is present
   d. Every time

10. While preparing the equipment to perform the venipuncture, the patient asks the phlebotomist what information the blood tests will give the physician. The proper course of action is to:
    a. Steer the conversation toward the weather or other neutral topic
    b. Explain the purpose of each test in layman terms so patient understands
    c. Tell the patient that protocol requires that they discuss it with their physician
    d. Tell the patient you do not know and steer the conversation to another topic

11. The phlebotomist had orders to draw an H & H on a trauma patient who had surgery earlier in the day and was directed by the nurse to an incorrect room. The phlebotomist whose shift was about to end went in, stated his name, and began the procedure. Lab results indicate a possible internal bleed. A blood transfusion was begun and the patient taken back into the OR. It was later discovered that a patient suffering from a massive GI bleed was incorrectly drawn in place of the trauma patient. Misidentification of this patient resulted in all of the following, *except:*
    a. Unnecessary treatment
    b. Firing of the nurse
    c. Incorrect diagnosis
    d. Firing of the phlebotomist

12. The phlebotomist enters the patient room and proceeds to verify the identity of the patient by:
    a. Asking the patient to state his name and compare lab requisition to armband
    b. Stating the patient's name and asking his social security number
    c. Showing the patient the printer label and asking if it is correct
    d. Comparing the requisition to the patient's arm band

13. The phlebotomist calls out the name of an outpatient and an elderly woman comes forward. The phlebotomist proceeds to verify the patient's identity by asking the patient to:
    a. State her date of birth
    b. State her name and date of birth
    c. State her name and physician
    d. State her name and age

14. The phlebotomist proceeds to identify a patient in the ER suffering from a broken leg by asking their name and date of birth. The name correctly matches the requisition but the date of birth is incorrect on the requisition and the ID band. The phlebotomist should:
    a. Assume that there is a clerical error and proceed with the venipuncture
    b. Assume the patient is in too much pain to remember and continue the procedure
    c. Verify the physician's name to confirm identity and continue the procedure
    d. Go to the triage desk to verify patient's identity and resolve the discrepancy

15. You arrive at the patient's room and begin the identification process only to find that the patient does not have his armband on,

it is lying on his nightstand. You explain that you must go find the nurse when he slips it back over his wrist. The phlebotomist should:

a. Continue with the identification process since the patient is now banded
b. Go to the nursing station and ask for the patient to be rebanded
c. Call down to the lab, explain what happened, and ask how to proceed
d. Ask for extra identification verifiers before performing venipuncture

16. The patient's arm is in a slightly bent position due to the bed being at a 45-degree incline. The *best* means by which a phlebotomist can better position the arm is to:
a. Lower the patient's bed flat
b. Place a blanket or towel under the arm
c. Ask the patient to hold their arm straight
d. Hold the patient's arm while performing the stick

17. The most important reason for explaining the procedure to the patient before performing the venipuncture is to:
a. Make the patient feel at ease
b. Help the patient feel in control
c. Adhere to hospital protocol
d. Gain informed consent

18. While verifying pretest preparation for a routine fasting blood draw, the patient confesses that she ate a candy bar around 2 AM that she had stashed in the nightstand. It is now 6 AM. How do you proceed?
a. Proceed with the collection, mark the tube nonfasting, document in the LIS
b. Check with the nurse to see if you should draw or reschedule the test
c. Tell the patient to hold off on breakfast until 10 AM and you'll come back then
d. Take the order back to the lab for tomorrow's morning draws

19. A competent and professional phlebotomist will try to:
a. Keep small talk to a minimum
b. Distract a nervous patient with small talk
c. Keep the conversation focused on the venipuncture process
d. Remain silent to ease the patient's anxiety

20. Proper tourniquet placement is:
a. Immediately above the puncture site
b. 1 to 2 inches above the puncture site
c. 3 to 4 inches above the puncture site
d. Three fingerwidths above the puncture site

21. The tourniquet should not be left on the arm longer than:
a. 30 seconds
b. 60 seconds
c. 2 minutes
d. 3 minutes

22. The phlebotomist was having difficulty getting blood flow into the tube after inserting the needle. Several attempts to adjust the needle were made until a slow stream of blood began to flow into the tube. Not wanting to lose the flow, the phlebotomist left the tourniquet on until the last tube filled. Possible consequences of leaving the tourniquet on too long that may compromise specimen integrity include all of the following, *except:*
a. Hemolysis
b. Petechiae
c. Hemoconcentration
d. Hematoma

23. Blood tests that may be affected by leaving the tourniquet on greater than 1 minute include all of the following, *except:*
a. Lactic acid
b. BUN
c. Potassium
d. Protein

24. When inspecting the antecubital fossa to select a vein for venipuncture, the order of selection is:
a. Basilic, cephalic, median cubital
b. Median cubital, cephalic, basilic
c. Cephalic, brachial, median cubital
d. Median cubital, brachial, cephalic

25. The purpose of palpating a vein is to determine all of the following characteristics of a suitable vein for venipuncture, *except:*
a. Bounciness
b. Rigidity
c. Depth
d. Direction

26. The phlebotomist was having great difficulty locating a vein so she used all of the following techniques *except:*
    a. Have the patient perform repeated fist clenching
    b. Gently massage the arm
    c. Apply a hot pack over the area
    d. Dangle the arm downward

27. The proper procedure to cleanse the selected venipuncture site with an antiseptic per CLSI is to:
    a. Vigorously rub the site
    b. Use concentric circles spiraling outward
    c. Use up and down swipes from left to right
    d. Dab with alcohol and wait 30 seconds

28. After cleansing the puncture site, the phlebotomist should wait 30 to 60 seconds before inserting the needle for all of the following reasons, *except to:*
    a. Avoid hemolysis of the specimen
    b. Prevent stinging at the point of needle entry
    c. Prevent hemoconcentration of the specimen
    d. Allow for maximum bacteriostatic action

29. When the palpated vein is deep within the tissue and not visible, how can the phlebotomist determine where to insert the needle?
    a. Clean a gloved finger and touch to locate it before insertion
    b. Use a pen to mark the area where the vein was felt
    c. Landmark the vein via a freckle, skin crease, etc.
    d. Stick in the general area and gently probe until located

30. A little old man covered in scabs was continuously picking at his wounds and came in for his regular PT test. He was a difficult draw. The phlebotomist selected and cleansed the site and the glove of her index finger. Just before needle insertion, the phlebotomist touched the selected site and then gently slid the needle into the vein. The patient ended up in ICU with septicemia originating at the venipuncture site, filed a lawsuit, and the hospital settled out of court. Why?
    a. Venipuncture protocol was followed but the hospital wanted to avoid the bad publicity of a trial
    b. Venipuncture protocol was not followed
    c. Settlement was cheaper than a lawsuit even though innocent
    d. Patient responsible for his own condition, hospital counsel was incorrect

31. The phlebotomist is called to ICU to pick up a CBC, electrolytes, and a PT that will be drawn by the nurse. On entry into the room, the phlebotomist notes that the nurse is completing the draw as she holds the CBC tube followed by the electrolyte tube upside down on the venous central line catheter using an adapter. How should the phlebotomist proceed?
    a. Request that all tubes be redrawn and explain why the tubes are unacceptable
    b. Begin labeling the tubes at the patient's bedside as the nurse finishes up
    c. Move to assist the nurse by inverting the tubes and handing her the next one
    d. Stand and wait until the nurse acknowledges the phlebotomist

32. All of the following measures should be performed to prevent movement of the needle in the patient's arm as the phlebotomist puts a tube on and takes it off of the needle, *except:*
    a. Use the flanges of the adapter to stabilize the needle
    b. Apply backward pressure on the adapter when inserting the tube
    c. Apply forward pressure on the adapter when removing the tube
    d. Anchor hand on patient's arm while pulling tube straight out of holder

33. The tourniquet should be removed:
    a. When the last tube has filled completely
    b. After the first tube begins to fill
    c. When the draw is half-way completed
    d. Before the first tube is engaged

34. The phlebotomist was so busy discussing the latest NFL football game with the patient that he failed to remove the tourniquet before removing the needle. As a result, the patient experienced the development of which of the following?
    a. Petechiae
    b. Hemolysis
    c. Hematoma
    d. Hemoconcentration

35. After removing an additive tube from the needle, the phlebotomist should be sure to mix the tubes by:
    a. Vigorous shaking 3 to 4 times
    b. Horizontal rocking 2 to 3 times
    c. Complete, gentle inversion 5 to 8 times
    d. Quarter inversions, left and right, 4 to 5 times

36. The last tube of blood collected should be removed from the needle/adapter unit before needle removal to prevent:
    a. Hematoma formation
    b. Blood dripping from needle tip
    c. Reflux of blood back into the vein
    d. Air from entering into the vein

37. The first thing that needs to be done immediately after the needle is removed from the arm and pressure is applied:
    a. Pick up the tubes to continue mixing
    b. Begin labeling the tubes
    c. Engage the needle safety device
    d. Discard the needle/adapter unit into a sharps container

38. After the needle is removed, pressure should be applied until:
    a. One minute has passed
    b. Platelet plug forms
    c. Blood flow slows
    d. The tubes are labeled

39. You have just removed the needle from the patient's arm for routine admissions testing on a new patient. The nurse comes into the room and asks you to leave so she can complete her admissions assessment in private. You should:
    a. Exit the room to finish up in the hallway
    b. Leave and return to the lab to finish up
    c. Call the lab and inquire how to handle the situation
    d. Tell the nurse you will leave as soon as the tubes are labeled

40. The phlebotomist performed a syringe draw using a 23-gauge needle for a CBC and electrolytes on a chemotherapy patient whose veins are very fragile. She transferred them into the appropriate tubes using a blood transfer device. The MLS told the phlebotomist that she needed to redraw the electrolytes because the specimen was hemolyzed. The cause of hemolysis is most likely due to:
    a. Pulling back on the syringe too quickly
    b. The patient's veins collapsing during the procedure
    c. Tube vacuum pulling the blood in too quickly
    d. Centrifuging of the specimen too long

41. Transferring blood from a syringe into the appropriate tube using a needleless blood transfer device requires:
    a. Using the same order as the routine venipuncture
    b. Using an alternate order to prevent microclot formation
    c. Does not matter; pushing the plunger prevents additive contamination
    d. Using the same order or alternate order as directed by lab protocol

42. If a needleless blood transfer device is not available, the phlebotomist should fill the tubes by:
    a. Placing the tubes in a rack and inserting the syringe needle into the tube stopper
    b. Holding the tubes in one hand using the other hand to insert the needle into tube stopper
    c. Leaving the blood in the syringe until she gets back to the lab to get a blood transfer device
    d. Calling to the lab to have a blood transfer device brought up to the patient's room

ANSWERS AND RATIONALES

1. **Answer: B**
   Rationale: All blood collections begin with a request for a blood test. Without a request, no blood test can be drawn. The other choices: knocking on the door, greeting the patient, and gaining the patient's consent are steps in the blood collection process.
   Text Reference: p. 129

2. **Answer: C**
Rationale: Requests for blood draws originate with a physician's order. The nurse may assess the need for a blood test but must gain the consent of the attending physician to do so. The physician must then follow-up with an order to document the request. The lab does not order blood tests and must have an order on hand before lab testing can be performed.
Text Reference: p. 129

3. **Answer: B**
Rationale: The minimum information to be included on a requisition includes patient demographics of name, DOB, sex, race, patient ID, name or code of physician, tests requested, and test status (i.e., STAT, fasting, timed, etc.)
Text Reference: p. 129

4. **Answer: C**
Rationale: The information on requisitions serves to correctly identify the patient; identifies the tests to be collected; and allows the phlebotomist to know what equipment is needed to perform the draw. The phlebotomist does not assess a patient's diagnosis.
Text Reference: p. 129

5. **Answer: A**
Rationale: A verbal request for lab testing must be followed up by a written order either in hard copy or electronic format.
Text Reference: p. 129 and Content Overview (earlier in this chapter)

6. **Answer: A**
Rationale: When lab requests are received, the phlebotomist must make sure that the necessary patient information is on the document or computer-generated request; check for duplicate orders and group them so collections can be performed in a single venipuncture; prioritize the requests as STAT, timed etc.; and make sure the necessary equipment and supplies are on the phlebotomy trays.
Text Reference: p. 130

7. **Answer: B**
Rationale: Barcoding patients allows for accurate and rapid connection between patients and any procedures performed in the hospital or lab, billing information, etc. It dramatically reduces the potential for error.
Text Reference: p. 129 and Chapter Overview (earlier in this chapter)

8. **Answer: C**
Rationale: STAT tests are medical emergencies and take priority over any other test. Next in line are timed tests followed by ASAP, then fasting. Routine tests are performed last.
Text Reference: p. 129 and Chapter Overview (earlier in this chapter)

9. **Answer: D**
Rationale: The phlebotomist should knock lightly on the door each time whether the door is open or closed. Knocking alerts the patient, the physician if present, and any visitors to the phlebotomist's arrival. It is a sign of respecting the patient's privacy and allows the patient time to prepare before anyone's entry into their room
Text Reference: p. 131

10. **Answer: C**
Rationale: Explaining the purpose of a laboratory test to patients is outside the scope of practice for a phlebotomist. The correct course of action is to tell the patient that protocol requires them to discuss any questions they may have regarding lab work or any other medical question with their physician.
Text Reference: p. 131

11. **Answer: B**
Rationale: The phlebotomist holds sole responsibility for verifying the identity of the patient and the requisition for blood collection and could be fired. The result was incorrect diagnosis and treatment, which included a blood transfusion and more surgery. The patient could have died. The fact that a nurse was said to have indicated an incorrect room is speculative at best. Placing blame does not absolve the phlebotomist of their duty to the patient.
Text Reference: p. 131

12. **Answer: A**
Rationale: Inpatient identity is verified by asking the patient to state his or her name and

then verifying it with the lab requisition. If the patient is unconscious, then a relative or nurse can assist in verifying the patient's identity.
Text Reference: p. 131

13. **Answer: B**
Rationale: Phlebotomists are required to verify two pieces of information from outpatients to confirm identity: name plus one other identifier, typically date of birth or a photo ID. A person who responds to a name being called may have heard incorrectly, thought it was their turn, etc., and responded. The patient must always state their name. Date of birth is an easy piece of information to verify. Stating the physician's name or one's age is not enough because patients may have the same name and the same physician or be of the same age.
Text Reference: p. 131 and Content Overview (earlier in this chapter)

14. **Answer: D**
Rationale: When the patient's identity cannot be confirmed with the requisition, the phlebotomist should stop the procedure and go ask the appropriate person to double check the information with what the patient states. The correct information should be reflected on a new order and new ID band. Never make assumptions when it comes to identifying a patient because it could lead to misdiagnosis, treatment, or death. Patients with the same name may also have the same physician.
Text Reference: p. 131

15. **Answer: B**
Rationale: If a patient's ID band has been removed, the patient must be re-banded by the nurse. The phlebotomist should not assume that the loose ID band belongs to the patient lying in the bed. The nurse should verify the patient when replacing the ID band.
Text Reference: p. 131

16. **Answer: B**
Rationale: The patient's arm should be in a straight position with the palm facing up. At times the patient's arm may need to be supported by having the patient make a fist with the other hand and placing it under the elbow or, for inpatients, placing

a pillow, blanket, or towel under the arm for support. The patient should not be asked to hold their arm straight without support nor should the phlebotomist attempt to hold it during the procedure. Both measures could result in a mishap with the patient needing to be restuck. Lowering the patient's bed flat may not be an option if the patient is uncomfortable or has breathing difficulties when lying flat. If the bed can be lowered, be sure to raise it after completion of the draw.
Text Reference: p. 132

17. **Answer: D**
Rationale: Informed consent cannot be given by the patient unless the procedure and reason for the venipuncture are fully explained to the patient. Failure to secure informed consent can lead to charges of assault and battery and/or a lawsuit.
Text Reference: p. 132 and Chapter 18

18. **Answer: B**
Rationale: The timeframe for refraining from food and beverage other than water is 8 to 12 hours. The patient is not fasting at this point in time. The correct course of action is to check with the nurse to see if the draw should performed or rescheduled. Patients should not be told to hold off on their meal until 4 hours later because they may become ill or medications to be taken with food may be delayed. Delaying the draw until the following day is a decision only the nurse or physician can make.
Text Reference: p. 132

19. **Answer: B**
Rationale: Small talk about the weather, sports, or other neutral subjects will distract a nervous patient and redirect their attention away from the venipuncture. Minimal or no talking or conversation centered around the venipuncture process may serve to heighten the patient's anxiety and progress toward the patient fainting.
Text Reference: p. 132

20. **Answer: C**
Rationale: Proper application of the tourniquet is 3 to 4 inches above the selected venipuncture site.
Text Reference: p. 134

21. **Answer: B**
    Rationale: The tourniquet should not be left on the arm longer than 1 minute or sample integrity and test results may be compromised.
    Text Reference: p. 134

22. **Answer: D**
    Rationale: Studies have documented that leaving the tourniquet on longer than 1 minute can result in possible hemolysis and hemoconcentration of the specimen. Petechiae may appear as well if the tourniquet is on too long and too tight.
    Text Reference: p. 134

23. **Answer: B**
    Rationale: Studies have documented that lactic acid, potassium, and protein results may be elevated due to prolonged tourniquet application, resulting in hemoconcentration of the blood at the venipuncture site. Extended tourniquet application may also add to potassium elevations as a result of hemolysis.
    Text Reference: p. 134 and Chapter Overview (earlier in this chapter)

24. **Answer: B**
    Rationale: The first choice in vein selection is the median cubital, second is the cephalic, and the last vein of choice is the basilic. Selection is based not only on size but location in the antecubital fossa, because the veins are anchored by tissue differently and locations of arteries and nerves may pose a problem in relation to vein locations. Each person's anatomy is slightly different, so proper palpation is required to select the best vein.
    Text Reference: p. 135

25. **Answer: B**
    Rationale: When determining which vein to select for venipuncture, the phlebotomist should assess the width, depth, direction, and feel of the vein. Veins are firm yet spongy or bouncy, not hard or rigid. Tendons or sclerotic veins are rigid and hard.
    Text Reference: p. 135

26. **Answer: A**
    Rationale: Repeated fist clenching can result in elevated potassium levels and should not be done when trying to locate a vein. Approved methods to assist in the location of difficult to find veins are: gently massaging the arm, applying a hot pack or warm towel over the area, and dangling the arm downward.
    Text Reference: p. 135

27. **Answer: B**
    Rationale: The proper way to cleanse the venipuncture site is to use 70% alcohol or other antiseptic using concentric circles that spiral outward.
    Text Reference: p. 136

28. **Answer: C**
    Rationale: After cleansing the site should be allowed to air dry for approximately 30 to 60 seconds to allow for maximum bacteriostatic action, prevent hemolysis of the specimen, and prevent stinging of the puncture site after needle insertion. Contact of 70% isopropyl alcohol with bacteria during that 30-to 60-second interval allows for penetration of the alcohol into the microorganism, allowing for dissolution of the cell membrane and hence death. Do *not* blow on the area to speed up evaporation or wipe the alcohol off. Hemoconcentration occurs as a result of prolonged tourniquet application.
    Text Reference: pp. 134, 136

29. **Answer: C**
    Rationale: When veins are not clearly visible it is difficult to determine where to insert the needle. Visually noting landmarks such as a freckle, mole, skin crease, etc., will provide a guide in these situations. You should never touch the site before needle insertion. You should not mark a vein with a pen as it may contaminate the field.
    Text Reference: p. 136 and Content Overview (earlier in this chapter)

30. **Answer: B**
    Rationale: Venipuncture protocol does *not* state anywhere that the phlebotomist can clean the index finger with alcohol and touch the puncture site before needle insertion. Protocol is violated when phlebotomists choose to do so and it puts the institution at risk for a lawsuit. It does not matter that

the patient may have picked at the wound and infected it. The phlebotomist touched it before insertion and may have contaminated the site and pushed bacteria into the vessel. Contributory negligence may be on the part of the patient, but the bigger issue is the failure to follow established protocol.
Text Reference: pp. 136-137

31. **Answer: A**
Rationale: The phlebotomist should request that all tubes be redrawn. Drawing tubes upside down on the needle results in contamination of the needle by the previous tube's additive. In addition, the order of draw was also incorrect—green top is drawn before lavender. Contamination of EDTA on the needle can increase K$^+$ levels. In addition, there is the risk of backflow of blood into the needle and the additive may enter into the patient's circulation. When performing any type of blood collection, the assembly should be angled downward to prevent these events from occurring.
Text Reference: p. 137

32. **Answer: D**
Rationale: The flanges of the adapter should be used to help stabilize the needle during the placement and removal of tubes on and off the needle. Fingers should be placed behind the flanges to apply backward pressure toward the phlebotomist as the tube is pushed onto the needle to prevent the needle from going through the vein. Fingers or a thumb should push gently against the bottom of the adapter along the flanges to create forward pressure as the tube is removed so that the needle is not pulled out of the vein.
Text Reference: p. 138

33. **Answer: B**
Rationale: The tourniquet should not be left on longer than 1 minute. It should be removed as soon as blood flow has been established with the first tube.
Text Reference: p. 138

34. **Answer: C**
Rationale: Failure to remove the tourniquet before removal of the needle may result in the formation of a hematoma. Petechiae can

result if the tourniquet is too tight and left on too long. Hemolysis and hemoconcentration affect the blood specimen if the tourniquet is left on too long and have nothing to do with the removal of the needle after tourniquet removal.
Text Reference: p. 138

35. **Answer: C**
Rationale: Additive tubes must be mixed per manufacturer specifications, which is typically 5 to 8 times by complete, gentle inversion. Vigorous shaking can result in hemolysis of the specimen. Horizontal or quarter inversions may not result in complete mixing of the blood with the anticoagulant.
Text Reference: p. 139

36. **Answer: B**
Rationale: The last tube of blood should be removed from the needle/adapter unit to prevent blood from dripping out of the needle tip and contaminating the patient's clothing, phlebotomy chair, floor, etc.
Text Reference: p. 139

37. **Answer: C**
Rationale: As soon as the needle is removed from the patient's arm, the needle safety feature should be activated to prevent accidental needlestick injury.
Text Reference: p. 140

38. **Answer: B**
Rationale: After the needle is removed, pressure should be applied for as long as it takes the platelet plug to form. The timeframe varies from person to person and takes up to 2 minutes or longer for persons on anticoagulants. A slow flow of blood at the puncture site indicates that the platelet plug has not fully developed. The phlebotomist may have labeled all tubes but hemostasis may not be complete. A gentle tug at the site can determine if the plug has fully developed. If pressure is released too soon, the patient may develop bruising or a hematoma.
Text Reference: p. 140

39. **Answer: D**
Rationale: All tubes must be labeled in the patient's presence whether outpatient or

in-patient. Tell the nurse you will leave as
soon as the tubes are labeled.
Text Reference: p. 140

40. **Answer: A**
Rationale: Pulling back too quickly on the
plunger of the syringe using a 23-gauge
needle may result in hemolysis of the RBCs
as the blood enters the lumen of the needle.
**Text Reference: p. 143 and Chapter 8
Chapter Overview**

41. **Answer: D**
Rationale: When transferring blood from a
syringe into the evacuated tubes, the order
of fill may be the same as the order of draw
for a routine venipuncture. Some institutions
require an alternate order of fill to prevent
microclot formation in the specimen and
require filling anticoagulated tubes first.

You should follow the protocol of your
institution.
**Text Reference: p. 143 and Chapter 9
Overview**

42. **Answer: A**
Rationale: If a needleless blood transfer device
is not available, the phlebotomist should use
the one-handed technique to fill the tubes by
placing them in a test tube rack and inserting
the needle into the stopper. The needle should
be removed by using a device other than the
hand to hold the tube down while withdrawing
the needle. Waiting for delivery of a device
or waiting to get back to the lab can result in
clot formation of the specimen, compromise
test results, and make it impossible to get the
specimen out of the syringe.
**Text Reference: p. 144 and Chapter 9
Overview**

DERMAL PUNCTURE
Pamela Primrose

INTRODUCTION

Dermal puncture is an alternative collection procedure used when minute amounts of blood are needed for testing, or for patients in whom venipuncture is inadvisable or impossible. It is the routine collection procedure for infants. In addition, it is the standard procedure for the bleeding time test and the ancillary blood glucose test. The depth of puncture must be carefully controlled to produce adequate flow while avoiding contact with underlying bone. Skin puncture devices deliver a precise incision; microsample containers, sized to fit the desired sample, collect the blood from the puncture site.

CONTENT OVERVIEW

Dermal Puncture
I. For the collection of capillary blood

Reasons for Performing Dermal Puncture
I. Venipuncture is impossible or inadvisable to do
II. Alternative to venipuncture for following:
   A. Bleeding time determinations
   B. Bedside glucose testing
   C. Alternative to arterial puncture
   D. Arterial blood gas (ABG) test using capillary blood

Procedure of Choice for Some Situations and Patients
I. Situations
   A. Patients requiring frequent blood tests—spares veins
   B. Glucose monitoring—small drop of blood
   C. One blood test ordered; dermal puncture appropriate option
   D. Patients on IV therapy—preserves veins for IV
II. Patients
   A. Geriatric
   B. Obese

C. Children under age of 2
   1. Easier
   2. Complications as a result of reduced blood volume from venipuncture
      a. Anemia
      b. Cardiac arrest
      c. Death
D. Medical conditions of patients
   1. Risk for thrombosis
   2. Risk for complications from deep venous puncture
      a. Hemorrhage
      b. Infection
      c. Organ/tissue damage
      d. Arteriospasm/cardiac arrest
   3. Injury from use of necessary restraints
   4. Burns or scars over venipuncture sites
   5. Swollen tissues
   6. Lymphatic drainage is compromised (i.e., mastectomy)

Tests Exempt from Dermal Puncture
I.   Blood cultures
II. Erythrocyte sedimentation rate
III. Coagulation tests

Differences Between Venous and Capillary Blood
I. Capillary blood composition
   A. Mixture of venous and arterial blood
   B. Warming of site increases arterial portion
   C. Tissue fluid—small amounts may be in sample; especially first drop
II. Test variances between collection methods
   A. Higher in capillary blood
      1. Hemoglobin
      2. Glucose
   B. Higher in venous blood
      1. Potassium
      2. Calcium
      3. Total protein
   C. Caution
      1. Cannot compare test results between techniques
      2. Repeated testing
         a. Requires use of same collection method

Equipment for Dermal Puncture

I.   Skin puncture devices
   A. Automatic puncture device
     1. Dimensions of puncture
       a. Predetermined depth
         i. Selection of depth of puncture criteria
           a) Age of patient
           b) Site of puncture: finger, heel
           c) Volume of blood needed
           d) Bone proximity
       b. Set width
       c. May be color coded for depths
       d. Examples
         i. Babies under 1 year: heel or big toe
           a) Depth 1 mm; width 2.5 mm—not to exceed 2 mm depth
           b) Preemie device: depth 0.85 mm; width 1.75 mm
         ii. Medium to high blood flow: depth 2 mm; width 1.5 mm
         iii. Single drop: depth 2.25 mm; 23-gauge puncture lancet
     2. Safety features
       a. Retractable blade
       b. Lock prevents reuse
       c. Prevents accidental stick

II. Lasette Laser lancing device
   A. Less pain
   B. Less bruising
   C. Cross-contamination prevented by use of single-use disposable lens cover
   D. Approved on patients >5 years old

III. Microsample containers
   A. Different sizes for various volumes
     1. Microcollection tubes (bullets)—most common
       a. Volume: up to 750 μL
       b. Types available
         i. Additives
         ii. Anticoagulants
         iii. Color coded same as tube stoppers
       c. Used for all types of dermal puncture collections
     2. Micropipettes
       a. Caraway or Natelson pipettes
         i. May include flea (metal filing) and magnet for mixing
       b. Plastic or glass capillary tube
         i. Glass poses sharps risk
         ii. OSHA recommends plastic
       c. Types
         i. Plain: blue band
         ii. Heparin-coated: yellow or green band
       d. Seal both ends
         i. Plastic caps preferred
       e. Can centrifuge, retrieve sample via syringe
       f. Volume: up to 470 μL
       g. Used for ABGs
     3. Capillary tubes (microhematocrit tubes)
       a. Small plastic tube
       b. Volume: up to 75 μL
       c. Types
         i. Plain: blue band
         ii. Heparin-coated: red or green band
       d. Seal same as micropipettes
       e. Not routiney used; example: plain or heparin-coated capillary tubes can be useful in checking POCT hematocrit
         i) Plain used with anticoagulated blood
         ii) Heparin used with capillary blood collection
     4. Dilution system with micropipette
       a. BD Unopette for CBCs

IV. Order of draw for dermal punctures
   A. Slides made first if needed
   B. EDTA microtainer tube drawn first
     1. Ensures adequate volume for accurate results
     2. Minimizes platelet aggregation
   C. Other additives such as heparin
   D. Clot microtainer tubes last
     1. Blood flow slows as platelets aggregate
     2. Not a problem for serum specimen

V.   Additional supplies
   A. Warming devices—increase circulation
     1. Types
       a. Towel or washcloth soaked in warm water
         i. Completely dry site before puncture
           a) Water hemolyzes cells
           b) Dilutes sample
       b. Commercial warming pack
         i. Wrap in towel and squeeze to activate

ii. Temperatures not to exceed 42° C
iii. Application time 3 to 5 minutes

Site Selection

I. General considerations
  A. Warm, healthy skin—no scars, cuts, rashes, bruises, edematous, etc.
  B. Avoid previous puncture sites
    1. Circulation compromised
    2. Lymphatic drainage compromised
  C. Easily accessible
  D. Good capillary flow
  E. Clearance above underlying bone
    1. Osteochondritis—inflammation of bone or cartilage
    2. Osteomyelitis—infection of bone or bone marrow; serious, sometimes fatal bone infection
II. Puncture depth and width
  A. Depth limits prevent inflammation and infection
    1. Depth ≤ 3 mm
    2. Heel puncture: maximum depth 2 mm
      a. Calcaneus (heel bone) close to surface
    3. Preemies: 0.65 to 0.85 mm
  B. Width limits
    1. Width = 2.4 mm
    2. Width more important than depth in achieving blood flow
      a. Capillary beds close to skin surface, especially in newborns
    3. Wider cut severs more capillaries
III. Dermal puncture sites in adults and older children
  A. Adults and children older than 1 year
    1. Fingertips of nondominant hand
    2. Best sites
      a. Palmar surface of distal segment middle and ring finger
      b. Thumb too callused
      c. Index finger has extra nerve endings—too painful
      d. Pinky—too little tissue; safety issue
      e. Big toe alternative option if fingers not available
      f. Never use earlobes
    3. Puncture site
      a. Near fleshy center of chosen finger
      b. Avoid edge—too bony
      c. Cut should be perpendicular to fingerprint ridges (whorls)
        i. Allows for nice drop formation
        ii. Lessens running into grooves

IV. Dermal puncture sites in infants
  A. Children under 1 year
    1. Performed in the heel
      a. Medial and lateral borders of plantar surface
      b. Center and posterior too close to calcaneus (heel)
      c. Arch too close to nerves, tendons
  B. Older infants—big toe if heel unacceptable

Dermal Puncture Procedure

I. Greet and identify patient
II. Assess need for dermal puncture
  A. Document on requisition: dermal puncture
III. Prepare to perform dermal puncture
  A. Wash hands, don gloves
  B. Assemble equipment
  C. Age appropriate
  D. Tests ordered
  E. Select and clean site
  F. Warm site first
    1. 3 to 5 minutes
    2. Temperature = 42° C
  G. Clean with 70% isopropyl alcohol
    1. Do not use povidone-iodine—elevates several test analytes:
      a. Acronym BURPP
        i. Bilirubin
        ii. Uric Acid
        iii. Phosphorus
        iv. Potassium
  H. Air dry completely to prevent problems from residual alcohol
    1. Stinging
    2. Contamination
    3. Hemolysis
    4. Prevents drop formation
  I. Gently massage finger proximal to puncture site – do not squeeze
    a. Increases blood flow
    b. Squeezing can hemolyze specimen
  J. Position and hold the area
    1. Hold firmly
      a. Finger: grasp between your thumb and index finger
      b. Heel: thumb in arch, hand over top of foot, index finger behind heel
      c. Palmar surface face up
  K. Make the puncture
    1. Perpendicular to fingerprints or heel lines
    2. Count to two before lifting device away

3. Ensures blade made puncture to full depth and retracts
4. Prevents scraping of skin if blade not retracted
L. Dispose of blade into sharps container
M. Failure to obtain blood—can try two times before getting someone else

IV. Prepare to collect sample
A. Wipe first drop off: prevents tissue fluid contamination
B. Finger in downward position: encourages blood flow by gravity
C. Alternate gentle pressure and release
D. Avoid constant massaging
1. Cuts off blood flow
2. Hemolysis
3. Tissue fluid contamination

V. Collect the sample
A. Microcollection tube slanted downward
1. Touch scoop to drop of blood—freely runs into tube
2. Do not scrape skin
a. Causes hemolysis
b. Activates platelets: site clots, reduce or no blood flow
c. Contaminates sample with epithelial cells
3. Tap lightly—moves blood to bottom
4. Collect amount indicated by tube markings
a. Overfilling can result in microclot formation
b. Underfilling can result in erroneous results to incorrect blood: anticoagulant ratio
5. Close lid
6. Invert 8 to 10 times if additives
B. Capillary tubes
1. Glass capillary tubes not routinely used
2. To reduce risk of blood-borne pathogen exposure OSHA recommends:
a. Using nonglass capillary tubes
b. Wrapping glass capillary tubes in puncture-resistant film
c. Using products that do not require pushing end of tube in putty to seal
d. Using products that allow blood HCT to be measured without centrifugation
3. Hold horizontally—prevents air bubbles
4. Touch to drop
5. Fill by capillary action

6. Do not touch skin
a. Contaminates specimen with tissue fluid
b. Same problems that occur with microcollection tube
C. Order of collection
1. Blood smears first: minimizes platelet aggregation at site
2. Platelet, CBCs, other hematology counts second
3. Other tests third (i.e., chemistry)

VI. Complete the procedure
A. Apply pressure with clean gauze
B. Bandage for older children and adults
C. No bandage for children under 2—choking hazard
D. Remove all equipment, supplies, etc.
E. Raise bed rails
F. Label tubes and place in carrier tube per institutional protocol
G. Thank patient

Other Uses for Dermal Puncture
I. Bleeding time test
A. Measures length of time required to stop bleeding after incision
B. Assesses overall integrity of primary hemostasis
1. Vascular system
2. Platelet function
C. Done before surgery
D. Abnormal results—requires further testing
1. Vascular disorders
2. Platelet disorders
3. Skin conditions
4. Medication interferences
a. Aspirin
b. Streptokinase
c. Ethanol
E. Results and complications
1. Normal bleeding time 2 to 10 minutes (depends on device)
2. Bleeding time greater than 15 to 20 minutes
a. Abnormal platelet plug formation
b. Test done incorrectly
i. Capillary scratched
ii. Technical error
c. Single incision: repeat on other arm
d. Double incision: times should be within several minutes of each other

3. Shortened bleeding time
    a. Test error: incisions too shallow
        i. Device lifted too soon
        ii. Interference of hair at site
II. Ancillary blood glucose test
    A. Performed at bedside
    B. Diabetes mellitus monitoring
    C. Dermal puncture
    D. Test strips vary by testing instrument—follow manufacturer instructions
    E. Calibrate machine before running patients
        1. Set schedule per manufacturer and institution
    F. Controls run per institution protocol: per shift, twice daily, etc.
        1. Run using same procedure as patient samples
    G. Calibration and control results critical for accurate results
        1. In range—OK
        2. Out of range—troubleshoot until values in range
    H. Record results

Bleeding Time Procedure
I. Assemble equipment
    A. Antiseptic materials
    B. Blood pressure cuff
    C. Automated bleeding time device
    D. Stopwatch or timer with second hand
    E. Filter paper
    F. Butterfly bandages
II. Prepare patient
    A. Explain procedure
    B. Note scarring may occur—especially in dark skinned persons
    C. Pretest assessment
        1. Medications patient is taking
            a. Aspirin or drugs that interfere with clotting
            b. Salicylates and aspirin
                i. Inhibit platelet function 7 to 10 days after last dose
            c. Ibuprofen
                i. Inhibits platelet function 24 hours
        2. Check institution's policy before proceeding with test
III. Position the arm, select the site, and clean the site
    A. Place arm on flat surface, volar side up
    B. Site selection
        1. 5 cm below antecubital fossa

2. Free of scars, hair, bruises
    3. Shave hairy arms
    C. Clean site and air dry as with all procedures
IV. Apply the blood pressure cuff
    A. 40 mm Hg
    B. Maintain pressure entire time—monitor and adjust as needed
    C. Wait 30 to 60 seconds to ensure steady pressure before making incision
V.   Position the device
    A. Parallel or perpendicular to antecubital crease
    B. Perpendicular—less scarring but less accurate
    C. Follow institution policy on placement
VI. Make the incision and start timing
    A. Press device on arm but no indentation
    B. Press trigger
    C. Start time simultaneously with depression of the trigger
    D. Remove device when blades retract
VII. Wick the blood away every 30 seconds
    A. Absorb with filter paper
    B. Touch edge of blood drop but not incision or skin
    C. Wick until drop disappears
    D. Two incisions—wick each drop independently of other
VIII. Complete the test
    A. Blood no longer absorbed by filter paper—bleeding stopped
    B. Record time
    C. Remove pressure cuff
        1. Attend to the patient
    D. Clean arm
    E. Apply butterfly bandage
    F. Instruct patient to leave bandage on for 24 hours to minimizes scarring
    G. Clean up supplies, etc.
    H. Thank patient

Ancillary Blood Glucose Test
I.   Perform routine dermal puncture per procedure
II. Collect the sample
    A. Collect free-falling drop of blood to cover appropriate area on strip
    B. Do not touch skin—contaminates strip
    C. Insert into instrument
III. Read and record the result
    A. Panic values: immediately report to nursing staff

CERTIFICATION PREPARATION QUESTIONS

1. The composition of capillary blood includes:
   a. Venous and capillary
   b. Arterial and capillary
   c. Venous and arterial
   d. Capillary and tissue fluid

2. Dermal punctures may be best for all of the following patients, *except*:
   a. Children
   b. Geriatric patients
   c. Anorexic patients
   d. Obese patients

3. Situations that may require dermal punctures include all of the following, *except*:
   a. Patients on IV therapy
   b. Patients with orders for only one blood test
   c. Patients at risk for arteriospasm or cardiac arrest
   d. Patients undergoing frequent coagulation testing

4. Which of the following tests can be performed on blood that is collected by dermal puncture?
   a. Erythrocyte sedimentation rate
   b. BUN
   c. Thrombin time
   d. Blood culture

5. All of the following test analytes are higher in venous blood than capillary blood, *except*:
   a. Glucose
   b. Potassium
   c. Calcium
   d. Total protein

6. During the course of a 5-hour glucose tolerance test (GTT), the phlebotomist began having difficulty getting a venous sample and switched over to dermal punctures to finish out the last three glucose tests. The phlebotomist's decision:
   a. Was appropriate because multiple venipunctures could compromise the integrity of the specimen
   b. Compromises the test interpretation because venous glucose levels are lower than capillary levels

   c. Was appropriate because glucose results are comparable between venous and capillary blood
   d. Compromises the test accuracy because less blood is available for testing by dermal puncture

7. Equipment for a dermal puncture to collect a sample for bilirubin testing on a newborn includes all of the following, *except*:
   a. Lancet
   b. Amber-colored microtainer tube
   c. Warming device
   d. Povidone-iodine

8. The dimensions of a dermal puncture are controlled by:
   a. Width of the blade
   b. Width, depth of the blade
   c. Pressure applied, depth of the blade
   d. Width, depth of the blade, pressure applied

9. Features of dermal puncture devices include all of the following, *except*:
   a. Retractable blade
   b. Single use
   c. Automatic puncture
   d. Uniform depth

10. The term "bullet" in blood collection refers to:
    a. Capillary tubes
    b. Microcollection tubes
    c. Micropipettes
    d. Microhematocrit

11. A flea or metal filing is used when collecting a:
    a. Unopette
    b. Microhematocrit
    c. Microcollection tube
    d. Natelson pipette

12. A dilution system that can be used for cell counts in hematology:
    a. Unopette
    b. Microhematocrit tube
    c. Bullet
    d. Caraway tube

13. The temperature of any warming device used for dermal punctures should not exceed:
    a. 36° C
    b. 42° C

c. 98.6° F

d. 101° F

14. Which of the following is needed when collecting a Caraway micropipette?
    a. Glass slide
    b. Unopette
    c. Plastic caps
    d. Bullet

15. All of the following are characteristic of a good dermal site, *except*:
    a. Good venous flow
    b. Clearance above underlying bone
    c. Easily accessible
    d. Warm, healthy skin

16. When performing a dermal puncture, the phlebotomist must be sure that the automatic device does not puncture the calcaneus located in the:
    a. Heel
    b. Middle finger
    c. Big toe
    d. Ring finger

17. If the bone is punctured during a dermal puncture procedure, it could result in an infection of the bone or bone marrow referred to as:
    a. Osteomyelitis
    b. Osteochondritis
    c. Osteitis
    d. Osteoma

18. The phlebotomist will be performing a dermal puncture on a preemie and selects a puncture device that has a puncture depth of:
    a. 1.8 to 2.4 mm
    b. 1.5 to 1.75 mm
    c. 0.65 to 0.85 mm
    d. 0.85 to 1.2 mm

19. The maximum depth of puncture for a heelstick is:
    a. 0.85 mm
    b. 1.5 mm
    c. 2.0 mm
    d. 2.4 mm

20. The width of a puncture should not exceed:
    a. 1.5 mm
    b. 1.75 mm

c. 2.0 mm

d. 2.4 mm

21. Puncture width plays a more important role in establishing blood flow in a dermal stick because:
    a. A wider cut severs more capillaries
    b. Newborns have fewer capillaries
    c. Adult capillaries are spread out
    d. Capillary depth varies across dermal bed

22. Dermal puncture sites in adults and children older than 1 year include all of the following, *except*:
    a. Middle finger
    b. Big toe
    c. Ring finger
    d. Thumb

23. When performing a dermal puncture on the finger, the puncture should be made:
    a. Horizontal to the whorls on the fleshy pad
    b. Parallel to the edge of the distal segment
    c. Perpendicular to the fingerprint ridges
    d. Parallel with the phalanges of the finger

24. Dermal punctures are performed on heels for children younger than 1 year because:
    a. It is difficult to keep their fingers extended
    b. It is easier to hold the heel during blood collection
    c. There is too little flesh on the fingers
    d. Tests results are more accurate from the heel

25. Dermal puncture sites on an infant include all of the following, *except*:
    a. Lateral arch of the plantar surface
    b. Medial border of the plantar surface
    c. Lateral border of the plantar surface
    d. Plantar surface of the big toe

26. Selection of the type of skin puncture device is determined by the:
    a. Phlebotomist's preference
    b. Age of the patient
    c. Supplies available
    d. Size of the microcollection tube

27. The acronym BURPP represents a collection of tests that:
    a. Cannot be performed using povidone-iodine
    b. Cannot be performed on capillary blood

c. Are performed using a Unopette
d. Means collect bullets: red, purple, pink

28. The phlebotomist is preparing the equipment for a dermal puncture to collect an H & H, BUN, and creatinine. She will collect the necessary specimens in the following order:
    a. Slides, gold, lavender
    b. Green, lavender
    c. Lavender, gold
    d. Green, gold

29. All of the following represent proper dermal puncture technique on an adult, *except:*
    a. Selecting middle or ring finger
    b. Cutting perpendicular to the fingerprints
    c. Wiping away the first drop
    d. Milking or massaging the finger

30. The first drop of blood must be wiped away after the puncture to:
    a. Remove the platelet plug
    b. Prevent tissue fluid contamination
    c. Allow for round drop formation
    d. Remove loose epithelial cells

31. Proper collection of microcollection tubes includes all of the following, *except*:
    a. Touching the scoop to the drop of blood
    b. Allowing blood to run freely into the tube
    c. Squeezing as you scrape upward to capture drop
    d. Tapping lightly to move blood into the tube

32. The phlebotomist was collecting a dermal puncture for a complete blood count (CBC) on a very lethargic, febrile newborn. She had a good flow going, so she filled the microtainer tube to the top because she knew from experience that often the technicians run the specimen several times to confirm any abnormal results. The CBC had to be recollected because:
    a. The extra time to fill the microtainer resulted in hemolysis of the specimen
    b. The specimen spilled when the aspirating needle displaced the extra blood
    c. Microclots had formed as a result of overfilling the microtainer tube
    d. The tech wanted to rerun the specimen again to recheck the first two results

33. Bandages should not be applied on children under the age of 2 years because:
    a. They can pull it off and may choke on it
    b. They don't need one as they quickly clot
    c. The adhesive irritates and tears the skin
    d. Bacteria may breed on the gauze

34. The proper technique for filling a hematocrit is by:
    a. Touching the drop and letting it fill by capillary action
    b. Angling the tube downward to let blood drip into it
    c. Placing the pipette directly on the skin as the drop forms
    d. Removing any air bubbles by flicking the tube

35. Screening test that involves the vascular system and platelet function to assess the overall integrity of primary hemostasis:
    a. Prothrombin time
    b. Bleeding time
    c. Thrombin time
    d. Platelet count

36. Normal bleeding time results fall within the range of:
    a. 1 to 2 minutes
    b. 2 to 10 minutes
    c. 6 to 12 minutes
    d. 15 to 20 minutes

37. An abnormal bleeding time test may indicate all of the following, *except*:
    a. Platelet disorder
    b. Skin condition
    c. Medication interference
    d. Secondary hemostasis disorder

38. The orientation of the blade on the arm that produces the most accurate results in a bleeding time test is:
    a. Diagonal to the antecubital crease
    b. 10 cm below the antecubital crease
    c. Perpendicular to the antecubital crease
    d. Parallel to the antecubital crease

39. During the bleeding time the blood pressure cuff must be inflated and maintained at a pressure of:
    a. 30 mm Hg
    b. 40 mm Hg

c. 50 mm Hg

d. 60 mm Hg

40. The phlebotomist is performing a bleeding time test and is ready to press the trigger of the cutting device and start the timer. She starts the timer:
    a. As soon as the first drop of blood appears
    b. Just before pressing the trigger of the device
    c. After the trigger is depressed and the device removed
    d. Simultaneously as she presses the trigger

41. Proper technique in wicking away the blood during a bleeding time includes all of the following, *except*:
    a. Touch filter paper edge to the surface of the drop
    b. Repeat the wicking process every 30 seconds
    c. Wick each incision simultaneously
    d. Continue to wick until the drop disappears

42. Before performing ancillary blood glucose testing, the phlebotomist must ensure that the instrument is operating properly by:
    a. Calibrating the reagent strips to the manufacturer's specifications
    b. Running controls the same as patient samples
    c. Comparing patient samples to previous results
    d. Troubleshooting abnormal patient results

ANSWERS AND RATIONALES

1. **Answer: C**
   Rationale: Capillaries are the bridge between arteries and veins and the blood in them consists of both arterial and capillary blood.
   Text Reference: p. 148

2. **Answer: C**
   Rationale: Dermal puncture is the preferred method of blood collection for children, especially those under the age of 2 who have smaller veins and blood volume considerations. Geriatric patients may have small, fragile, and difficult to find veins. Obese patients may also have veins that are difficult to find. Being anorexic poses no notable problem in finding veins and they may in fact be quite visible.
   Text Reference: p. 148

3. **Answer: D**
   Rationale: Patients on IV therapy or those receiving chemotherapy intravenously need to save their veins for treatment. Some patients are at risk for serious complications that are associated with deep vein puncture that include arteriospasm and cardiac arrest along with hemorrhage, infection, and anemia. If a patient has only one blood test ordered and it is dermal puncture appropriate, this procedure can be an option. Dermal puncture is not an appropriate method of blood collection for coagulation testing.
   Text Reference: p. 148

4. **Answer: B**
   Rationale: Blood cultures, coagulation tests, and sedimentation rates cannot be performed on blood from dermal punctures. BUN is a chemistry test that can be performed when collected by dermal puncture.
   Text Reference: p. 149

5. **Answer: A**
   Rationale: The levels of many analytes are the same in both venous and capillary blood but not all. Potassium, calcium, and total protein have higher reference values in venous blood than capillary blood. Glucose and hemoglobin are higher in capillary blood versus venous blood.
   Text Reference: p. 149

6. **Answer: B**
   Rationale: The interpretation of the test may be compromised because venous glucose levels are lower than capillary levels. When repeated blood determinations are required, it is important to use the same collection technique each time because test results obtained from two different collection techniques cannot be compared.
   Text Reference: p. 149

7. **Answer: D**
   Rationale: The antiseptic of choice for dermal punctures is 70% isopropyl alcohol. Povidone-iodine is not recommended for

dermal punctures because it interferes with test results for bilirubin, uric acid, phosphorus, and potassium. Bilirubin needs to be protected from light so an amber-colored microcollection tube is appropriate. Warming devices enhance blood flow and the lancet is necessary to make the puncture.
Text Reference: pp. 149, 153

8. **Answer: B**
Rationale: The dimensions of the dermal puncture are controlled by the width and depth of the blade. The device is to be placed firmly over the puncture site without an indentation that would arise from applying pressure.
Text Reference: p. 149

9. **Answer: D**
Rationale: Features of dermal puncture devices include automatic puncture device with a retractable blade, or a laser lancing device and single use. Dermal puncture devices do not have a uniform depth. The depth varies for infants, children, and adults.
Text Reference: p. 149

10. **Answer: B**
Rationale: The term "bullet" is another name for a microcollection tube.
Text Reference: p. 150

11. **Answer: D**
Rationale: A flea or metal filing is used to mix blood that has been collected in a micropipette, such as a Caraway or Natelson pipette.
Text Reference: p. 150

12. **Answer: A**
Rationale: A Unopette is a dilution system collected by dermal puncture using a calibrated capillary pipette in a holder that is designed to draw up a measured amount of blood that can then be dispensed into the diluent of the Unopette reservoir for the correct dilution for the specified test.
Text Reference: p. 150

13. **Answer: B**
Rationale: The temperature of warming devices for dermal punctures should not exceed 42° C.
Text Reference: p. 151

14. **Answer: C**
Rationale: Collection of a Caraway or Natelson micropipette requires the use of plastic caps to seal the sample. A bullet is a microcollection tube, a Unopette is a dilutions system for hematology testing. Glass slides are used when collecting a CBC via dermal puncture.
Text Reference: p. 150

15. **Answer: A**
Rationale: A good dermal site is free of scars, cuts, bruises, etc.; is easily accessible; warm and healthy; and has enough clearance between the underlying bone and the tissue to be punctured. You want good capillary flow near the surface of the skin. You do not want to puncture a vein, especially in a child or infant, because it may cause excessive bleeding during the procedure. In addition, the test results may be interpreted incorrectly as the blood would be venous and not capillary.
Text Reference: p. 151

16. **Answer: A**
Rationale: The calcaneus refers to the heel bone.
Text Reference: p. 151

17. **Answer: A**
Rationale: Puncture of the bone during a dermal puncture could potentially result in an infection of the bone or bone marrow, referred to as osteomyelitis. Osteochondritis is an inflammation of the bone or cartilage; osteitis is inflammation of the bone; and osteoma is a bone tumor.
Text Reference: p. 151

18. **Answer: C**
Rationale: The recommended depth for a preemie is 0.65 to 0.85 mm to minimize the risk of puncturing the calcaneus.
Text Reference: p. 151

19. **Answer: C**
Rationale: The maximum depth of puncture for a heelstick is 2 mm because the calcaneus may lie close to the surface on the foot.
Text Reference: p. 151

20. **Answer: D**
    Rationale: The width of a dermal puncture should not exceed 2.4 mm. This width is adequate in establishing good capillary blood flow for blood collection.
    Text Reference: p. 151

21. **Answer: A**
    Rationale: Width of a puncture is more important in determining blood flow because it severs more capillaries, thereby producing greater blood flow.
    Textbook Reference: p. 151

22. **Answer: D**
    Rationale: Dermal puncture sites in adults and children over the age of 1 year include the middle and ring fingers or the big toe if the fingers cannot be used. The thumb is too calloused and may not produce good blood flow; the index finger has extra nerve endings and is more painful; and the pinky finger does not have enough tissue for a safe puncture.
    Text Reference: p. 152

23. **Answer: C**
    Rationale: The puncture site should be made perpendicular to the whorls or ridges of the fingerprint, which allows for a cleaner drop of blood to form. Cutting parallel with the fingerprint results in blood flow into the grooves, poor drop formation, and a mess.
    Text Reference: p. 152

24. **Answer: C**
    Rationale: Children under the age of 1 do not have enough tissue on their fingers to safely perform a dermal puncture. The heel is the site of choice for this age group.
    Text Reference: p. 152

25. **Answer: A**
    Rationale: Dermal puncture sites on the plantar surface include the medial and lateral borders. In an older infant, if the heel is unacceptable due to bruising and too many puncture wounds from the previous draw, then the big toe may also be used. The arch is too close to tendons and nerves and must not be used.
    Text Reference: p. 152

26. **Answer: B**
    Rationale: The age of the patient will be the determining factor in the type of skin puncture device selected. The depth of the device varies between infants, children, and adults. In addition, laser devices are only approved for those over the age of 5 years. The tests ordered also influence the type of device depending on if it is for glucose monitoring or if you need to collect multiple samples.
    Text Reference: pp. 151, 153

27. **Answer: A**
    Rationale: BURPP stands for bilirubin, uric acid, phosphorus, and potassium. These are all tests that cannot be drawn from a dermal puncture if povidone-iodine is used as the antiseptic.
    Text Reference: p. 114

28. **Answer: C**
    Rationale: The order of draw for a dermal puncture differs from that for a routine venipuncture. EDTA tubes must be drawn first to minimize the effect of platelet aggregation that begins at the puncture site. Other additives come second, with serum samples last. Slides are not needed for an H & H.
    Text Reference: p. 157 and Content Overview (earlier in this chapter)

29. **Answer: D**
    Rationale: Proper dermal puncture technique on an adult includes selecting the middle or ring finger, making the puncture perpendicular to the fingerprints, and wiping away the first drop of blood. Constant milking or massaging the finger cuts off blood low, causes hemolysis, and introduces tissue fluid into the sample.
    Text Reference: pp. 155-156

30. **Answer: B**
    Rationale: The first drop of blood must be wiped away to prevent tissue fluid and or residual antiseptic from contaminating the specimen. Cutting perpendicular to the fingerprints allows for better drop formation. Loose epithelial cells will be removed during the cleansing process and will not affect the sample unless the skin is scraped during collection.
    Text Reference: p. 156

31. **Answer: C**
Rationale: Collecting blood into microcollection tubes requires that the droplet be formed by gentle pressure; the scoop is touched to the drop to allow it to run freely into the tube. Tapping lightly moves the blood to the bottom of the tube as you collect it. Squeezing and scraping result in hemolysis, tissue fluid, and epithelial cell contamination of the specimen.
Text Reference: p. 156

32. **Answer: C**
Rationale: Overfilling anticoagulated tubes can result in microclot formation because of the improper blood to anticoagulant ratios.
Text Reference: Chapter Overview (earlier in this chapter)

33. **Answer: A**
Rationale: Bandages should not be used on children under the age of 2 years because they could remove the bandage and choke on it.
Text Reference: p. 158

34. **Answer: A**
Rationale: A hematocrit should be filled by lightly touching the drop of blood with the hematocrit tube held horizontally to prevent air bubble formation and allowing the tube to fill by capillary action in one smooth action. Forming a large drop of blood allows the tube to fill completely with one drop.
Text Reference: p. 156

35. **Answer: B**
Rationale: The bleeding time is a test used to assess the overall integrity of primary hemostasis because it involves platelets and the vascular system. Prothrombin time and thrombin time are used to assess secondary hemostasis. Platelets are only one component of assessing primary hemostasis as injury to the tissue activates a series of responses that result in balanced vasoconstriction and vasodilation, production and processing of VWF, etc.
Text Reference: p. 159

36. **Answer: B**
Rationale: The normal reference range for a bleeding time is 2 to 10 minutes.
Text Reference: p. 159

37. **Answer: D**
Rationale: Abnormal results may be due to platelet or vascular disorders, skin conditions, or medications that interfere with clotting, such as aspirin, streptokinase, or ethanol. The bleeding time test is an assessment of primary hemostasis and platelet function.
Text Reference: p. 159

38. **Answer: D**
Rationale: Making the incisions for the bleeding time 5 cm below and parallel to the antecubital crease produces more accurate results.
Text Reference: p. 161

39. **Answer: B**
Rationale: The blood pressure cuff is inflated to a pressure of 40 mm Hg and maintained throughout the duration of the bleeding time test.
Text Reference: p. 161

40. **Answer: D**
Rationale: The trigger of the cutting device should be depressed simultaneously with the start of the timer in the bleeding time procedure. Starting the timer after depression of the cutting device produces falsely elevated times.
Text Reference: p. 162

41. **Answer: C**
Rationale: If two incisions are made, then wicking of each incision must be done independently of the other. The clotting time for both incisions must be within several minutes of each other otherwise the test must be repeated on the other arm.
Text Reference: pp. 159, 162

42. **Answer: B**
Rationale: Ancillary blood glucose test instruments are calibrated on a regularly scheduled basis using calibrators supplied by the manufacturer. Control solutions are run using the same procedure as patient samples on a daily basis per institutional protocol. If calibration results and control results are incorrect, then troubleshooting is required to identify and correct the problem before the instrument can be used.
Text Reference: p. 159

VENIPUNCTURE COMPLICATIONS

Tina Lewis

INTRODUCTION

Although most venipuncture collections are routine and are completed without problems, complications can arise. Many factors can interfere with the collection of blood, but most complications can be dealt with by knowing what to expect and planning ahead. Complications include problems with access to the patient, site selection, site cleaning, tourniquet application, sample collection, completion of the procedure, and sample integrity. In addition, patients may experience long-term health-related complications from venipuncture. Specimens may be rejected for a variety of reasons and thus require a redraw. By learning the most common complications and the best approaches for preventing or overcoming them, you will be better prepared in your work as a phlebotomist.

CONTENT OVERVIEW

Factors That Prevent Access to the Patient
I. Location of patient
    A. STAT, timed tests must be drawn—locate patient and proceed to area to draw blood
    B. If rescheduling required—tell nurse
II. Identification of patient
    A. Requisition must match identification band
    B. Discrepancies resolved before drawing blood
    C. Arm band must be on patient—nurse affixes
    D. Blood bank specimens—special identification armbands and labels
    E. Special situations—follow hospital protocol for identification
       1. Emergency requisitions
       2. ER collections
       3. Phoned orders
       4. Requisitions picked up at site

Barriers to Communicating with Patients
I. Sleeping or unconscious patients
    A. Gently wake sleeping patient
    B. Talk to unconscious patient as if awake

II. Presence of physician or clergy
    A. Return later if test not STAT or timed
    B. STAT or timed tests—respectfully interrupt
III. Visitors present
    A. Greet same as patient
    B. Explain your presence
    C. Request visitors to step out
IV. Apprehensive patient
    A. Engage in distracting conversation
    B. Request assistance by nurse or other phlebotomist if necessary
V. Language problems
    A. Difficulty getting informed consent
    B. Request translator
    C. Demonstrate what you need to do and possibly get informed consent
VI. Patient refusal
    A. Patient retains the right to refuse any treatment or test
    B. Explain tests needed for treatment
    C. If still refuses, document refusal on form and in computer
    D. Inform health care provider (i.e. physician, nurse, etc.)

Problems in Site Selection—Avoid the Following Sites
I. Occluded veins (sclerosed veins)
    A. Hard, cordlike
    B. Due to chemotherapy, disease, inflammation, repeated venipuncture
    C. Susceptible to infection due to impediment of blood flow
    D. Blood from these sites—erroneous results
II. Hematomas
    A. Causes
       1. Needle going through vein
       2. Partial entry of bevel into vein
       3. Failure to apply pressure after draw
    B. Do not draw blood from hematoma
       1. Blood not fresh
       2. Blood flow into vein constricted
       3. Erroneous test results
    C. Draw below the hematoma
III. Edematous tissue
    A. Tissue swollen
    B. Accumulation of tissue fluid
    C. Erroneous test results

IV. Burns and scars
   A. Susceptible to infection
   B. Painful
   C. Difficult to penetrate
V. Mastectomies
   A. Lymphostasis on side of mastectomy due to removal of lymph nodes
   B. Alter test results
   C. Painful to patient
   D. Increased risk of infection
VI. Disruption of skin integrity
   A. Skin rashes
   B. Lesions
   C. New tattoos
   D. Unhealed incisions
VII. Difficulty finding a vein
   A. Check the other arm
   B. Enhance vein prominence
      1. Massage site upward from wrist
      2. Dangle arm downward
      3. Apply heat
      4. Rotate wrist
      5. Tap site with index and middle fingers
   C. Use blood pressure cuff—requires special training
      1. Pressure below systolic but above diastolic: range of 60 to 80 mm Hg
      2. Requires taking patient's blood pressure first
   D. Use alternative sites
      1. Hand—decrease needle gauge; use smaller tube, syringe, or butterfly
      2. Foot—usually requires physician permission
      3. Leg—usually requires physician permission

Problems Associated with Cleaning the Site
I. Alcohol *cannot* be used in collection of blood alcohol
   A. Use soap/water or other nonalcoholic antiseptic solution
II. Alcohol is not recommended by itself as antiseptic for blood cultures
III. Povidone-iodine is not used for dermal punctures because it can cause an increase in bilirubin, uric acid, phosphorus, and potassium
IV. Allergies to iodine require the use of alternatives, such as chlorhexidine gluconate
V. Chlorhexidine gluconate cannot be used in children under the age of 2 months

Problems with Tourniquet Application
I. Hemoconcentration
   A. Tourniquet application should *not* exceed 1 minute
      1. Plasma filters into tissues
      2. Results in increased proportion of cells in vein
      3. Affects large molecules—plasma proteins, enzymes, lipids
      4. Increases cell counts, iron, calcium levels
      5. Alters potassium and lactic acid levels via another mechanism
   B. Patient should *not* pump fist
   C. Other causes—occluded veins, prolonged IV therapy, dehydration
II. Formation of petechiae
   A. Small, nonraised red spots
   B. Appear on tourniquet application
   C. Indicates capillary wall or platelet disorder
   D. Site may bleed excessively after venipuncture
      1. Apply pressure until bleeding stops per routine venipuncture procedure
III. Tourniquet tied too tightly
   A. Numbness of arm
   B. Pinching of skin
IV. Latex allergy
   A. Ask *all* patients if they have a latex allergy
   B. Use nonlatex gloves and tourniquet

Complications During Collection
I. Change in patient status
   A. Syncope (fainting)
      1. Skin cold, damp, clammy
      2. Immediately remove tourniquet and needle, apply pressure
      3. Have patient lower head, cool cloth to forehead, emesis basin as needed
      4. Document incident
   B. Seizures
      1. Immediately stop procedure
      2. Do *not* put anything in patient's mouth
   C. Nausea and vomiting (emesis)
      1. Reassure patient
      2. Give emesis basin
      3. Instruct patient to breathe slowly and deeply
      4. Cool cloth to forehead
II. Hematoma—see above
   A. Remove tourniquet and needle immediately
   B. Apply pressure, cold pack to reduce swelling and pain

III. Lack of blood flow
   A. Defective evacuated tubes—vacuum depleted
      1. Always have extra tubes within reach
   B. Improperly positioned needle
      1. Bevel is stuck to the vein wall—rotate needle
      2. Needle is passed through both sides of the vein—slowly pull back on the needle
      3. Needle not advanced far enough into vein—slowly advance needle
      4. Tube too large for vein, causing the excessive vacuum to pull vein onto bevel and block blood flow—use smaller tube
IV. Collapsed vein
   A. Result of too much vacuum on small vein from tube—use smaller tubes
   B. Result of pulling back too quickly on syringe plunger—pull back slowly
   C. Immediately remove tourniquet and needle—select another vein
V. Inadvertent puncture of the artery
   A. Blood may be bright red
   B. Spurts or pulses into tube
      1. Apply pressure to the site for 5 minutes or until bleeding stops after draw complete
   C. Label specimen as an arterial sample and deliver to lab
VI. Needle unscrews from barrel during collection—withdraw immediately
VII. Failure to collect on first attempt—ask patient's permission to redraw; limit two tries
   A. Use new needle and tubes
   B. Go below previous stick or choose new vein, arm
   C. Two misses requires a different phlebotomist to perform puncture

Problems in Completing the Procedure
I. Patient requests
   A. Request for water—ask nurse—patient may be on fluid restrictions
   B. Request for change in bed position—ask nurse
II. Prolonged bleeding
   A. Bleeding usually stops within 5 minutes
   B. Aspirin or anticoagulant therapy prolongs bleeding
   C. Apply pressure until bleeding stops to prevent compartment syndrome
   D. Inform nurse of excessive times

Factors That Affect Sample Integrity
I. Hemolysis
   A. Destruction of RBCs
   B. Release of hemoglobin and cellular contents into plasma
   C. Causes
      1. Too small needle for vein size
      2. Using needle ≥ 23 gauge
      3. Small needle, large vacuum tube
      4. Small needle for transferring blood from syringe into tube
      5. Vigorous mixing or shaking of tube
      6. Frothing of blood into syringe
      7. Pulling back too quickly on syringe plunger
      8. Blood entering tube from syringe incorrectly—not running down side of tube
      9. Forcing blood from syringe into tube
   D. Interferes with test results—increased results (see Box 11-2 on p. 178 in textbook)
      1. Potassium
      2. Lactate dehydrogenase (LD/LDH)
      3. Aspartate aminotransferase
II. Blood drawn from hematoma—affects test results due to old blood: see previous discussion
III. Short draw resulting in incorrect anticoagulant to blood ratio, QNS, etc.
IV. Patient position
   A. Upright position results in fluid shift into tissues; increases some analytes by 5% to 8%
      1. Protein
      2. H & H
      3. Enzymes
      4. Calcium
      5. Iron
      6. Hormones
   B. Have patient sit for 15 to 30 minutes before the draw
V. Reflux of anticoagulant
   A. Flow of blood from tube into needle and patient's vein
   B. Tube contents come into contact with stopper during blood collection
   C. Can result in transfer of anticoagulant into patient resulting in cascade of issues
      1. Adverse reactions to anticoagulant
      2. Loss of additive can alter results
      3. Contamination of next tube

D. Prevention
  1. Keep tube angled downward below site
  2. Fill tube from bottom up
  3. Remove last tube before removing tourniquet or needle

Long-Term Complications Associated with Venipuncture
  I. Anemia
    A. Blood loss of 4 to 7 mL/day can result in anemia
    B. Use small volume tubes
  II. Hematoma—see previous discussions
  III. Compartment syndrome
    A. Large volume of blood leaks into tissues
    B. Swelling, pain, burning, numbness
    C. Risk permanent nerve damage
  IV. Nerve damage
    A. Contact with needle during venipuncture
    B. Do not probe excessively
    C. Avoid using basilic vein
  V. Infection
    A. Use proper aseptic technique
    B. Keep bandage on 15 minutes

Specimen Rejection
  I. No requisition
  II. Unlabeled or mislabeled specimens
  III. Incompletely filled tubes
  IV. Defective tubes
  V. Collection in wrong tube
  VI. Short draw
  VII. Hemolysis
  VIII. Clotted blood in anticoagulant specimen
  IX. Contaminated specimens
  X. Improper special collection and/or handling (i.e., patient not fasting, exposure of specimen to light, etc.)

Specimen Recollection
  I. Site not properly cleaned (i.e., blood culture)
  II. Use of the wrong antiseptic (i.e., alcohol used for blood alcohol collection)
  III. Incomplete drying of antiseptic resulting in hemolysis and contamination of specimen
  IV. Powder from gloves
  V. Microscopic clots in an anticoagulated specimen
  VI. Contaminated specimens and containers (i.e., blood on outside of tube)
  VII. Improper special handling (i.e., not on slushy ice solution, exposure to light)

CERTIFICATION PREPARATION QUESTIONS

1. When entering a patient's hospital room to collect a sample it is found that the patient does not have on an ID band. You notify the nursing station and are told that the person is the correct patient. What is the proper means for identifying the patient at this point?
   a. Ask the patient for their name to confirm
   b. Ask a family member to confirm patient's ID
   c. Ask a nurse to attach a new ID band to the patient
   d. Look around the room to see if the ID band can be located

2. The patient is sleeping when you enter to draw a timed blood specimen. How should you proceed?
   a. Proceed with the collection quietly so the patient is not disturbed
   b. Gently wake the patient before proceeding with the collection
   c. Ask the nurse to page you when the patient is awake
   d. Turn the lights on; make a lot of noise, while calling out the patient's name

3. The phlebotomist arrives at the patient's room to find a clergyman visiting. In what instance would it be appropriate to interrupt a patient when in the presence of clergy or physician?
   a. Routine sample collection
   b. STAT sample collection
   c. Timed sample collection
   d. Both b and c

4. A phlebotomist returns later in the day to draw a timed blood collection from a patient who had consented to have blood drawn in the morning but has now refused. All of the following must be done when a patient refuses a blood draw, *except*:
   a. Explain that the procedure is necessary for treatment
   b. Document the patient's refusal on the request
   c. Notify the health care provider of the refusal
   d. Use the blood from the morning draw

5. A phlebotomist must draw blood from an unconscious patient. Which of the following is the correct approach once identification has been confirmed?
   a. Begin the procedure without disturbing the patient
   b. Communicate to the patient each step of the process
   c. Get a nurse to document consent and witness the procedure
   d. Wait until a family member arrives to give consent

6. You arrive at the patient's room for a timed draw only to find the patient is missing. The nurse states that the patient is having a radiographic procedure done and will not return for at least 2 more hours. How would you proceed?
   a. Return to the lab, document the patient's location, and cancel the order
   b. Put the lab request back in the stack for the next batch of timed tests
   c. Document the delay and reschedule the draw as soon as the patient returns
   d. Tell radiology to stop by the lab before returning the patient to his/her room

7. A patient who requires a blood alcohol level has a wrist band confirming an allergy to iodine. What is the proper cleansing agent to use?
   a. Alcohol
   b. Betadine
   c. Chlorhexidine gluconate
   d. B and C

8. The medical term for "fainting" is
   _____.
   a. Emesis
   b. Syncope
   c. Petechiae
   d. Fatigue

9. Due to the increased risk in latex allergies, the phlebotomist must do which of the following routinely as a part of venipuncture collection?
   a. Ask all patients whether they have a latex allergy
   b. Use a vinyl tourniquet on all patients
   c. Use vinyl gloves on all patients
   d. None of the above

10. When the phlebotomist is encountering difficulty locating a vein for specimen procurement, all of the following techniques should be used, *except*?
    a. Check the other arm or alternate locations
    b. Massages the arm in the downward position
    c. Apply heat to the site for 3 to 5 minutes
    d. Have the patient open and close their hand

11. The term lymphostasis is defined as:
    a. The lack of lymph nodes
    b. The lack of lymph fluid movement
    c. Increased lymphocyte count
    d. Decreased lymphocyte count

12. The medical term for nausea and vomiting is
    _____.
    a. Syncope
    b. Vertigo
    c. Emesis
    d. Petechiae

13. When inserting the needle into a hand vein using a winged infusion set, the correct angle of entry is _____.
    a. 10 to15 degrees
    b. 20 to 25 degrees
    c. 30 to 35 degrees
    d. 45 degrees

14. Which of the following could not cause lack of blood flow when attempting to draw blood?
    a. Defective evacuated tubes
    b. Improper needle position
    c. Anticoagulant therapy
    d. Missing the vein

15. A phlebotomist must redraw a patient that was reported to be a difficult draw due to veins that collapse during venipuncture. Which of the following techniques could the phlebotomist use to minimize the likelihood of collapsing a vein?
    a. Threading the needle up into the vein
    b. Probing to find the vein in the antecubital fossa
    c. Increasing the angle of entry when performing the puncture
    d. Pulling back on the needle after insertion and repositioning

16. You must redraw a patient for a potassium level because the first specimen was hemolyzed. Knowing that the patient is a difficult draw, which of the following would you do to prevent hemolysis of the sample?
    a. Use a 22-gauge needle with a 7-mL tube
    b. Draw blood into a syringe while quickly pulling on the plunger
    c. Force the blood from a syringe into a vacuum tube
    d. Use a winged infusion needle for a routine venipuncture

17. Which of the following tests would not be affected by hemolysis?
    a. Potassium
    b. LD/LDH
    c. Cholesterol
    d. AST

18. Application of a tourniquet too tightly can cause which of the following?
    a. Decreased arterial blood flow
    b. Numbing of the arm
    c. Nerve damage
    d. All of the above

19. Which of the following tests are not affected by patient position?
    a. Protein
    b. Potassium
    c. Enzymes
    d. Cell counts

20. Reflux or the flow of blood from the collection tube back into the needle and into the patient's vein can be prevented by all of the following, *except*:
    a. Keeping the patient's arm in a downward position
    b. Filling tubes from the bottom upward
    c. Preventing contact of the needle with blood in the tube
    d. Removing the tourniquet after the tube is removed

21. Which of the following would be a reason for specimen rejection?
    a. Tube labeled using a black marker pen
    b. Improper specimen handling after collection
    c. Specimen delivered via pneumatic tube system
    d. Tube is wrapped in aluminum foil

22. When the blood oozes from the vein into the surrounding tissue a(n) _____ is formed.
    a. Hematoma
    b. Edema
    c. Occlusion
    d. Infection

23. Proper identification of patients is critical in expediting patient care. Which of the following could impede patient identification?
    a. Emergency requisitions
    b. Telephone orders
    c. Collection during trauma situations
    d. All of the above

24. Which of the following departments requires special identification bands for patients?
    a. Hematology
    b. Blood bank
    c. Chemistry
    d. Microbiology

25. Bright red blood is spurting into the tube causing you to suspect that you may have punctured an artery during your venous draw. How should you proceed?
    a. Immediately stop the procedure and apply pressure
    b. Redraw the specimen from a vein
    c. Complete the draw and label the specimen *arterial*
    d. Both a and b

26. Small, nonraised red spots that appear on the skin when the tourniquet is applied are known as _____.
    a. Petechiae
    b. Hematoma
    c. Edema
    d. Scleroderma

27. Your patient begins to have a seizure during a blood draw. Which of the following techniques should be avoided in a patient who has a seizure during blood collection?
    a. Remove tourniquet
    b. Remove needle
    c. Place something in the patient's mouth
    d. Apply pressure to the site

28. Povidone-iodine is not recommended for cleansing the site for dermal puncture when collecting which of the following tests?
    a. Blood cultures
    b. Alcohol
    c. Bilirubin
    d. Calcium

29. Which of the following medication therapies can cause potential for prolonged bleeding?
    a. Aspirin therapy
    b. Heparin therapy
    c. Coumadin therapy
    d. All of the above

30. All of the following may result in the formation of a hematoma during a blood collection procedure, *except*:
    a. Excessive probing
    b. Failure to remove the tourniquet before removing the needle
    c. Application of pressure to the site with the arm out straight
    d. Needle passing through both sides of the vein

31. To avoid the potential for infection after blood collection, a bandage should be placed over the site of puncture for at least _____.
    a. 15 minutes
    b. 10 minutes
    c. 5 minutes
    d. Until the bleeding has ceased

32. A condition in which pressure within the tissue prevents blood from flowing freely in the blood vessels is known as _____.
    a. Falconi syndrome
    b. Contraction syndrome
    c. Compartment syndrome
    d. Fall syndrome

33. Why would a phlebotomist want to avoid using the basilic vein whenever possible?
    a. Using this site may increase risk of infection
    b. There is increased risk of damaging a nerve or hitting the brachial artery
    c. Specimens drawn from this vein are often hemolyzed
    d. Only a small gauge needle can be used to access this vein

34. A phlebotomist is having difficulty drawing blood on a patient. How many attempts may the phlebotomist make at blood collection at one time on this patient?
    a. Four
    b. Three
    c. Two
    d. One

35. A phlebotomist is unable to collect blood on the first attempt. How should they proceed?
    a. Contact the nurse and have the test cancelled
    b. Use a new needle, tube, and site location and make a second attempt
    c. Call another phlebotomist in to attempt collection
    d. Attempt collection again using the same needle, tube, and site location

36. Which of the following may be used in conjunction with a winged infusion set to collect blood?
    a. Vacutainer tube
    b. Syringe
    c. Blood culture bottle
    d. All of the above

37. Which of the following is *not* a reason to avoid drawing through scars or burns?
    a. Scars and burns usually overlay arteries
    b. Scars and burns are susceptible to infection
    c. Scarred or burned areas may be painful
    d. Scarred or burned areas may be difficult to palpate and stick

38. During venipuncture site selection, which of the following would *not* preclude selection of a particular site?
    a. Slight edema of an arm
    b. New sleeve tattoo on entire arm
    c. Veins feel cordlike and hard
    d. Appearance of petechiae on tourniquet application

39. The phlebotomist must discontinue the blood collection if any of the following occurs, *except*:
    a. Hematoma
    b. Needle unscrews from the Vacutainer holder
    c. Blood appears to be arterial blood
    d. Patient becomes weak and nauseous

40. Phlebotomists can experience communication problems with patients who are hearing impaired or who do not speak English. Why must a phlebotomist ensure a patient can thoroughly understand their intentions and instructions?
    a. If a patient cannot understand the phlebotomist, they cannot give informed consent
    b. It may cause problems with casual conversation
    c. Patients must understand in order to assist the phlebotomist with blood collection
    d. None of the above

41. Which of the following would *not* be a potential cause for development of an occluded or sclerosed vein?
    a. Inflammation
    b. Chemotherapy
    c. Palpation
    d. Repeated venipuncture

42. Permission from a physician is required to draw blood from an arm on the same side as a mastectomy because:
    a. Risk of infection is higher
    b. Lymphostasis may adversely affect test results
    c. Injury can result from tourniquet application
    d. All of the above

43. A patient who has been in the hospital for several weeks has developed hematomas and oozing puncture sites over the antecubital area on the only arm available for performing venipunctures. The best site for venipuncture is now:
    a. Above the hematomas and oozing puncture sites
    b. Off to the side of hematomas and oozing puncture sites
    c. To go through the hematomas and oozing puncture sites
    d. Distal to the hematomas and oozing puncture sites

ANSWERS AND RATIONALES

1. **Answer: C**
   Rationale: A phlebotomist must have an identification band attached to the patient to properly identify the patient before sample collection.
   Text Reference: pp. 168-169

2. **Answer: B**
   Rationale: A phlebotomist should always gently wake a sleeping patient so that they are not startled out of a deep sleep to explain what needs to be done and gain the consent of the patient to do the procedure.
   Text Reference: p. 169

3. **Answer: D**
   Rationale: Timed and STAT samples should not be delayed for physicians or clergy. Routine samples should be collected at a later time after the physician or clergy member leaves the patient's room.
   Text Reference: p. 169

4. **Answer: D**
   Rationale: All of the items listed should be carried out in the order listed if a patient refuses to have blood drawn. Blood from the morning draw is not appropriate because the physician wants to know the status of the patient at the specified time of day. Certain blood analytes fluctuate at different times of the day (i.e., diurnal variation, diet, medication, etc.) and require collection and analysis at specified times.
   Text Reference: p. 169

5. **Answer: B**
   Rationale: If the patient is unconscious, the phlebotomist should proceed as if the patient was awake. Communicate all intentions, actions, and instructions just as if the patient was able to respond. Unconscious patients may still be able to hear.
   Text Reference: p. 169

6. **Answer: C**
   Rationale: Any delay in collection of timed specimens must be accounted for by documenting according to laboratory/hospital protocol. Some procedures cannot be interrupted for a blood draw, such as radiographic procedures, while others do not pose a problem, such as physical therapy. In this case, as soon as the patient returns, the nurse should notify the lab for collection

of the specimen. Notation of the original collection time along with actual time drawn should be appropriately recorded according to lab protocol.
Text Reference: p. 168

7. **Answer: C**
Rationale: Alcohol can never be used as an antiseptic agent when collecting blood alcohol samples. Betadine contains iodine and could not be used in this instance. The sample should be collected using chlorhexidine gluconate.
Text Reference: p. 171

8. **Answer: B**
Rationale: The term syncope is the medical term for fainting.
Text Reference: p. 171

9. **Answer: A**
Rationale: Although the use of vinyl gloves and tourniquets is occurring more commonly in health care settings, they are more costly. Therefore, it is more cost-efficient for the phlebotomist to ask all patients about latex allergies and use vinyl products only when necessary if the facility still employs the use of latex gloves and tourniquets.
Text Reference: p. 171

10. **Answer: D**
Rationale: Any of the techniques listed can be used to increase the chance of a successful site location except for fist clenching, which can result in hemoconcentration.
Text Reference: p. 170

11. **Answer: B**
Rationale: Lymphostasis or lack of fluid movement resulting in edema is found in patients who have had removal of lymph tissue on the side of a mastectomy. As a result, test results may be affected and the risk of infection is increased if venipuncture is performed on that arm.
Text Reference: p. 170

12. **Answer: C**
Rationale: The medical term for nausea and vomiting is emesis.
Text Reference: p. 171

13. **Answer: A**
Rationale: Inserting a winged infusion into a hand vein at an angle of greater than 10 to 15 degrees could cause the needle to pass through the vessel entirely. Also, due to the lack of fatty tissue in the hand and the fact that the veins lay near the skin surface, there would be potential for hitting some other anatomic structure other than a vein.
Text Reference: p. 173

14. **Answer: C**
Rationale: Anticoagulant therapy typically thins the patient's blood and causes blood to flow more easily. This therapy will not impede blood flow; however, it could cause the patient to bleed around the puncture site more freely.
Text Reference: pp. 176-177

15. **Answer: A**
Rationale: Threading the needle up the vein minimizes collapsed veins and the likelihood of blowing the vein. Probing, increased angle entry, and pulling back on the needle and repositioning could increase the risk of collapsing the vein.
Text Reference: p. 177

16. **Answer: D**
Rationale: Using a winged infusion set for routine venipuncture would not cause hemolysis in and of itself. Hemolysis could occur using a winged infusion needle if there were other complicating factors such as those listed in options a-c.
Text Reference: p. 177

17. **Answer: C**
Rationale: Hemolysis is caused by the destruction of red blood cells, resulting in the release of hemoglobin and cellular components into the plasma. Cholesterol is a lipid found in the plasma and is not affected by the destruction of red blood cells. All of the other tests listed are severely affected by hemolysis.
Text Reference: pp. 177-178

18. **Answer: D**
Rationale: Application of the tourniquet too tightly can cause the arterial blood flow to the area below the tourniquet to

be decreased or even cut off. Numbing of the arm and nerve damage can be caused by the tourniquet being tied too tightly or leaving a tourniquet applied for too long of a time period.
Text Reference: p. 171

19. **Answer: B**
Rationale: Potassium is the only test listed above that is not affected in some manner by patient position. For tests that may be significantly affected by patient position the physician may request that the patient lie down before sample collection. Being in an upright position may result in a shift of extracellular fluid volume into the tissues. As a result, protein and protein-bound substances move into the vascular space, resulting in a 5% to 8% increase in hemoglobin, hematocrit, calcium, iron, enzymes, hormones, etc. It may take 15 minutes for redistribution and stabilization of extracellular fluid volumes and electrolytes in the vascular space when a patient moves from standing to sitting positions.
Text Reference: p. 178

20. **Answer: D**
Rationale: The medical term associated with the flow of blood back into the collection needle and then into the patient's vein is reflux. Reflux can only occur if there is contact between blood in the tube and the needle. Prevention of reflux can be achieved by making sure the arm is at a slight downward slant so that the tubes fill from the bottom up.
Text Reference: p. 178

21. **Answer: B**
Rationale: Improper specimen handling such as transporting a tube at an incorrect temperature, for example, is grounds for specimen rejection. Pneumatic tube systems are used frequently in larger facilities for transportation of specimens. All tubes should be labeled by the phlebotomist in some appropriate manner. The permanent laboratory marker is acceptable provided that all the appropriate labeling information is recorded on the tube. Specimens that need protection from light may be wrapped in aluminum foil.
Text Reference: p. 179

22. **Answer: A**
Rationale: Edema is the swelling of tissues due to fluid. An occlusion occurs when the vein is blocked for some reason and blood is unable to flow. An infection may occur anytime proper disinfecting techniques are not used. A hematoma is the result of leakage of blood from the vein into the surrounding tissues.
Text Reference: pp. 170, 177-178

23. **Answer: D**
Rationale: Emergency requisitions are often filled out quickly and not checked for accuracy. Telephone orders to the lab still require a permanent written requisition and increase the risk for identification problems. Trauma situations require immediate care and often non–lifesaving measures such as ID band identification may be delayed because of emergency medical procedures. Follow your facility's policy for patient identification in emergency situations. Regardless of any situation, the patient identification and the requisition must match identically to proceed with sample collection.
Text Reference: pp. 168-169

24. **Answer: B**
Rationale: The American Association of Blood Banks requires special identification for patients receiving blood transfusions. Those identification bands are attached to the patient when the specimen for testing is collected.
Text Reference: p. 169

25. **Answer: C**
Rationale: A specimen accidentally drawn from an artery can still be submitted to the lab for testing. The specimen must be labeled as *arterial* because there are differences between arterial and venous blood for some tests. The phlebotomist, *not* the patient, *must* apply pressure over the puncture site for 5 minutes or until bleeding stops.
Text Reference: p. 177

26. **Answer: A**
Rationale: Petechiae are small red raised spots. These spots appear when the patient has a capillary wall or platelet disorder. The appearance of petechiae also indicates that

the patient may bleed excessively after the collection procedure.
Text Reference: p. 171

27. **Answer: C**
Rationale: If a patient has a seizure during a collection procedure, the procedure should be stopped immediately. Removal of the tourniquet and needle, and application of pressure to the site are required. Never place anything in the patient's mouth because this may cause injury.
Text Reference: p. 171

28. **Answer: C**
Rationale: CLSI does not recommend the use of povidone-iodine for dermal punctures; however it is not prohibited in all circumstances. Povidone-iodine is not recommended in dermal punctures because it may elevate test results for bilirubin, uric acid, phosphorus, and potassium.
Text Reference: p. 171

29. **Answer: D**
Rationale: All of the medications listed above are used as anticoagulants in many patients and may result in prolonged bleeding after blood collection.
Text Reference: p. 177

30. **Answer: C**
Rationale: The proper procedure for ceasing blood flow after a venipuncture is to apply pressure to the site with the arm extended straight out. Each of the other situational issues listed could cause potential hematoma formation.
Text Reference: pp. 170, 176-178

31. **Answer: A**
Rationale: Not bandaging a puncture site may result in the introduction of bacteria directly into nonintact skin. Leaving the bandage on for too long may cause irritation to the skin surrounding the site if the patient has allergic reactions to adhesives of any type. The appropriate time for application of a bandage is 15 minutes.
Text Reference: p. 179

32. **Answer: C**
Rationale: Patients on large doses of Coumadin or those with bleeding problems (i.e., hemophilia) may experience bleeding

into the tissues. Small amounts result in formation of a hematoma, larger volumes lead to compartment syndrome. Compartment syndrome is the condition in which pressure within the tissues prevents blood flowing freely in the blood vessels. This may cause swelling and pain, and can cause permanent damage to the nerves and other tissues.
Text Reference: p. 179

33. **Answer: B**
Rationale: Nerves in the antecubital area can be damaged by excessive or blind probing. Since the basilic vein is more difficult to access, it is recommended that the phlebotomist avoid this vein whenever possible.
Text Reference: p. 179

34. **Answer: C**
Rationale: At most institutions, only two attempts at blood collection are permitted.
Text Reference: p. 177

35. **Answer: B**
Rationale: Most institutions allow the phlebotomist to make two attempts at collection at any one time. The phlebotomist must use a new needle, tube, and site location when attempting the second time.
Text Reference: p. 177

36. **Answer: D**
Rationale: Any of the devices can be attached to a winged infusion set to perform blood collection.
Text Reference: p. 174

37. **Answer: A**
Rationale: Dependent on the location of the scar or burn it may overlay an artery; however, this is not a reason to avoid any site location since arteries are present in many locations that are acceptable for blood collection.
Text Reference: p. 170

38. **Answer: D**
Rationale: Any site that exhibits edema, hematomas, sclerosed or cordlike veins, and new tattoos should not be used as a site for venipuncture. Petechiae may appear as small, round, flat red spots, indicating intradermal hemorrhage that can result for a number of reasons ranging from medication,

impaired blood coagulation, or trauma. They would appear on tourniquet application at any site but do not interfere with specimen collection or specimen integrity.
Text Reference: pp. 169-171

39. **Answer: C**
Rationale: The development of a hematoma indicates that the needle has punctured through the venous wall or come out of the vein, causing blood to flow into the tissue. Possible nerve compression or compartmental syndrome may result depending on the extent of tissue infiltration. If a needle becomes disengaged from the needle holder, the draw must be stopped because the phlebotomist no longer has control of the needle and injury could occur. Weakness and nausea may be signs of syncope and the draw should be discontinued. Accidental puncture of an artery can still proceed. The phlebotomist must label the specimen as *arterial* and apply pressure on the site for a minimum of 5 minutes until bleeding stops.
Text Reference: pp. 171, 176-177

40. **Answer: A**
Rationale: Patients must give informed consent for the phlebotomist to perform any collection procedure. If the patient is unable to understand the phlebotomist, the phlebotomist must not perform the procedure until such time as the patient does understand. The phlebotomist must make sure the patient hears and understands what is being communicated. The phlebotomist may also need the assistance of a translator.
Text Reference: p. 169

41. **Answer: C**
Rationale: Occluded or sclerosed veins may occur for various reasons. However, palpitation of the vein should not cause these conditions. In addition to the other conditions listed, inflammation and disease may also cause sclerosed or occluded veins. Veins of this nature are susceptible to infection and since blood flow is impaired to these areas, samples from these areas could produce erroneous results.
Text Reference: p. 169

42. **Answer: D**
Rationale: Due to the lymphostasis, the risk of injury from tourniquet application, and the risk of infection in the arm, a physician must be granted permission for venipuncture from an arm on the same side that a mastectomy has been performed.
Text Reference: p. 170

43. **Answer: D**
Rationale: Blood flow would be least affected by a hematoma or oozing puncture sites distal to those areas. Sticking in, above, or beside a hematoma or an oozing puncture site is not only painful to the patient but can compromise the integrity of the specimen. Blood from the hematoma is not fresh venous blood and may be hemolyzed and possibly occlude blood flow to the vein, thereby yielding erroneous results. Tissue fluid from oozing puncture sites can also compromise specimen integrity.
Text Reference: pp. 170, 176-178

BLOOD COLLECTION IN SPECIAL POPULATIONS

Tina Lewis

INTRODUCTION

Four special populations—pediatric patients, geriatric patients, patients requiring chronic blood draws, and patients in the emergency room or intensive care unit—have special needs and require special knowledge and procedures to collect blood safely and considerately. In young children, loss of blood volume and the child's fear of the procedure are paramount concerns; in geriatric patients, skin changes and the possible presence of hearing loss or mental impairment are important considerations. Patients with certain diseases require regular blood tests for an extended or indefinite period, and the sites commonly used for drawing blood may become damaged from overuse. Patients in the emergency room or intensive care unit have vascular access devices or intravenous lines in place. Only specially trained personnel can draw blood from these devices on a physician's order, but the phlebotomists may be called to assist in the draw or handle the samples during and after collection. Each of these special populations requires approaches and equipment beyond those needed for routine blood collection. By understanding these special requirements, you will gain the skills you need to collect blood from the widest possible patient population.

CONTENT OVERVIEW

Pediatric Patient

I. Special physiologic considerations
   A. Lower blood volume in children requires small volume draws
   B. Dermal puncture is the recommended collection procedure, if possible
   C. Newborns have increased RBC count and lower plasma volume and may need larger volumes of blood drawn for adequate serum/plasma levels for testing
   D. Newborns and children are more susceptible to infection
   E. Anemia may result from repeated draws
   F. Record time and volume of blood drawn
   G. Anxiety and prolonged crying may elevate WBC, result in left shift, and increase pH values

II. Special psychological considerations
   A. Children have different levels of understanding, ability to cooperate, and anxiety
      1. Prepare your materials/supplies so the child does not see them
      2. Perform procedure in a room other than the child's hospital room
      3. Use a soothing tone and be friendly
      4. Explain the procedure in terms a child can understand
      5. Do not say "It will not hurt"; say "will hurt a little"
      6. Give the child choices, if possible—can say "ouch," cry, or yell, but hold arm still
      7. Use shortest and smallest needle gauge and hide needle as long as possible and distract child while inserting needle
      8. Talk to child during procedure to let them know how much longer it will take to complete
      9. Praise or reward the child

III. Involvement of parents and siblings
   A. Assess the situation to determine if parents or siblings will help or hinder the procedure completion
   B. Ask parents, siblings to step out of room if necessary

IV. Identification of newborns
   A. Use hospital ID number
   B. Do not use patient's name

V. Supplies
   A. Be prepared
   B. Use age-appropriate collection devices (e.g., small-gauge needles, butterfly needles, pediatric tubes)

VI. Anesthetics
   A. Topical anesthetics (EMLA) may be used
   B. Not recommended for phenylketonuria (PKU) testing

VII. Immobilization of infants and children
   A. Use appropriate age-dependent restraining techniques to ensure patient safety during draw

B. Examples
   1. Blanket to tightly wrap other arm and legs in as restraint
   2. Seated in lap of parent or assistant who holds other arm and body
   3. Restrained while lying down, etc.
VIII. Pediatric dermal puncture
   A. Use heel puncture for children less than 1 year of age
   B. Sites include middle and ring finger or big toe per facility policy (See Chapter 10, pp. 151-152)
IX. Special considerations
   A. ID band must be present on infant
   B. Keep equipment out of patient's reach
   C. Warm heel before collection attempt
   D. Avoid using adhesive bandages
   E. Remove all equipment at completion
   F. Document collection in nursery log
X. Special dermal puncture procedures
   A. Neonatal bilirubin
      1. Protect sample from light
         a. Turn off bilirubin lights before draw
         b. Use amber-colored container
         c. Foil wrap specimen if no amber-colored container available
      2. Hemolysis falsely lowers bilirubin results
      3. Collection time must be recorded to track the rate of bilirubin increase
   B. Newborn (NBS-newborn screening)
      1. Required by U. S. law
         a. Hypothyroidism
         b. PKU
      2. Other neonatal screens designated by each state, such as:
         a. Galactosemia
         b. Homocystinuria
         c. Maple syrup disease
         d. Biotinidase deficiency
         e. Sickle cell anemia
      3. Collection:
         a. Capillary stick on special filter paper
         b. Dorsal hand vein not recommended as phenylalanine levels differ between capillary and venous samples
         c. Follow dermal collection procedures for NBS
            i. Apply large drop of blood evenly distributed on circle
            ii. Apply to one side of filter paper

iii. Blood visible on both sides
iv. Air-dry in horizontal position, R.T., away from sunlight
XI. Venipuncture in newborns
   A. Dorsal hand veins
      1. Children under 2 years including newborns
      2. 23-gauge butterfly needle
      3. Once blood flow established
         a. Release hold on collection needle
         b. Fill collection containers
      4. Apply pressure to site after withdrawing needle
   B. Scalp punctures
      1. Require specialized training
      2. Used only when other venipuncture sites are not accessible

Geriatric Patients
I. Physical changes
   A. Skin becomes less elastic and thinner
   B. Blood vessels more fragile
   C. Arteries closer to surface
II. Common disorders
   A. Hearing loss
   B. Unclear speech
   C. Arthritis
   D. Anticoagulation therapy
   E. Poor nutrition and dehydration
   F. Tremors
III. Mental impairment
   A. Forgetfulness
   B. Confusion
   C. Dementia
IV. Special considerations for blood collection
   A. Identification of patient—rely on ID bracelet
   B. Limiting blood loss to prevent anemia
   C. Application of tourniquet—over clothing to limit bruising
   D. Locating a vein
      1. Place arm on pillow
      2. Grip washcloth
      3. Support sides of arm with rolled towels
      4. Gently massage, do *not* slap arm to improve blood flow
      5. Look for veins in unusual places
   E. Performing the puncture
      1. Anchor vein along sides to prevent rolling
      2. Use smaller gauge needle
      3. Do not probe
      4. Apply pressure longer

Patients Requiring Blood Draws for Extended Periods of Time

I. Conditions
   A. Hepatitis C infection
   B. HIV
   C. Chronic infections
   D. Leukemia
   E. Terminal cancers
   F. Sickle cell disease
   G. IV drug use
II. Venipuncture considerations
   A. Rotate sites
   B. Use smallest gauge needle consistent with tests required
   C. Use alternate sites (i.e., forearm, underside of arm, wrist, hand, fingers)

Special Equipment Used in the Intensive Care Unit and Emergency Room

I. Types of vascular access devices
   A. Central line/central venous catheter
      1. Broviac
      2. Groshong
      3. Hickman
      4. Triple lumen
   B. Implanted port
   C. Peripherally inserted central catheter (PICC)—not used for blood draws
   D. Arterial line—most commonly used is radial artery (alternate sites: brachial, axillary, and femoral arteries)
   E. Heparin or saline lock
   F. Arteriovenous (AV) shunt
II. Drawing from a vascular access device
   A. Only done by specially trained personnel with a physician's order
      1. Never use syringe larger than 20 mL
      2. For noncoagulation specimens, discard 2 times the dead space
      3. For coagulation specimens, discard 6 times the dead space—approximately 5 mL
      4. First sample collected should not be used due to the anticoagulant and/or flush in the line or port
      5. Check for correct order of draw
III. Working with intravenous lines
   A. Use arm without IV if possible, otherwise follow established guidelines
   B. Have nurse turn off IV drip before the draw for a minimum of 2 minutes
   C. Apply tourniquet distal to IV insertion site
   D. Select a vein distal to the IV insertion site and in a different vein

E. Discard the first 5 mL of blood
F. Note on requisition that sample was drawn from an arm with an IV

CERTIFICATION PREPARATION QUESTIONS

1. Which of the following represents the correct ratio of plasma to red blood cells in newborns?
   a. 40% plasma, 60% red blood cells
   b. 60% plasma, 40% red blood cells
   c. 45% plasma, 55% red blood cells
   d. 60% plasma, 45% red blood cells

2. Monitoring the amount of blood drawn from patients who require repeated blood draws is important for all patients but is even more important for children because:
   a. Children have a lower blood volume than adults
   b. You may be able to use previously drawn specimens
   c. Children are more difficult to draw than adults
   d. Parents may object to their child having numerous draws

3. Which of the following represents a safe percentage of blood volume that can be removed from an infant in a 24-hour time period?
   a. 2%
   b. 5%
   c. 7%
   d. 10%

4. You must draw blood for a complete blood count (CBC) ordered daily on a 2-year-old child with leukemia. Which of the following techniques is most commonly used for blood collection in pediatric patients?
   a. Vacutainer collection
   b. Syringe collection
   c. Winged infusion set
   d. Dermal puncture

5. In general, the patient populations that are more susceptible to infection and thus require extra precaution to prevent exposure of this group to potential sources of infection include all of the following, except:
   a. Infants and small children
   b. Geriatric patients
   c. Newborns
   d. Teens

6. Performing blood collection on pediatric patients is quite challenging and requires the patience and understanding of the phlebotomist. All of the following considerations may cause difficulty in pediatric blood collection, *except*:
   a. Children differ in levels of understanding
   b. Children have less of an ability to cooperate
   c. Children have higher anxiety about medical procedures
   d. Children do not have the capacity to make choices

7. A 4-year-old outpatient requires a blood draw for collection of a CBC and venous blood gases. The child had been crying excessively before your arrival. Which of the following laboratory values may be elevated because of prolonged stress or crying by an infant or child if you were to proceed with the draw?
   a. White blood cell count
   b. pH level
   c. Both a and b
   d. None of the above

8. Which of the following is an appropriate measure that can reduce anxiety in a child during blood collection?
   a. Collect blood in patient's hospital room if possible
   b. Tell the child that "it will not hurt"
   c. Maintain an authoritative manner during collection
   d. Prepare your supplies outside of the child's field of vision

9. Older children have the ability to better understand what a venipuncture entails. Therefore, which of the following is the most important point to emphasize with the child?
   a. Telling the child it will not hurt very much
   b. Explaining all the different tube colors that you will be drawing
   c. Telling the child they can choose a special sticker as a reward for being brave
   d. Emphasizing the necessity to hold still during the procedure

10. Proper identification procedures for adults may differ from children and infants. Which of the following methods is correct for identification of a newborn?
    a. Identify based on sex and last name (i.e., Baby Girl Smith)
    b. Identify based on identification number of the baby
    c. Identify based on identification number of the mother
    d. Identify based on social security number

11. The most commonly used anesthetic used during blood collection procedures is:
    a. Alcohol
    b. Iodine
    c. EMLA
    d. Betadine

12. To maximize the chances of adequate blood collection from an infant using dermal puncture, which of the following steps should the phlebotomist perform?
    a. Warm the heel for 3 to 5 minutes
    b. Milk foot from the toes toward the heel
    c. Use a tourniquet just above the ankle
    d. Wipe away the first drop of blood

13. Which of the following statements is true regarding bilirubin?
    a. Bilirubin must be protected from light
    b. Bilirubin causes hemolysis when in excess
    c. Bilirubin is removed from the body via the pancreas
    d. Bilirubin is collected in a tan color stopper tube

14. Which of the following test(s) are required to be performed by law on all newborns in the United States?
    a. PKU
    b. Ammonia
    c. Glucose
    d. Hepatitis B virus (HBV)

15. Which of the following sites is preferred for venous blood collection in pediatric patients under the age of 2 years, requiring a large amount of sample?
    a. Planar side of heel
    b. Distal phalanx of finger
    c. Dorsal surface of the hand
    d. Viable scalp veins

16. The steps involved in performing a dorsal hand vein draw on infants involve all of the following, *except*:
    a. Using the infant ID band to identify the patient

b. Applying a tourniquet 2 to 3 inches above the hand
c. Cleansing the area with isopropyl alcohol
d. Inserting a 23-gauge needle into the dorsal hand vein

17. A dorsal hand vein is not recommended for neonatal screening collections for the following reason:
a. It is too difficult to control the amount of blood application to the circles
b. A newborn's hand veins are too tiny for a 23-gauge needle
c. Reference values for neonatal tests are based on capillary blood not venous blood
d. The sample may become hemolyzed because of the smaller gauge of the needle

18. As a phlebotomist you are making frequent trips to the local nursing home to collect blood draws. You notice that this group of patients exhibits more anxiety than other patient populations that you typically draw. Which of the following may lead to increased anxiety in geriatric patients during blood collection procedures?
a. Geriatric patients feel less in control
b. Geriatric patients may have hearing loss
c. Geriatric patients have chronic conditions
d. All of the above

19. As people age there are a number of physiologic changes that occur within the body that can present problems during a venipuncture procedure. Which of the following physical changes does not cause difficulty in blood collection in the geriatric patient?
a. Incontinence
b. Reduced skin collagen
c. Arteries are close to surface
d. Fragile blood vessels

20. Some medical conditions require that the patient undergo repeated blood testing to monitor his or her medical state. Which of the following conditions does not require repeated blood draws for an extended period of time?
a. HIV infection
b. Hypothyroidism
c. Sickle cell disease
d. Leukemia

21. The geriatric population may exhibit varying degrees of mental impairment. Which of the following conditions is common in geriatric patients?
a. Dementia
b. Forgetfulness
c. Confusion
d. All of the above

22. Geriatric patients are at risk for which of the following as a result of venipuncture procedures:
a. Blood volume related anemia
b. Development of petechiae
c. Edema from a tight tourniquet
d. Arthritis from clenching fist

23. Which of the following techniques can be used to reduce the potential for bruising in geriatric patients?
a. Gentle pressure when milking the finger
b. Application of tourniquet over clothing
c. Both a and b
d. None of the above

24. The best area for site selection in a geriatric patient is:
a. Hand
b. Wrist
c. Antecubital fossa
d. Forearm

25. Which of the following statements about bilirubin is *not* true?
a. Bilirubin is a breakdown product of red blood cells
b. Bilirubin is produced by the kidneys
c. Bilirubin in excess can cause jaundice
d. Bilirubin in excess can lead to brain damage

26. Why is it important to keep equipment out of the reach of pediatric patients?
a. To avoid injury to the patient
b. To keep the equipment sterile
c. To allow parents to assist in the process
d. To keep the child from breaking anything

27. Which of the following is *not* considered a prenatal screening test?
a. Homocystine
b. Galactose
c. Alkaline phosphatase
d. PKU

28. What is the appropriate needle gauge to use when routinely performing venipuncture for collection of a large blood volume on an infant?
    a. 25-gauge
    b. 23-gauge
    c. 21-gauge
    d. 18-gauge

29. Which of the following is *not* a type of central venous catheter (CVC)?
    a. Groshong
    b. Broviac
    c. PICC
    d. Triple lumen

30. Which type of vascular access device is surgically placed under the skin and connected to an indwelling line?
    a. PICC
    b. CVC
    c. Hickman
    d. Implanted port

31. Which of the following devices is not typically used for the drawing of blood due to the tendency for the tubing to collapse upon aspiration?
    a. PICC
    b. CVC
    c. Hickman
    d. Implanted port

32. Why must a phlebotomist discard the first sample drawn from a heparin or saline lock?
    a. Risk of sample clotting in line
    b. Presence of antibodies in tubing
    c. Potential dilution of the specimen
    d. Reduce risk of infection in the catheter

33. Which of the following devices is an artificial connection between an artery and a vein?
    a. Saline lock
    b. Arterial line
    c. Arteriovenous shunt
    d. PICC

34. Which of the following represents the order of blood draw when drawing blood from a vascular access device (VAD)?
    a. Anticoagulated tubes, clotted tubes, blood culture tubes
    b. Anticoagulated tubes, blood culture tubes, clotted tubes

    c. Blood culture tubes, clotted tubes, anticoagulated tubes
    d. Blood culture tubes, anticoagulated tubes, clotted tubes

35. A phlebotomist needs to draw blood from a patient who has an IV line in place in both arms. Correct procedure includes all of the following, *except*:
    a. The site of the venipuncture should be distal to the IV
    b. IV turned off for at least 2 minutes before the draw
    c. The first 5 mL of blood should be discarded
    d. The order of draw is reversed to avoid the dilution effect

36. Which of the following arteries is most commonly used for placement of an arterial line?
    a. Brachial artery
    b. Radial artery
    c. Axillary artery
    d. Femoral artery

37. Which of the following AV shunts consists of a fistula that may never be used for phlebotomy purposes?
    a. External shunt
    b. Internal shunt
    c. PICC
    d. Groshong

38. When drawing blood from a patient's arm containing an IV, which of the following is true?
    a. A discard tube of at least 2 mL must be drawn
    b. The patient must be instructed to keep their fist open
    c. The phlebotomist must identify the draw location on the requisition
    d. Wait 10 minutes after IV turned off if using the same vein for the draw

39. As the phlebotomist at your lab, you routinely go to area nursing homes to collect blood draws. The challenges you are faced with from this population of patients includes all of the following, *except*:
    a. Veins easily roll
    b. Veins are more elastic
    c. Arthritis may impede access to veins
    d. Arteries are close to the surface

40. Which of the following conditions often effect elderly patients and may cause complications when trying to collect a blood sample?
    a. Parkinson disease
    b. Down syndrome
    c. Hashimoto thyroiditis
    d. Tay-Sach disease

41. You enter a patient's room and observe that they have a VAD. How should you proceed?
    a. Get the nurse to draw the blood specimens for you
    b. Call the doctor and request permission to draw blood through the VAD
    c. Call the lab to send another phlebotomist to assist you with the collection
    d. Proceed with the collection because it is an internal AV shunt and is easy to stick

42. A maximum of 3% has been set as a safe volume for withdrawal of blood in an infant in 24 hours. You check the log and note that a baby weighing 3.2 kg with an approximate blood volume of 80 mL/kg has already had 2.4 mL of blood drawn today. You need to collect another specimen. Can you draw the baby's blood?
    a. Yes, because the maximum blood withdrawal allowed for this baby is 7.68 mL
    b. Yes, because the maximum blood withdrawal allowed for this baby is 9.6 mL
    c. No, because the maximum blood withdrawal for this baby is already 2.4 mL
    d. No, because the maximum blood withdrawal for this baby has been exceeded at 0.096 mL

43. Restraining a child during a blood collection procedure may be necessary. Which of the following are acceptable?
    a. Lay the child down and lean over the child
    b. Seat the child on parent's lap and have the parent hug the child's body
    c. Hold the child's unused arm securely in either position
    d. All of the above
    e. None of the above because restraint nullifies child's consent

44. You are called to the nursery for a STAT draw on a newborn. While preparing your materials you note that you do not have a heel-warmer packet and neither does the nursery. How should you proceed?
    a. Fill a latex or vinyl glove with hot water and place it on the baby's heel
    b. Wet a small towel or washcloth and place in the microwave to heat it
    c. Proceed without a heel-warmer but double stick the heel for greater blood flow
    d. Call down to the lab for STAT delivery of a heel-warmer to the nursery

ANSWERS AND RATIONALES

1. **Answer: A**
   Rationale: Newborns have a higher proportion of red blood cells than adults and a lower proportion of plasma—40% plasma, 60% red blood cells. Adults have a ratio of 45% red blood cells and 55% plasma.
   Text Reference: p. 185

2. **Answer: A**
   Rationale: The younger the child, the lower the blood volume. Therefore, special consideration must be taken when drawing blood from infants and small children because they have lower blood volumes and can tolerate less blood being removed at one time. Parents may object if they are not kept apprised of the child's need for repeated blood draws, but it is not the reason for monitoring the amount of blood drawn from children.
   Text Reference: pp. 184-185

3. **Answer: B**
   Rationale: Due to overall lower blood volume in infants, it is safe to remove only 5% of the infant's blood volume in a 24-hour period. The preferred maximum is 3% or less with no more than 10% in a 1-month period.
   Text Reference: p. 184

4. **Answer: D**
   Rationale: Due to the necessity to minimize blood loss in infants, dermal puncture is the most common technique used in pediatric patients. The type of test and the amount of blood required for testing determine the appropriateness of a dermal puncture versus a venipuncture on pediatric patients. In this case, a child with leukemia may also suffer

from anemia, so minimizing the amount of blood drawn each day is important.
Text Reference: p. 185

5. **Answer: D**
Rationale: Due to the immaturity of the immune system, newborns and pediatric patients are more susceptible to infections. Any patient that suffers from a compromised immune system is susceptible to infection. Geriatric patients are also susceptible to infections due to disease or loss of immune function due to the aging process.
Text Reference: pp. 185, 190

6. **Answer: D**
Rationale: There are several special psychological considerations that may make pediatric collection more challenging and often more difficult. Giving children age-appropriate choices increases their feelings of control.
Text Reference: pp. 185-186

7. **Answer: C**
Rationale: It is very important to try to keep the patient calm during blood collection if possible. Pediatric patients who have stressful collection procedures often have inaccurate test results such as WBC and pH values.
Text Reference: p. 185

8. **Answer: D**
Rationale: Preparing all of your supplies before entering the collection area will minimize the time the child has to be anxious before collection. However, having an assistant lab person assemble equipment while you explain the procedure will allow for parents who are present to observe proper assembly of materials, etc. Whenever possible, remove the patient from the hospital room to minimize anxiety. Never tell the patient "it will not hurt." Misleading the child will make the child distrust not only the phlebotomist but other health care professionals and often make care and treatment more difficult. When collecting blood from pediatric patients, it is best to maintain calm and cheerful mannerisms.
Text Reference: pp. 185-186

9. **Answer: D**
Rationale: Explaining to the child the importance of holding still during the procedure and what may happen if they do not may gain their cooperation. You should never tell a child it will not hurt. Offering a reward such as a sticker should never be contingent on their not crying, etc. Being scared, crying, or even yelling are normal reactions and should be allowed and the child should be told it is alright—they can cry or yell but should hold still while doing so.
Text Reference: pp. 185-186

10. **Answer: B**
Rationale: Each patient in the hospital including newborns has unique identification numbers that are specific to that particular patient. Only the patient identification number can be used to positively identify the correct patient. Phlebotomists should be especially careful of collection of samples from twins.
Text Reference: p. 186

11. **Answer: C**
Rationale: The question is referring to the most common topical anesthetic (EMLA) used to numb the patient's skin in the area of blood collection. Phlebotomists should read each question carefully. The other answers listed are antiseptics not anesthetics.
Text Reference: p. 186

12. **Answer: A**
Rationale: The optimal collection site for infants is the heel. Fingertips are not used in infants and small children. Warming the heel for 3 to 5 minutes increases blood circulation in the area of collection and maximizes the chance of adequate blood collection. Wiping away the first drop of blood does not impact adequate blood flow.
Text Reference: p. 187

13. **Answer: A**
Rationale: Bilirubin is a substance produced by the normal breakdown of red blood cells. It is removed from the body by the liver and is light sensitive. When in excess, bilirubin can cause the patient to become jaundiced and may cause permanent brain damage to the basal ganglia and auditory nerves if levels get too high. Ultraviolet light treatment

can be used to breakdown excess bilirubin in newborns.
Text Reference: p. 187

14. **Answer: A**
Rationale: U.S. law mandates screening of all newborns to detect metabolic disorders that may cause severe brain damage, including PKU and thyroid testing. Other additional newborn screening tests are designated by each state.
Text Reference: p. 188

15. **Answer: C**
Rationale: When a larger volume of blood is needed from a pediatric patient under the age of 2 years, it is preferred to use the dorsal surface of the hand for collection. The scalp vein can be used if no other vein is accessible. Collection of blood from the scalp vein requires additional training and expertise.
Text Reference: p. 188

16. **Answer: B**
Rationale: All steps are required with the exception of tourniquet application. The dorsal hand vein technique does not require the use of a tourniquet in the procedure.
Text Reference: pp. 188-189

17. **Answer: C**
Rationale: Although some books say dorsal hand vein collection of newborn screens is permitted, recent studies have shown that PKU levels differ between venous and capillary blood. Reference values are based on capillary values.
Text Reference: p. 188

18. **Answer: D**
Rationale: Geriatric patients experience anxiety levels greater than those of the average adult for many reasons. These patients feel less in control for many reasons. They may be unable to hear or see the phlebotomist well. They may also have other medical conditions or use medication that may cause them to be more anxious about the blood collection procedure.
Text Reference: pp. 189-190

19. **Answer: A**
Rationale: The capability of the geriatric patient to control urinary functions typically

does not impact the blood collection process.
Text Reference: p. 190

20. **Answer: B**
Rationale: Hypothyroidism typically requires blood collection only for a short period of time until a therapeutic medication level can be acquired. The other conditions listed require ongoing therapy and monitoring of blood values.
Text Reference: p. 191

21. **Answer: D**
Rationale: Mental impairment of geriatric patients is common and may include one or more of the conditions listed.
Text Reference: p. 190

22. **Answer: A**
Rationale: Geriatric patients often have an increased incidence of blood draws in comparison to the average adult patient. Therefore, these patients do have an increased risk of volume loss–related anemias.
Text Reference: pp. 189-190

23. **Answer: C**
Rationale: Geriatric patients bruise very easily due to the decreased elasticity of the blood vessels. In addition, many geriatric patients may be undergoing anticoagulant therapy, which may also increase the risk of bruising. The procedures listed cannot guarantee bruising will not occur; however, these methods can reduce the risk of bruising.
Text Reference: p. 190

24. **Answer: C**
Rationale: The antecubital fossa is usually but *not* always the best area for blood collection in geriatric patients for various reasons. The phlebotomist should look in other locations to find the most reasonable collection site.
Text Reference: p. 191

25. **Answer: B**
Rationale: Bilirubin is a normal breakdown product of red blood cells; in excess it can lead to jaundice and brain damage. It is not produced in the body by the kidneys; however, the kidneys may help to excrete excess bilirubin via urine.
Text Reference: p. 187

26. **Answer: A**
    Rationale: The equipment used for blood collection has the potential to cause injury to a pediatric patient. Most tubes used today are plastic; however, needles and antiseptics may be potentially harmful to the patient and must be removed and discarded after the procedure.
    Text Reference: pp. 186-187

27. **Answer: C**
    Rationale: Prenatal testing may be done for galactosemia, homocystinuria, maple syrup disease, and biotinidase deficiency, along with hypothyroidism and PKU disease. Alkaline phosphatase is a routine chemistry test performed as part of a basic metabolic, complete metabolic, and a liver profile.
    Text Reference: p. 188

28. **Answer: B**
    Rationale: Typically, routine venipunctures requiring a larger blood volume than what could be obtained via dermal puncture on newborns are performed using a 23-gauge needle. Use of a smaller gauge needle could increase the risk of hemolysis. Use of a larger gauge needle would likely cause damage to the vessel and surrounding tissue.
    Text Reference: p. 188

29. **Answer: C**
    Rationale: PICC lines are inserted by threading the catheter into the central vein after insertion into a peripheral vein, which is accessed from the antecubital area. CVCs are inserted directly into the large veins emptying into the heart directly. Groshong, Boviac, triple lumen, and Hickman catheters are all types of CVCs.
    Text Reference: pp. 191-192

30. **Answer: D**
    Rationale: Implanted ports are chambers that are located under the skin and connected to an indwelling line. These devices are surgically implanted and allow venous access by using a noncoring needle through the skin into the chamber, through a self-sealing septum.
    Text Reference: p. 191

31. **Answer: A**
    Rationale: PICC lines are not used for drawing blood on a routine basis. The tubing is easily collapsed and the application of too much suction on aspiration may lead to damage of the PICC line.
    Text Reference: p. 191

32. **Answer: C**
    Rationale: Saline and heparin locks are flushed on a routine basis by nursing personnel to keep the peripheral catheter device from clotting off. The phlebotomist must discard the first sample collected from the device to avoid the potential of contamination or dilution of the sample to be used for testing.
    Text Reference: p. 192

33. **Answer: C**
    Rationale: An arteriovenous (AV) shunt is an artificial connection between an artery and a vein. AV shunts are used for dialysis patients to provide access for blood removal, purification, and return.
    Text Reference: p. 192

34. **Answer: D**
    Rationale: When drawing blood from a VAD, remember to discard the first sample collected from the device to avoid contamination and/or dilution. Blood culture tubes should be drawn first, followed by anticoagulated tubes, and lastly, clotted tubes.
    Text Reference: p. 192

35. **Answer: D**
    Rationale: Many inpatients commonly have IV lines in place. However, any time the sample can be drawn from a location other than the arm containing the IV, this is the preferred choice. If there are multiple IV lines or the only available draw site is in the same arm as the IV line, then the phlebotomist must follow the appropriate steps to ensure that a valid sample is collected.
    Text Reference: pp. 192-193

36. **Answer: B**
    Rationale: The radial artery is the most commonly used artery for placement of an arterial line. However, any of the other arterial sites listed may be used as alternative sites when necessary.
    Text Reference: p. 192

37. **Answer: B**
Rationale: An external AV shunt consists of a cannula with a rubber septum. A needle can be inserted through the septum to withdraw blood. An internal shunt has a permanent internal connection between the artery and the vein called a fistula. The fistula should never be used for blood collection.
Text Reference: p. 192

38. **Answer: C**
Rationale: When blood is drawn from a site containing an IV, the phlebotomist must note on the requisition that the blood was drawn from an arm containing an IV.
Text Reference: pp. 192-193

39. **Answer: B**
Rationale: Blood vessels are very narrow and less elastic in the elderly, making penetration difficult. Veins roll more easily than those of normal adult patients because of loss of muscle tissue. Immobilization of the vein should be done on both sides of the vein instead of directly on it. Arteries are close to the surface and must not be mistaken for veins. Arthritis may prevent the patient from fully straightening out the arm, thereby preventing easy access to the antecubital area.
Text Reference: p. 190

40. **Answer: A**
Rationale: Parkinson disease is just one of several diseases and conditions that may cause complications during sample procurement from a geriatric patient. Other conditions include stroke, hearing loss, heart attacks, and many other nonspecific conditions.
Text Reference: p. 190

41. **Answer: A**
Rationale: Only trained personnel such as nurse can draw blood from a VAD. Permission for trained personnel to draw blood from a VAD must be documented.
Text Reference: p. 192

42. **Answer: A**
Rationale: $80\,mL/kg \times 3.2\,kg \times 0.03 = 7.68\,mL$, which is the maximum safe volume of blood withdrawal from this baby in a 24-hour period.
Text Reference: p. 185

43. **Answer: D**
Rationale: Laying a child down or seating a child in a parent's lap while restraining the free arm are both acceptable methods of immobilizing infants and children for their safety during a blood collection procedure. Because children are minors and unable to give informed consent, the parent's consent must be obtained before performing any procedure on a child or infant.
Text Reference: pp. 186-187

44. **Answer: D**
Rationale: You should never fill a latex or vinyl glove with hot water or warm a towel or cloth in a microwave because you cannot control the temperature of the make-shift warmer and may burn the delicate skin of a newborn. Proceeding without a heel-warmer may result in multiple sticks on the newborn's heel in order to collect enough blood for the test due to decreased circulation in cooler extremities. Calling down to the lab for a runner to deliver a heel-warmer is the best choice.
Text Reference: p. 187

ARTERIAL BLOOD COLLECTION

Tina Lewis

INTRODUCTION

Arterial blood is collected to determine the level of oxygen and carbon dioxide in the blood and measure the pH. Arterial collection is much more dangerous to the patient than venous collection, and it requires in-depth training beyond routine phlebotomy skills. It is usually performed by physicians, nurses, respiratory therapists (RTs), medical laboratory scientists/technicians (MT/MLS, MLT), and in some areas of the country, trained phlebotomists. Depending on hospital/laboratory protocol, phlebotomists occasionally are asked to perform or assist with this procedure, and because of the ongoing changes in health care delivery, it is likely that at some point you will have to collect an arterial sample. However, you will not be permitted to participate in actual arterial collection before you receive specialized training at a health care institution. Arterial collection is most often performed in the radial artery, where collateral circulation from the ulnar artery can make up the loss to the supplied tissues. Arterial samples must be processed very quickly after collection to minimize changes in analyte values.

CONTENT OVERVIEW

Composition of Arterial Blood
I.   Rich in oxygen and electrolytes
II. Uniform composition throughout body

Purpose of ABG Testing
I.   Measures concentration of oxygen, carbon dioxide, bicarbonate, and pH.
II. Most often used for ammonia and lactic acid levels in addition to arterial blood gas (ABG) measurements
III. Measures gas exchange ability in the lungs along with the buffering capacity of the blood.
IV. Normal blood pH 7.35 to 7.45
     A. Acidosis—pH less than 7.35
     B. Acidosis—pH greater than 7.45

V.   Conditions resulting in abnormal ABG values
     A. Chronic obstructive pulmonary disease (COPD)
     B. Lung cancer
     C. Diabetic coma
     D. Shock
     E. Cardiac or respiratory failure
     F. Neuromuscular disease

Arterial Blood Gas Testing
I.   Equipment for arterial puncture
     A. Heparinized syringe and needle
        1. Use a solution of sodium heparin with a concentration of 1000 U/mL
        2. Calculate the volume of heparin needed. Use 0.05 mL heparin solution for each milliliter of blood to be drawn.
        3. Draw up heparin into syringe that is glass or gas-impermeable plastic
        4. Rotate the liquid in the syringe to coat the barrel
        5. Expel the excess heparin and air
     B. May use treated, prepackaged syringes
     C. Needle size: 21 to 22 gauge, 1 to 1½ inches long depending on artery used
     D. Antiseptic—use two because the risk of infection is greater in arterial draws
        1. Alcohol
        2. Povidone-iodine or chlorhexidine
     E. Lidocaine anesthetic injected subcutaneously; optional
     F. Safety equipment and personal protective equipment (PPE)
     G. Luer tip to prevent exposure of specimen to air
     H. Other equipment
        1. Transport container
        2. Crushed ice
        3. Ice and water—slurry of ice
        4. Gauze pads
        5. Pressure bandages
        6. Thermometer to take patient's temperature
        7. No tourniquet needed
II. Site selection
     A. Radial artery
        1. Artery of choice

B. Brachial artery
1. Large
2. Easy to palpate and puncture
3. Deep and near median nerve
4. Risk of hematoma and bleeding
C. Femoral artery
1. Largest artery used
2. Good when cardiac output is low and other sites unavailable
3. Requires advanced training, usually a doctor
   a. Poor collateral circulation
   b. Increased risk of infection
   c. Puncture may dislodge plaque from wall of artery
D. Dorsalis pedis artery
1. Alternate adult site
2. Performed by qualified, trained personnel
E. Umbilical artery
1. Alternate infant site
2. Performed by qualified, trained personnel
F. Scalp artery
1. Alternate infant site
2. Performed by qualified, trained personnel
III. Testing collateral circulation
A. Modified Allen test
1. Negative result: no color after 5 to 10 seconds—do not use artery
2. Positive result: color appears within 5 to 10 seconds—OK to proceed
B. Review Procedure 13-1, p. 199
IV. Radial artery puncture
A. Prepare patient and examine requisition
1. Take and record patient temperature if facility protocol requires it
2. Document oxygen received and device used to deliver oxygen
3. Patient should be in respiratory steady state for at least 30 minutes
B. Choose and prepare site
1. Perform modified Allen test
2. Clean site first with alcohol and then povidone-iodine
3. Inject local anesthetic if allowed
C. Perform puncture inserting needle at 45- to 60-degree angle with bevel up and facing upper arm
D. Withdraw needle, expel any air in needle, engage safety device, cap off syringe with Luer tip cap, apply pressure, and ice syringe

E. Examine and bandage puncture site for complete hemostasis generally after 5 minutes or 15 minutes for patients on anticoagulant therapy. If still bleeding continue with pressure until bleeding stops, then, check for pulse distal to site
F. Dispose of needle in sharps and other trash per protocol of facility
G. Label and deliver to lab immediately
H. Analyze ABGs according to lab protocol and syringe type
1. Plastic syringe—do not ice; deliver to lab and analyze within 30 minutes
2. Glass syringe—put on slurry of ice if delay in transport; analyze within 1 hour

Arterial Puncture Complications
I. Arteriospasm
A. Spontaneous constriction of artery
B. Occurs in response to pain
C. Prevents oxygen from getting into tissues
II. Nerve damage
A. Result of inadvertent contact of needle with nerve
B. More likely to occur during arterial puncture because of depth of vessel
III. Hematoma
A. Results from inadequate pressure after arterial puncture
B. More likely in elderly due to less elasticity in vessels—don't close as readily after puncture
IV. Thrombosis
A. Clot in artery may occur after arterial puncture
V. Hemorrhage
A. Patients on anticoagulant therapy
B. Patients with bleeding disorders
VI. Infection
A. Due to contaminants entering vascular system
B. Microorganisms easily carried throughout body—may not encounter immune system cells and be destroyed
VII. Sampling error
A. Using too much heparin—lowers pH value
B. Using too little heparin—specimen clots
C. Insufficient mixing—clots
D. Air bubbles in syringe—decrease CO_2 levels

E. Improper plastic syringe—atmospheric gas diffuse into specimen, specimen gases diffuse out
F. Improper anticoagulant—pH altered by EDTA, oxalates, citrates
G. Puncture of vein instead of artery—values incorrect
H. Atmospheric exposure of sample alters values

VIII. Specimen rejection
A. Inadequate specimen volume
B. Clotting
C. Improper or absent labeling
D. Use of wrong syringe
E. Air in sample
F. Failure to ice sample
G. Delay in specimen delivery

Capillary Blood Gas Testing

I. Used when arterial collection is not possible or not recommended.
II. Most commonly used in pediatric patients (i.e., neonatal intensive care unit [NICU])
III. Mixture of blood from the vessels located in the dermal layer (i.e., capillaries, venules, arterioles, tissue fluid, and it is exposed to air during collection
IV. Capillary blood gas collection procedure via heel stick
A. Warm site for 5 to 10 minutes to 40° C to 42° C so blood is similar to arterial blood
B. Collect sample in heparinized glass pipette that may contain metal filing (i.e., flea)
  1. Fill tube completely, no air bubbles
  2. Mix blood with heparin using a magnet to pull flea back and forth
C. Seal both ends of tube with plastic caps
D. Mix well again and transport to lab on ice slurry if delay in transport anticipated.

CERTIFICATION PREPARATION QUESTIONS

1. An arterial blood specimen would be collected to assess all of the following analytes, *except:*
   a. Oxygen
   b. Carbon dioxide
   c. Carbon monoxide
   d. Bicarbonate

2. All of the following statements are true about arterial blood collection and testing, *except:*
   a. Is more dangerous than venous blood collection

   b. Requires additional, specialized training
   c. Can be performed by a MLS or MLT
   d. Requires use of EDTA coated syringe

3. Assessment of the patient before arterial blood gas collection may include all of the following, *except:*
   a. Patient temperature at the time of the draw
   b. Amount of oxygen patient is receiving
   c. Device use to deliver oxygen to patient
   d. Lung capacity of patient

4. The most frequently used artery for arterial blood gas collection is:
   a. Radial artery
   b. Ulnar artery
   c. Femoral artery
   d. Brachial artery

5. Which of the following laboratory tests is *not* routinely performed on arterial blood?
   a. Arterial blood gases
   b. Ammonia
   c. Ferritin
   d. Lactic acid

6. A disadvantage of using the brachial artery in an arterial blood gas draw includes all of the following, *except:*
   a. Insufficient collateral circulation
   b. Risk of puncturing the median nerve
   c. Difficult to compress
   d. Risk of hematoma or bleeding

7. Equipment used in the collection of arterial blood gases includes commercially prepared syringes that come with all of the following, *except:*
   a. Heparin coated syringe
   b. Luer cap for the syringe hub
   c. Safety needle
   d. Lidocaine anesthetic

8. The best choice of needle for a radial arterial blood gas draw is:
   a. 22-gauge, 1-inch
   b. 20-gauge, 1½-inch
   c. 18-gauge, 1-inch
   d. 25-gauge, 1½-inch

9. The physician suspects the diabetic patient may be in metabolic acidosis and orders

ABGs to check pH and other blood gas values. Which of the following values represent normal arterial blood pH?
a. 7.00 to 8.00
b. 7.35 to 7.45
c. 7.50 to 7.75
d. 7.20 to 7.30

10. The purpose of the Allen test before collection of an arterial blood gas is to:
a. Measure the pulse rate in the radial artery
b. Locate the position, depth, and width of the radial artery
c. Assess collateral circulation in the radial artery
d. Locate the pulse point before collection

11. A positive Allen test is evidenced when:
a. Ulnar pulse rate synchronizes with the radial pulse
b. Pulse rate increases in the radial artery
c. Color appears in the hand within 5 to 10 seconds
d. Strong pulse can be felt when hand color is blanched

12. Which of the following statements is *not* true?
a. ABGs measure the gas exchange ability of the lungs
b. ABGs measure the amount of carbon monoxide in the blood
c. ABGs measure the amount of oxygen in the blood
d. ABGs measure the amount of carbon dioxide in the blood

13. What is the anticoagulant used in the collection syringe for ABG collection?
a. EDTA
b. Sodium citrate
c. Heparin
d. Sodium oxalate

14. Acceptable antiseptic(s) used in performing arterial blood draws is (are)
a. Alcohol
b. Chlorhexidine
c. Alcohol and povidone-iodine
d. All of the above

15. Why is lidocaine used in collection of ABGs?
a. To prevent infection
b. To prevent swelling
c. To lessen pain
d. To amplify vein size

16. It would be advisable to wear which of the following types of PPE (personal protective equipment) when performing a blood collection procedure during which spraying of blood might be anticipated such as ABG collection?
a. Gloves, gown, respirator
b. Gloves, gown, face protection
c. Gown, face protection, respirator
d. Gloves, face protection, respirator

17. Which of the following types of equipment will *not* be used during ABG collection?
a. Gauze pads
b. Pressure bandages
c. Butterfly closure
d. Heparinized syringe

18. Why is a tourniquet not used when collecting arterial blood gases?
a. May compromise the sample
b. Arteries are easily visible
c. May cause elevations in potassium
d. Arterial blood is under pressure

19. Which of the following transport mechanisms may be required when collecting ABGs?
a. Transported on ice slurry
b. Protect sample from light
c. Protect from light and put on ice
d. Keep sample at 37° C

20. Where is the radial artery located?
a. Only in the antecubital fossa
b. Along the thumb side of the wrist
c. Along the smallest finger side of the wrist
d. Inguinal area at juncture of thigh and groin

21. Which of the following arteries that are typically used for arterial puncture carries an increased risk of complications from the procedure such as increased risk of infection or dislodging of plaque from arterial walls?
a. Radial artery
b. Brachial artery
c. Femoral artery
d. Umbilical artery

22. Which of the following arterial puncture sites do *not* require highly trained personnel such as a physician for specimen collection?
a. Femoral artery
b. Dorsalis pedis artery
c. Umbilical artery
d. Radial artery

23. All of the following are potential complications of arterial blood collection, *except:*
    a. Nerve damage
    b. Thrombosis
    c. Hematoma
    d. Petechiae

24. The formation of a clot within the artery or vein is known as a:
    a. Hemorrhage
    b. Hematoma
    c. Thrombosis
    d. Arteriospasm

25. The MLS receives an arterial sample on ice and checks the collection time to see if the ABG analysis should be run. The analysis may be run if it is within what timeframe from time of draw?
    a. Within 5 to 10 minutes
    b. Within 15 to 20 minutes
    c. Within 30 to 45 minutes
    d. Within 1 hour

26. An ABG sample transported to the laboratory at room temperature must be analyzed within:
    a. 5 minutes
    b. 30 minutes
    c. 30 to 45 minutes
    d. 1 hour

27. Which of the following is *not* a source of error when collecting ABGs?
    a. Using too much heparin
    b. Transporting ABGs in a plastic syringe at room temperature
    c. Insufficient mixing of sample and anticoagulant
    d. Air bubbles entering the syringe

28. Which of the following would *not* cause an ABG specimen to be rejected on receipt to the laboratory?
    a. Clotting of specimen
    b. Improper labeling of syringe
    c. Transporting glass syringe in an ice slurry
    d. Inadequate volume for testing

29. Capillary blood gas testing is most commonly performed on what type of patient?
    a. Geriatric patient
    b. Cardiac patient
    c. Pediatric patient
    d. Diabetic patient

30. Which of the following statements *is* true regarding the potential for nerve damage during arterial blood collection?
    a. Caused by inadvertent contact with a nerve
    b. Less likely to occur with arterial puncture
    c. More likely to occur with venipuncture draws
    d. Increase occurs when surface arteries used

31. The proper angle of penetration for a radial arterial blood gas draw is:
    a. 15°
    b. 20°
    c. 45°
    d. 90°

32. The acceptable angle of insertion for a femoral arterial blood draw is:
    a. 30°
    b. 45°
    c. 60°
    d. 90°

33. You perform an arterial puncture and are unsure if your specimen is arterial. What should you look for to determine the source of your specimen?
    a. Bright cherry-red color
    b. Dark reddish-blue color
    c. Pulsation as blood enters syringe
    a. Both b and c

34. Examination of the arterial puncture site includes checking the pulse after completion of the draw at a point:
    a. Proximal to the site
    b. Distal to the site
    c. Medial to the site
    d. Trans at the ulnar site

35. A low pH indicates which of the following?
    a. Acidosis
    b. Alkalosis
    c. Bicarbonate imbalance
    d. Decreased CO_2

36. When performing capillary blood gas collection, the phlebotomist uses what to close the ends of the capillary collection tube?

a. Plastic wrap
b. Plastic caps
c. Metal fleas
d. Foil

37. When performing a radial artery puncture, the bevel of the needle should be:
    a. Facing up and toward the fingertips
    b. Facing up and toward the upper arm
    c. At a 90° angle to the wrist and toward the fingertips
    d. Angled downward toward the upper arm

38. Why is it important to properly warm the heel for 5 to 10 minutes before collecting capillary blood gases?
    a. To enhance the visibility of the capillaries
    b. To increase arterial blood flow to the area
    c. To make the blood content similar to arterial blood
    d. Both b and c
    e. All of the above

39. Before the collection of capillary blood gas samples, a small metal device is sometimes placed in the heparinized capillary tube to assist with mixing. The device is known as what?
    a. A gnat
    b. A flea
    c. A bead
    d. A bug

40. Which of the following anticoagulants does *not* alter the pH of the sample collected?
    a. EDTA
    b. Oxalates
    c. Citrate
    d. Heparin

41. The purpose of sealing the ABG syringe or capillary sample is to:
    a. Prevent air contamination of the sample
    b. Prevent the sample from leaking out of the syringe or capillary tube
    c. Prevent air bubbles from forming
    d. All of the above

42. Before collection of ABGs, the patient must be in a respiratory steady state. Which of the following defines a respiratory steady state?
    a. The patient has received a steady amount of oxygen before collection of the sample
    b. Oxygen has been turned off for 15 minutes before the arterial draw to assess lung function
    c. The patient has received a specified amount of oxygen and refrained from exercise for 20 to 30 minutes
    d. The patient's temperature and respiration rate are normal at a specified amount of oxygen therapy

43. Before collection of ABGs, all of the following must be recorded by the phlebotomist, *except:*
    a. Weight and height of patient
    b. Flow rate of oxygen therapy
    c. Mode of oxygen therapy
    d. Steady respiratory status

ANSWERS AND RATIONALES

1. **Answer: C**
   Rationale: Arterial blood is collected not only to determine the amount of oxygen in the blood but also to monitor the amount of carbon dioxide and bicarbonate in the patient's blood. Carbon monoxide is not a part of the ABG test.
   Text Reference: p. 196

2. **Answer: D**
   Rationale: Arterial blood gases require the use of a heparinized syringe. Arterial blood collection is more dangerous than venous blood collections because of the potential for life-threatening complications to occur. Arterial blood collection is performed by health care personnel who have been specially trained in the collection of ABGs. Usually, arterial blood draws are completed by a trained respiratory therapist, MT/MLS, MLT, phlebotomist, a nurse, or a physician.
   Text Reference: p.196

3. **Answer: D**
   Rationale: ABGs measure the amount of oxygen, carbon dioxide, pH, and bicarbonate levels in the blood. It is important to accurately record how much oxygen the patient is receiving, its mode of delivery, and length of time the patient has been in a respiratory steady state in order to assess the lungs' capacity to oxygenate blood and the efficacy of oxygen therapy, if any. Changes in

arterial oxygen and carbon dioxide levels can be altered if the patient hyperventilates, holds his or her breath, cries, etc.
Text Reference: p. 201

4. **Answer: A**
Rationale: Arterial collection is most often performed from the radial artery where collateral circulation from other arteries can make up for the blood loss to the supplied tissues.
Text Reference: p. 198

5. **Answer: C**
Rationale: Ferritin levels are typically performed on plasma or serum collected from venous blood. Arterial blood is the preferred sample for ABGs. Ammonia levels in venous blood differ from arterial levels for a number of reasons beyond the scope of this discussion. However, the use of a tourniquet to collect a blood sample artificially increases the ammonia level, thus arterial blood is preferred. Venous lactic acid levels are very similar to arterial blood. If ABGs are ordered along with lactic acid for the diagnosis of critically ill patients that present in the emergency room (ER), only one draw would be necessary.
Text Reference: p. 196

6. **Answer: A**
Rationale: The brachial artery has less collateral circulation than the radial artery, but it is adequate. The location of the brachial artery is deep and close to the median nerve. Compression of the brachial artery is difficult and poses a greater risk of hematoma and bleeding at the puncture site.
Text Reference: p. 198

7. **Answer: D**
Rationale: Commercially prepared kits for ABGs typically include a special heparinized syringe, safety needle, and Luer cap or other closure device at a minimum. Lidocaine anesthetic is not included in every hospital protocol for the collection of ABGs and thus would not be included in the kit. Administration of an anesthetic is an optional step. Some kits also provide alcohol and povidone-iodine ampules.
Text Reference: p. 197

8. **Answer: A**
Rationale: For a radial arterial blood gas draw, the best choice would be a 21- or 22-gauge, 1-inch needle. Needles that are 1½ inches are used primarily for femoral arterial draws. Larger needle gauges may prevent entry into the artery and smaller needle gauges may result in hemolysis of the specimen.
Text Reference: p. 196

9. **Answer: B**
Rationale: The blood pH range is very narrow, between the values of 7.35 to 7.45. A diabetic patient in metabolic acidosis would have a pH below the normal range.
Text Reference: p. 196

10. **Answer: C**
Rationale: The Allen test assesses the adequacy of collateral circulation in the radial artery. If the Allen test is negative, then circulation to the hand is inadequate and the radial artery should not be used. If the Allen test is positive then adequate circulation is present and the radial artery can be punctured.
Text Reference: pp. 198-199

11. **Answer: C**
Rationale: Compression of both the radial and ulnar arteries causes the hand to blanch as blood flow is blocked. On release of the ulnar artery, blood flow returns to the hand if collateral circulation is adequate. Hand color is restored within 5 to 10 seconds.
Text Reference: p. 199

12. **Answer: B**
Rationale: Carbon monoxide is not one of the tests measured in ABGs. The purpose of ABGs is to measure the amount of carbon dioxide in the blood in addition to the amount of oxygen and the ability of the lungs to exchange gases.
Text Reference: p. 196

13. **Answer: C**
Rationale: The syringe must be prepared using a heparin anticoagulant. Use of the other anticoagulants alters the specimen pH.
Text Reference: p. 197

14. **Answer: D**
Rationale: Under normal circumstances the appropriate cleaning techniques would be

to use both alcohol and povidone-iodine because of the increased risk of infection. However, all of the antiseptics listed are considered acceptable. Follow your facility's protocol and procedure for performing arterial blood draws.
Text Reference: p. 197

15. **Answer: C**
Rationale: Lidocaine is a type of anesthetic used locally at the site of ABG collection. Arterial blood draws can be painful and lidocaine can reduce the pain during collection. The use of lidocaine is optional. Some facilities use lidocaine routinely as a part of the procedure, whereas other facilities do not use it at all.
Text Reference: p. 197

16. **Answer: B**
Rationale: The minimum PPE for blood collection is gloves. A properly performed ABG collection typically does not yield blood spray for someone with experience. However, arterial blood may spray out of the puncture due to arterial pressure depending upon the skill level of the phlebotomist. A gown and face shield should also be used in procedures in which blood spray may be anticipated. Some facilities require goggles and mask, or face shield for all blood draws. Follow your facility protocol and procedures for PPE when performing ABG collection and other blood collection procedures.
Text Reference: p. 197

17. **Answer: C**
Rationale: Butterfly closures are used for closure of the skin when there is an incision and would not be of any use during an arterial blood collection.
Text Reference: p. 197

18. **Answer: D**
Rationale: Arterial blood is already under pressure. Therefore, there is no need to increase vessel pressure to facilitate arterial blood collection.
Text Reference: p. 197

19. **Answer: A**
Rationale: According to CLSI, arterial samples should be delivered to the lab and analyzed within 30 minutes of collection if plastic syringes are used. Glass syringes may require storing the specimen on a slurry of ice if transport to the lab is delayed but they should be delivered and analyzed within 1 hour of collection. Follow the protocols of your institution.
Text Reference: p. 200

20. **Answer: B**
Rationale: The radial artery may be accessed from the antecubital fossa; however, this is not the only place nor is it the best place for locating the artery. The artery is best accessed in the wrist on the thumb side.
Text Reference: p. 198

21. **Answer: C**
Rationale: The femoral artery is the largest artery used for collection of arterial blood gases. Due to the increased risk of infection and the risk of dislodging plaque from arterial walls, this procedure is only performed by a physician.
Text Reference: p. 198

22. **Answer: D**
Rationale: The radial artery is the most common artery used for this type of specimen collection and is routinely performed by trained personnel such as an MT/MLS, MLT, respiratory technician, nurse, and phlebotomist depending on the facility. The other sites require special training and qualifications for specimen collection from these areas.
Text Reference: p. 198

23. **Answer: D**
Rationale: All of the complications listed above could potentially occur with collection of arterial samples except for petechiae, which form on tourniquet application due to a platelet or bleeding disorder. In addition, hemorrhage, infection, and arteriospasm may also occur when collecting ABG samples.
Text Reference: p. 200

24. **Answer: C**
Rationale: Thrombosis is the formation of a clot within the artery or a vein. Thrombosis is a potential complication of the arterial puncture collection procedure.
Text Reference: p. 200

25. **Answer: D**
Rationale: Specimens that are transported to the laboratory on ice must be tested within 1 hour of collection.
Text Reference: p. 200

26. **Answer: B**
Rationale: Samples not transported as recommended in an ice slurry must be analyzed preferably within 5 to 10 minutes but not longer than 30 minutes of the collection time to provide accurate results.
Text Reference: p. 200

27. **Answer: B**
Rationale: Transportation of the ABG specimen drawn in a plastic syringe at room temperature is the appropriate transport recommendation to the laboratory. Any of the other conditions may cause an error in test results.
Text Reference: p. 200

28. **Answer: C**
Rationale: Transportation of the specimen in an ice slurry is the appropriate transport recommendation for ABGs drawn in glass syringes. Clotting, improper labeling, and inadequate volume of blood for testing can cause the specimen to be rejected on receipt in the laboratory.
Text Reference: p. 200

29. **Answer: C**
Rationale: Capillary blood gas testing is performed when an arterial sample collection is not possible or recommended. Pediatric patients are the patient population that requires the collection of capillary blood gases, particularly those pediatric patients in the neonatal intensive care unit (NICU) and newborn nursery.
Text Reference: p. 200

30. **Answer: A**
Rationale: Nerve damage is caused by inadvertent contact with a nerve during the puncture. Nerve damage is more likely to occur during ABG collection as a result of the depth the needle must travel through the tissue to reach the vessel.
Text Reference: p. 200

31. **Answer: C**
Rationale: The acceptable angle of needle insertion when performing a radial ABG is between 45° and 60° above the plane of the skin. Some references say between 30° and 45°. So an average angle would be around 45°.
Text Reference: p. 201

32. **Answer: D**
Rationale: Due to the depth of the femoral artery, the acceptable angle of insertion for a femoral arterial blood draw is 90°.
Text Reference: p. 198

33. **Answer: C**
Rationale: Arterial blood is pumped into the syringe in a pulsating mode as blood is pumped through the arteries. Color of arterial blood is not completely reliable due to inadequate lung function of some patients resulting in blood that appears darker in color than normal oxygenated blood that typically appears bright red.
Text Reference: p. 202

34. **Answer: B**
Rationale: The pulse must be checked distal to the arterial puncture to ensure adequate blood flow is present after the puncture. If the pulse is weak or absent then damage to the artery or the presence of a thrombus may be obstructing the flow of blood. The nurse should be immediately notified so that the doctor can order the proper protocol to restore circulation.
Text Reference: p. 202

35. **Answer: A**
Rationale: Normal blood pH is 7.35 to 7.45. A decrease in pH below 7.35 indicates acidosis. Values above 7.45 would indicate an alkalosis of the blood.
Text Reference: p. 196

36. **Answer: B**
Rationale: The phlebotomist may use plastic caps that are designed to work with the capillary tube. The tube must be sealed to prevent contamination of the specimen from the air.
Text Reference: p. 203

37. **Answer: B**
    Rationale: The proper insertion of the needle in a radial artery puncture is facing up and toward the upper arm facing the arterial blood flow into the hand.
    Text Reference: p. 201

38. **Answer: D**
    Rationale: Warming the heel for 5 to 10 minutes before the stick serves to maximize the arterial characteristics of the capillary blood and enhance blood flow to the area.
    Text Reference: p. 200

39. **Answer: B**
    Rationale: A flea is the appropriate term. The flea is used in *some* capillary arterial blood gas collection products to assist in mixing the sample with the anticoagulant. Mixing can also be achieved by rolling the capillary tube between the hands.
    Text Reference: p. 200

40. **Answer: D**
    Rationale: The use of any other anticoagulant besides heparin may cause an alteration in blood pH. The use of these anticoagulants would be a basis for the specimen to be rejected.
    Textbook Reference: p. 200

41. **Answer: A**
    Rationale: To preserve the integrity of the sample, it must be protected from exposure to atmospheric gases after collection by sealing the ends of the capillary tube and covering the end of the syringe.
    Text Reference: p. 200

42. **Answer: C**
    Rationale: It is not only important that the patient be in a respiratory steady state when the ABG collection is begun, but also that the patient remains in this state throughout the collection process. Keep patient calm to prevent hyperventilation, crying, or holding breath which would alter oxygen and carbon dioxide levels.
    Text Reference: p. 201

43. **Answer: A**
    Rationale: The amount of oxygen intake of the patient room air versus oxygen at a flow rate of 100%, etc., will affect the results of the ABGs and the mode of delivery (i.e., nasal canula). The patient must be at a steady respiratory status for at least 20 to 30 minutes before drawing ABGs.
    Text Reference: p. 201

SPECIAL COLLECTIONS AND PROCEDURES

Tina Lewis

INTRODUCTION

Although routine venipuncture is the most common procedure you will perform as a phlebotomist, special collecting or handling procedures are needed in situations for samples that involve one or more special circumstances. Fasting specimens, timed specimens, blood cultures, and blood donor specimens all require special handling, which may involve keeping the sample warm, cool, or away from light, or providing immediate delivery or legal documentation.

CONTENT OVERVIEW

Factors that Influence Blood Composition

I. Age
  A. Various test values vary with age (i.e., organ function declines, values elevated)
II. Altitude
  A. Higher altitudes result in higher red blood cell (RBC) counts due to decreased oxygen
III. Dehydration
  A. Hemoconcentration due to loss of fluids
IV. Environment
  A. Altitude—high
    1. Increases RBCs, hemoglobin (Hgb), and hematocrit (Hct)
V. Gender
  A. Values differ between sexes for various tests
  B. Hgb, Hct, RBC higher in males versus females
VI. Pregnancy
  A. Affects lab values due to increased fluid retention—dilution effect
VII. Stress
  A. Anxiety, crying, etc., increases white blood cell (WBC) count
  B. Hyperventilation alters ABG values (i.e., decreased pH, decreased pCO_2)
VIII. Diet
  A. Fatty meal results in elevation of triglycerides

B. Carbohydrate meal—good or bad carbs results in elevated glucose level for several hours
C. Nonfasting blood draw affects LDL/HDL levels, triglycerides, glucose
  1. Fasting required for these tests
IX. Diurnal variation
  A. Normal fluctuations of body chemistry
    1. Cortisol twice as high in morning versus afternoon
    2. Blood draws may be scheduled for diurnal peak and trough
  B. 12-hour fast required—glucose, triglycerides
X. Drugs—examples:
  A. Aspirin increases bleeding times
  B. Insulin decreases glucose levels—timed draws to monitor therapy
XI. Exercise
  A. Short-term: increases various analytes
    1. Enzymes such as muscle creatinine kinase (MCK)
    2. WBCs
    3. Creatinine
    4. Fatty acids
  B. Long-term: increases various analytes
    1. Sex hormones
    2. Aldolase
    3. Many of the same values increased in short-term exercise
XII. Body position
  A. Gravity induces fluid shift on standing
  B. Affects enzymes, albumin, blood cells
XIII. Smoking: increases various analytes
  A. Catecholamines
  B. Cortisol
  C. WBCs
  D. Mean corpuscular volume (MCV)
  E. Hgb
  F. Alters ABGs

Fasting Specimens and the Basal State

I. Diurnal variation
  A. Normal daily fluctuations in body chemistry
  B. Related to body cycles
    1. Hormonal cycles
    2. Sleep-wake cycles
    3. Other regular patterns of change

II. Basal state
   A. Body's state after 12 hours of fasting and abstention from strenuous exercise
      1. Normal reference values
         a. Based on the basal state
         b. Most routine phlebotomy rounds are scheduled for early morning draws when patients are more likely to be in a basal state
      2. Fasting specimens
         a. Glucose and triglycerides require a 12-hour fast—no food, caffeine, nicotine
            i. Caffeine and nicotine are metabolic stimulants and alter the basal state
         b. Water is allowed
         c. Regular medications taken or withheld per physician's instruction
         d. Must confirm with patient if they are fasting

III. Timed specimens
   A. Medication levels
      1. Change over time and must monitor
      2. Examples: digoxin, levodopa
   B. Change in patient condition
      1. Due to illness, injury, accident, surgery
      2. Example: Decrease in hemoglobin
   C. Normal diurnal variation at different times of the day
      1. Levels higher and lower depending on time of day
      2. Example: Cortisol higher in morning, lower in afternoon

IV. 2-hour postprandial test (i.e., diabetes mellitus)
   A. Compare FBS with glucose level 2 hours after eating full meal or ingesting a standardized dose of glucose
   B. Interpretation
      1. Normal: glucose levels normal at 2 hours
      2. Abnormal: glucose levels elevated at 2 hours; indicative of diabetes mellitus

V. Oral glucose tolerance test
   A. Timed testing: fasting, ½ hr, 1 hr, 2 hr, 3 hr, etc.
   B. Use same method of collection (i.e., venipuncture or dermal puncture for all samples)
      1. Venous blood glucose lower than capillary blood glucose
   C. Use same anticoagulant and specimen type
      1. Plasma and serum values 12% to 15% higher than whole blood glucose values

D. Urine may be collected at the same time
E. Ingest glucose solution within 5 minutes
F. Diagnose diabetes mellitus and other carbohydrate metabolism disorders
G. Hyperglycemia 3-hour oral glucose tolerance test (OGTT)
H. Hypoglycemia 5-hour OGTT
I. Gestational diabetes 1-hour OGTT

VI. Other tolerance tests
   A. Epinephrine tolerance test
      1. Mobilization of glycogen from liver
   B. Glucagon tolerance test
      1. Mobilization of glycogen from liver
   C. Lactose tolerance test
      1. Test for presence of lactase

VII. Diurnal variation
   A. Hormones (cortisol, testosterone, estradiol, progesterone)
   B. Serum Iron
   C. Glucose
   D. White blood cells, especially eosinophils

VIII. Therapeutic drug monitoring (TDM)
   A. Some drugs have a shorter half-life than others and require more frequent monitoring of peak and trough levels to be drawn
      1. Digoxin
      2. Procainamide
      3. Gentamicin
      4. Tobramycin
      5. Vancomycin
      6. Theophylline
      7. Dilantin
      8. Valproic acid

Blood Cultures

I. Purpose
   A. Ordered to test for the presence of microorganisms
      1. Septicemia—any pathogenic organism
      2. Bacteremia—bacterial infection
      3. Fever of unknown origin

II. Types of collection containers
   A. Long-necked bottles
      1. Vacutainer/needle
   B. Shorter bottles
      1. Winged infusion device
   C. Standard evacuated tubes (SPS anticoagulant)
   D. Sizes
      1. Standard
      2. Pediatric—ratio of blood to culture media important

E. Activated charcoal or antimicrobial removal device (ARD) to absorb antibiotics

F. Blood-to-broth ratio 1:3 to 1:5 is recommended
  1. Adults: 20–30 mL; 10–15 mL aerobic, 10–15 mL anaerobic
  2. children: recommend 6 mL—doubles detection rate versus collecting 2 mL

III. STAT and timed
  A. Just before spike in temperature if predictable
  B. Timed regular intervals (i.e., hourly)
  C. Just before antibiotic administration

IV. Multiple sites
  A. To differentiate skin contaminant from true pathogen
  B. Must be cultured from two different sites to be considered pathogen

V. Site preparation—disinfect with following according to facility protocol:
  A. Alcohol, povidone, iodine
  B. Povidone-iodine
  C. Benzalkonium chloride (BZK)
  D. Chlorhexidine
  E. One-step Medi-flex ChloraPrep applicator
  F. ChloraPrep Triple Swabsticks (chlorhexidine gluconate 2% w/v and isopropyl alcohol 70% v/v
    1. Do not use in children less than 2 months of age or weighing less than 750 g
    2. Infants 2 months and older use chlorhexidine gluconate per clinical and laboratory standards (CLSI)
  G. Under 2 months or less than 750 g—can use prepackaged sterile 70% alcohol prep, allow to air dry and repeat
  H. Air dry 1 minute after disinfecting

VI. Sample collection—set of 2
  A. Anaerobic sample—first sample
  B. Aerobic sample—second sample
  C. Anticoagulated tube—only one sample required
  D. Syringe draw—first sample transfer is anaerobic
  E. Butterfly infusion set—aerobic first, then anaerobic

Blood Donor Collection

I. Regulated by the AABB and the FDA
II. Screening process—records retained for 5 years
  A. Registration
  B. Age minimum—17 years old, 16 in some states
  C. Weight minimum—110 pounds
  D. Time between donations—8 weeks
  E. Interview and medical history
    1. Rejection examples: exposure to HIV or hepatitis; current drug use; cardiovascular conditions
  F. Physical examination
    1. Weight
    2. BP
    3. Pulse
    4. Hemoglobin (copper sulfate or automated) or spun hematocrit

III. Collection procedure
  A. Collection of one "unit" (405 to 495 mL [i.e., ½ L)
  B. Clean site by scrubbing with soap and water followed by 2% iodine or povidone-iodine swab stick or chlorhexidine as directed by facility protocol. Available are ChloraPrep Triple Swabsticks (chlorhexidine gluconate 2% w/v and isopropyl alcohol 70% v/v).
  C. Collection via large antecubital vein into sterile plastic bag via 16- or 18-gauge needle
  D. Remove needle and apply firm pressure until bleeding ceases
  E. Bandage site

IV. Autologous donation
  A. Donate every 72 hours if health good
  B. Hemoglobin greater than 11 g/dL

V. Therapeutic phlebotomy
  A. Polycythemia
  B. Hemochromatosis

Special Specimen Handling

I. Cold agglutinins—antibodies
  A. RBCs stick together (agglutinate) at room temperature in response to infection (i.e., *Mycoplasma pneumonia*)
  B. Prewarm tube to 37° C for 30 minutes
  C. Wrap in heel-warmer pack to keep warm until analyzed

II. Cryofibrinogen and cryoglobulin
  A. Same collection method as cold agglutinins

III. Chilled specimens: 1° to 5° C, transport to lab ASAP
  A. Arterial blood gas—if transport delay for glass syringe
  B. Ammonia

C. Lactic acid
D. Pyruvate
E. Glucagon
F. Gastrin
G. Adrenocorticotropic hormone (ACTH)
H. Parathyroid hormone

IV. Light-sensitive specimens—wrap in aluminum foil or use amber-colored microtube
A. Bilirubin
B. Beta-carotene
C. Vitamin A, beta-carotene
D. Vitamin B_6
E. Porphyrins

V. Time sensitive specimens—analyte unstable or volatile; test immediately after collection
A. Ammonia
B. Lactate
C. Platelet aggregation
D. Brain natriuretic peptide (BNP)
E. Prostatic acid phosphatase
F. ACTH
G. Aldolase

VI. Legal and forensic specimens—alcohol, drugs, DNA, paternity
A. Chain of custody requirements—NIDA (National Institute on Drug Abuse) has established these requirements:
1. Purpose and procedure of test must be explained to patient
2. Patient must sign a consent form
3. Patient must present picture ID
4. Specimen must be labeled correctly
5. Specimen must be sealed so as to identify any attempt at tampering
6. Specimen must be placed in a locked container for transport to testing site
7. Signatures required when specimen exchanges hands—person delivering and person receiving

VII. Legal alcohol collection
A. Do not clean site with alcohol. Use sterile soap, water, or other nonalcoholic antiseptic solution
B. Full tube draw required
C. Do not uncap sample

Blood Smears

I. Feathered edge, no holes, no streaks, etc.
II. Differential count—identify different types of WBCs, RBC morphology, platelet morphology
III. Reticulocytes
A. Assess percentage of reticulocytes released into peripheral blood from bone marrow
B. Used to access bone marrow response to blood loss, therapy, etc.

IV. Malaria smear—*Plasmodium*
A. 2 to 3 regular smears
B. 1 thick smear
C. Draw during or just before febrile state

CERTIFICATION PREPARATION QUESTIONS

1. The normal daily fluctuations in body chemistry related to hormonal cycles, sleep-wake cycles, and other regular patterns of change are known as:
   a. Therapeutic drug monitoring
   b. Hyperglycemia
   c. Diurnal variation
   d. Septicemia

2. By definition, the basal state of the body is the body's state after abstention from exercise and fasting for _____ hours.
   a. 6
   b. 12
   c. 20
   d. 24

3. All of the following factors influence blood composition, *except*:
   a. Age
   b. Stress
   c. Diet
   d. Height

4. The phlebotomist must check the fasting status of the patient before performing the venipuncture. Which of the following substances is *not* prohibited during a fasting period?
   a. Caffeine
   b. Water
   c. Nicotine
   d. Glucose

5. Which of the following ordered tests is usually drawn as a timed specimen?
   a. Cholesterol
   b. Triglycerides
   c. Digoxin
   d. CBC

6. Which of the following tests are used to test for diabetes mellitus?
   a. 2-hour postprandial test
   b. Epinephrine tolerance test
   c. Lactose tolerance test
   d. Glucagon tolerance test

7. An abnormally elevated blood sugar is found in which of the following condition(s)?
   a. Hyperglycemia
   b. Hypoglycemia
   c. Hyperlipidemia
   d. Hyperhidrosis

8. Which of the following tests is used to diagnose hypoglycemia?
   a. Glycohemoglobin
   b. 3-hour OGTT
   c. 5-hour OGTT
   d. Epinephrine tolerance test

9. When testing a 2-hour postprandial sample for glucose, the patient who is diabetic would have a glucose level that is:
   a. Higher than normal reference range
   b. Lower than normal reference range
   c. Identical to normal reference range
   d. Identical to the baseline sample value

10. How long must a patient fast before beginning an oral glucose tolerance test?
    a. 2 hours
    b. 6 hours
    c. 10 hours
    d. 12 hours

11. During glucose tolerance testing, the patient must be instructed to drink the standardized glucose solution within _____ minutes?
    a. 5
    b. 10
    c. 15
    d. 20

12. You have discovered that your GTT patient has just vomited in the waiting room not more than 20 minutes after ingesting the glucose solution. How should you proceed?
    a. Stop the test, document, and send the patient home
    b. Give the patient another dose of the glucose solution and continue test

c. Continue the test but document the time the patient vomited
d. Call the physician to see if the test should be continued or rescheduled

13. To maintain constant drug levels and make sure that a drug does not reach toxic levels in a patient, the phlebotomist may be called to perform blood collection for _____.
    a. Lipid monitoring
    b. Therapeutic drug monitoring
    c. Drug screening
    d. Toxicology

14. A blood infection by a pathogenic microorganism is known as _____.
    a. Septic shock
    b. Septicemia
    c. Bacteremia
    d. Fever of unknown origin

15. The nursing station calls the laboratory with orders for a set of blood cultures to be drawn. The nurse is newly licensed and wants to confirm the optimal time that they should be collected. You tell the nurse that the most optimal collection time for retrieval of a bacterial sample in the bloodstream is:
    a. In the morning when temperature is normal
    b. In the evening when temperature is elevated
    c. Just before temperature spike
    d. After medication to reduce the fever

16. The level of a drug that is drawn 30 minutes before the administration of the next dose is known as the:
    a. Peak level
    b. Trough level
    c. Therapeutic level
    d. None of the above

17. Blood cultures are drawn at timed intervals from multiple sites for all the following reasons, *except*:
    a. Increase the likelihood of retrieving pathogens
    b. Decrease the number of false positive tests
    c. Retrieve different organisms colonizing various vessels

d. Verify presence of known contaminant at two different sites

18. When collecting blood cultures the phlebotomist uses a butterfly winged infusion device. Which sample is typically drawn first?
    a. Anaerobic bottle
    b. Aerobic bottle
    c. Anticoagulated tube
    d. SST tube

19. All of the following antiseptic solutions are acceptable when preparing a venipuncture site for collection of blood cultures, *except*:
    a. Alcohol and povidone-iodine
    b. Povidone-iodine
    c. Isopropyl alcohol
    d. Soap and water

20. Which of the following organizations regulates and safeguards the collection procedures for blood donor collections?
    a. U.S. Food and Drug Administration
    b. Drug Enforcement Agency
    c. Centers for Disease Control and Prevention
    d. Occupational Health and Safety Administration

21. Which of the following must a blood donor provide on his or her registration?
    a. Name
    b. Address
    c. Date of birth
    d. All of the above

22. The phlebotomist will be performing blood donor draws at the local university and will be involved with screening the potential donors. Which of the following is *not* a reason for donor rejection during blood donor collection procedures?
    a. Exposure to HIV
    b. Exposure to hepatitis
    c. Race/ethnicity
    d. Drug consumption

23. The blood donor is screened for hemoglobin levels using this solution _____.
    a. Copper sulfate
    b. Copper oxalate
    c. Sodium sulfate
    d. Sodium oxalate

24. A first-time blood donor wants to know how much blood will be taken during the procedure. The phlebotomist states that the average volume of a "unit" of blood is:
    a. 250 mL
    b. 350 mL
    c. 450 mL
    d. 550 mL

25. The minimum gauge needle used for collection of blood for blood donation is _____ in size.
    a. 22 gauge
    b. 21 gauge
    c. 20 gauge
    d. 18 gauge

26. The donation of blood by a patient for his or her own use at a later time is known as:
    a. Directed donation
    b. Therapeutic phlebotomy
    c. Autologous donation
    d. None of the above

27. You have a patient with polycythemia vera who comes in on a regular basis to have blood drawn. The removal of blood from a patient's system to aid in treatment of a particular disorder is known as _____.
    a. Directed donation
    b. Therapeutic phlebotomy
    c. Autologous donation
    d. None of the above

28. The phlebotomist has just completed the collection of a specimen for cold agglutinins. What special collection and/or transport measures must be taken by the phlebotomist after collection of this sample?
    a. The specimen must be protected from light
    b. The specimen must be transported on ice
    c. The specimen must be collected in a prewarmed tube
    d. The specimen must be collected in a heparinized syringe

29. Which of the following specimen collections does not require the collection of the sample in a prewarmed tube?
    a. Cryoglobulin
    b. Sedimentation rate
    c. Cold agglutinins
    d. Cryofibrinogen

30. Which of the following sample collections does *not* require transportation of the sample to the laboratory in a chilled environment?
    a. Ammonia
    b. Vitamin A
    c. Gastrin
    d. Parathyroid hormone

31. The phlebotomist has just collected a specimen that needs to be protected from light during transportation to the laboratory. Which of the following specimens did the phlebotomist collect?
    a. Alkaline phosphatase
    b. Lactate dehydrogenase
    c. Beta-carotene
    d. Triglycerides

32. Which of the following specimens is *not* a time-sensitive specimen collection and does not need to be delivered to the lab immediately?
    a. Ammonia
    b. Glucagon
    c. Lactate
    d. Aldolase

33. Which of the following samples is *not* collected for use as evidence in a legal proceeding?
    a. Alcohol
    b. DNA analysis
    c. PKU testing
    d. Drug testing

34. The phlebotomist is called to the ER to pick up forensic specimens for a sexual assault. The most important concept the phlebotomist must adhere to in handling forensic specimens is proper:
    a. Specimen volume
    b. Specimen transportation
    c. Chain of custody
    d. Temperature of specimen

35. Collection of specimens for blood alcohol should be obtained using any of the following antiseptics, *except*:
    a. Soap and sterile water
    b. Iodine
    c. Cyclohexadiene
    d. Alcohol

36. Which of the following statements is *not* true regarding the collection of blood alcohol specimens?
    a. The site must not be cleaned with alcohol
    b. The patient must recline during blood collection
    c. Tubes must be filled as full as the vacuum tube will allow
    d. Specimen should remained capped until testing

37. Which of the following cells is *not* found on a normal peripheral blood smear?
    a. White blood cells
    b. Red blood cells
    c. Platelets
    d. Mast cells

38. Which of the following criteria is evaluated to determine if a peripheral blood smear is of adequate quality?
    a. The slide has a feathered edge
    b. The slide has no holes
    c. The slide has no streaks
    d. All of the above

39. When making a smear for examination for malaria, the phlebotomist should prepare which of the following?
    a. Three normal and one thick blood smear
    b. One normal and one thick blood smear
    c. Three wedge and one thick blood smear
    d. Two wet mounts and two normal blood smears

40. When should the phlebotomist draw a specimen for examination for malaria?
    a. On the patient's arrival at the facility
    b. Just before the patient's febrile episode
    c. 72 hours after onset of symptoms
    d. After chills and shaking subside

ANSWERS AND RATIONALES

1. **Answer: C**
   Rationale: Diurnal variation can influence the composition of blood. Most specimen collections should be scheduled when the patient is in the basal state.
   Text Reference: p. 207

2. **Answer: B**
   Rationale: In order for the body to be in the basal state, which is usually when most patients are scheduled for laboratory blood work, the patient must fast and refrain from exercise for 12 hours.
   Text Reference: p. 207

3. **Answer: D**
   Rationale: All of the factors above except height influence blood composition along with altitude, dehydration, environment, gender, pregnancy, diurnal variation, drugs, exercise, body position, and smoking.
   Text Reference: p. 207

4. **Answer: B**
   Rationale: Water is the only substance that the patient may be permitted to intake during a fasting period without impacting blood composition. Many physicians will even ask that the patient refrain from drinking water as well to avoid confusion in the patient in regard to liquid consumption.
   Text Reference: p. 207

5. **Answer: C**
   Rationale: Many medication levels are drawn as timed specimens such as digoxin. Other timed specimens include hemoglobin levels used to monitor internal bleeding, cortisol, and other hormone levels.
   Text Reference: p. 208

6. **Answer: A**
   Rationale: Both the 2-hour postprandial and oral glucose tolerance tests are used to aid in the diagnosis of diabetes mellitus.
   Text Reference: p. 208

7. **Answer: A**
   Rationale: Hyperglycemia by definition is the abnormal elevation in blood sugar usually caused by diabetes.
   Text Reference: p. 208

8. **Answer: C**
   Rationale: The 5-hour OGTT is used to diagnose hypoglycemia. Glycohemoglobin is used to monitor long-term glucose uptake. The 3-hour OGTT is most commonly used for hyperglycemia testing and epinephrine tolerance is used to

determine the body's capability to mobilize glycogen from the liver.
Text Reference: p. 208

9. **Answer: A**
   Rationale: In patients with diabetes, the 2-hour postprandial sample will show an increase in glucose that is higher than the normal glucose value. The 5-hour OGTT is used to diagnose hypoglycemia.
   Text Reference: p. 208

10. **Answer: D**
    Rationale: Patients are instructed to eat high-carbohydrate meals for several days and then fast for 12 hours before testing.
    Text Reference: p. 208

11. **Answer: A**
    Rationale: In order for the test to be administered correctly, the patient must consume the standardized glucose solution within 5 minutes.
    Text Reference: p. 208

12. **Answer: D**
    Rationale: If the patient vomits the glucose solution, it will invalidate the test results. Depending on the length of time between ingestion of the glucose solution and the episode of vomiting, a little or a lot of the solution may have been absorbed. The physician should be the one to make the decision to continue or reschedule the test.
    Text Reference: p. 209

13. **Answer: B**
    Rationale: Because people metabolize and excrete drugs at different rates, a standardized dose may not be beneficial to the patient. Therapeutic drug monitoring is used to ensure that the patient is receiving the appropriate amount of a drug for therapeutic purposes but not so much that the drug is toxic or dangerous to the patient. Also, TDM is used to ensure that therapeutic drugs actually reach a level in the plasma at which a patient will actually benefit from the drug.
    Text Reference: p. 210

14. **Answer: B**
    Rationale: Septicemia is the infection of the blood by a pathogenic microorganism.

Bacteremia refers specifically to a bacterial infection.
Text Reference: p. 210

15. **Answer: C**
Rationale: The most optimal time for retrieval of a microorganism in the blood is just before the time when the patient's temperature spikes. By recording patient temperatures, the spikes may be predicted and the phlebotomy may be scheduled accordingly.
Text Reference: p. 210

16. **Answer: B**
Rationale: The peak level is the highest level of the drug in the patient's blood, which will occur some time after the drug is administered. The lowest level of the drug in the blood is the trough level, which is drawn 30 minutes before the administration of the next drug dose.
Text Reference: p. 210

17. **Answer: C**
Rationale: Blood cultures have a low potential for organism retrieval and a high potential for contamination and therefore false positive results. By collecting multiple samples at various intervals, there is an increased chance of obtaining a sample containing the microorganism.
Text Reference: p. 210

18. **Answer: B**
Rationale: The aerobic blood culture bottle is drawn first. Anaerobic organisms cannot tolerate air. The first sample that is drawn has the most exposure to air because of the air in the tubing and is therefore best suited for aerobic culture. Syringe draws require the anaerobic bottle to be filled first. It is not recommended that blood culture bottles be drawn directly via a Vacutainer device and needle because of possible reflux of media into the patient. It is also difficult to accurately judge the sample volume.
Text Reference: p. 211

19. **Answer: D**
Rationale: In preparation of a blood culture collection site, the phlebotomist can cleanse the site with any of the antiseptics listed except soap and water. If the patient is allergic to iodine or iodine-based solutions, the phlebotomist should then use alcohol two times to cleanse the site. There are prepackaged swabs, such as Medi-flex ChloraPrep Triple applicator (chlorhexidine gluconate 2% w/v and isopropyl alcohol 70% v/v) or povidone-iodine triple prep.
Text Reference: p. 212

20. **Answer: A**
Rationale: The U.S. Food and Drug Administration along with the American Association of Blood Banks are responsible for the regulation and safeguarding of blood donor collection procedures.
Text Reference: p. 211

21. **Answer: D**
Rationale: During blood donor registration the potential donor must include his or her name, address, date of birth, and a written consent. All of this information must be retained for 5 years.
Text Reference: p. 211

22. **Answer: C**
Rationale: The race of the donor is irrelevant when collection of blood is for donation. All donors are considered unless they meet other qualifications for donor rejection.
Text Reference: p. 211

23. **Answer: A**
Rationale: A copper sulfate solution is used to determine hemoglobin levels of blood donors as a screening mechanism. Blood that sinks in copper sulfate because it is weighted by hemoglobin is acceptable for donation. Some donor centers use spun hematocrits.
Text Reference: p. 211

24. **Answer: C**
Rationale: The average volume of a unit of blood is 405 to 495 mL or approximately one half a liter (i.e., 450 mL).
Text Reference: p. 211

25. **Answer: D**
Rationale: The needle used for collection of blood for blood donation is a 16- or

18-gauge needle. The large needle size prevents hemolysis of the red blood cells during collection.
Text Reference: p. 211

26. **Answer: C**
Rationale: When a patient donates blood for his or her own personal use at a later date, the donation is known as an autologous donation. A directed donor is a person who donates blood for use by a person of their choosing for a specified purpose (usually for a family member or friend).
Text Reference: p. 213

27. **Answer: B**
Rationale: Therapeutic phlebotomy is used as part of a treatment protocol for disorders such as polycythemia and hemachromatosis. These units of blood are removed from the patient and cannot be used for transfusion to any other individual.
Text Reference: p. 213

28. **Answer: C**
Rationale: The specimen must be collected in a prewarmed tube and also must be transported to the lab in a warm environment. The specimen may be wrapped in an activated heel warmer for transport to the lab to keep the specimen warm.
Text Reference: pp. 213-214

29. **Answer: B**
Rationale: Sedimentation rate specimens are drawn in a lavender top EDTA tube and do not require prewarming of that tube. Cryoglobulin, cold agglutinins, and cryofibrinogen require collection in a prewarmed tube and transportation in a warm environment.
Text Reference: pp. 213-214

30. **Answer: B**
Rationale: Ammonia, gastrin, and parathyroid hormone require chilling during transportation to the laboratory. Vitamin A does require special transportation procedures; however, it does not require chilling. Vitamin A requires protection from light during transport to the lab.
Text Reference: p. 214

31. **Answer: C**
Rationale: Beta-carotene along with bilirubin, vitamin A, vitamin B_6, and porphyrins must all be light protected during transportation to the laboratory.
Text Reference: p. 214

32. **Answer: B**
Rationale: Glucagon specimens require chilling during transportation to the laboratory but are not time sensitive. Ammonia, lactate, and aldolase along with platelet aggregations, BNP, PAP, and ACTH specimens are all time sensitive and must be analyzed as soon as possible. Therefore, those samples must be transported to the laboratory immediately.
Text Reference: p. 215

33. **Answer: C**
Rationale: PKU testing is a legally required test performed on all infants as part of the metabolic screening test; however, it is not a test used for evidence in a legal proceeding.
Text Reference: pp. 214-215

34. **Answer: C**
Rationale: Specimen volume and transportation protocols must be followed; however, the most important concept in handling forensic specimens is the chain of custody protocol. The protocol ensures that the sample is always in the custody of a person legally entrusted to be in control of it.
Text Reference: p. 215

35. **Answer: D**
Rationale: Using alcohol to cleanse the site may alter the test result and render the test inadmissible in any legal proceeding surrounding the patient's condition at the time of blood collection.
Text Reference: p. 215

36. **Answer: B**
Rationale: Patient position does not impact blood alcohol concentration and therefore is not a true statement. The site must not be cleansed with alcohol; the tube must be completely filled so that alcohol does not escape into the space between the cap and the surface of the blood; and the tube

should remain uncapped to prevent the loss of alcohol. Violation in any of these areas would compromise the integrity of the specimen and render it inadmissible.
Text Reference: p. 215

37. **Answer: D**
Rationale: Mast cells are basophils that have moved into tissue and therefore would not be present on a normal peripheral blood smear.
Text Reference: pp. 100-104, 215

38. **Answer: D**
Rationale: The attributes of a good slide include a good feathered edge with no holes or streaks in the smear. In addition, the slide should not be too thick or too long. The slide also should not be too short or to thin.
Text Reference: p. 214

39. **Answer: A**
Rationale: Since malaria is a difficult disease to diagnose, the optimal sample for organism retrieval would be for the phlebotomist to collect three normal smears and then one thick blood smear for review by the technologists.
Text Reference: pp. 216, 218

40. **Answer: B**
Rationale: The best chance of isolating the malarial organisms is just before the start of the patient's febrile episode. These episodes are cyclic and are dependent on the type of malarial organism infecting the patient.
Text Reference: pp. 216, 218

SPECIAL NONBLOOD COLLECTION PROCEDURES

Tina Lewis

INTRODUCTION

A phlebotomist is rarely just a phlebotomist today. In addition to collecting blood, you may be called on to collect nonblood specimens, assist the nurse or physician in doing so, or instruct patients regarding the procedures for collecting or handling such specimens. Nonblood specimens can provide valuable information about a patient's health or disease state. Each of the specimen types discussed in this chapter review is collected to provide special information about physiologic processes occurring in the body or about the presence of infection or foreign substances. Strict adherence to collection protocols is as important for these procedures as it is for blood collection. Nonblood specimens include urine, feces, semen, and other bodily fluids. Special handling procedures are needed for some specimens to maintain sterility, preserve specimen integrity, or ensure chain of custody.

CONTENT OVERVIEW

Urine Specimens
I. What is the test?
   A. Called urinalysis or UA
      1. Must be delivered to lab within 1 hour of collection
      2. Can delay delivery if refrigerated
   B. Test included
      1. Physical
      2. Chemical
      3. Microscopic
         a. Some labs perform on every specimen
         b. Some labs perform only if chemical analysis is abnormal
II. Why collect a urine specimen?
   A. Provides valuable insight into the inner workings of the body
      1. Prerenal conditions
      2. Renal conditions
      3. Postrenal conditions
III. Types of urine specimens
   A. Random specimen
      1. Screening sample
   B. First morning specimen
      1. Pregnancy test
   C. Timed specimen—2 hour, 12 hour, 24 hour with refrigeration or preservative
      1. Proteins (i.e., creatinine)
      2. Hormones
      3. Creatinine clearance test
IV. Urine preservatives
   A. Refrigeration
   B. Boric acid
      1. Allows for urine to remain at room temperature
      2. Provides comparable results with refrigerated urine
      3. One of the most common preservatives
   C. Tartaric acid
      1. Allows for urine to remain at room temperature
      2. Provides comparable results with refrigerated urine
      3. One of the most common preservatives
   D. Hydrochloric acid
   E. Thymol
   F. Nitric acid
   G. Acetic acid
   H. Toluene
V. Collection procedures for urine specimens
   A. Midstream clean catch
      1. Clean genitalia using sterile soap, specially prepackaged towelettes, etc.
         a. Women spread labia, begin cleansing at urethra moving outward
         b. Men pull back foreskin if uncircumcised, begin cleansing at urethra moving outward
      2. Collect sample—do not touch inside of container with hand
         a. Void into toilet
         b. Move container into flow collecting midstream until 3/4 full
         c. Void final portion into toilet
      3. Complete procedure
         a. Seal container with lid
         b. Refrigerate or add preservative as required for test
         c. Label with name, date, time of collection

B. Pediatric collection
  1. Collect by attaching a soft, clear self-adhesive plastic bag over child's genital area
  2. Collection is non-sterile
C. Catheter collection
  1. Collection by physician, nurse, other trained personnel
  2. Insertion of catheter into bladder through urethra
  3. Used when patient unable to collect clean-catch specimen for C & S
VI. Suprapubic aspiration
  A. Collected by physician
  B. Cases of suspected anaerobic infection or cytologic cell examination
VII. Urine samples for drug testing
  A. Random clean-catch sample into chemically clean container
  B. Chain of custody guidelines followed—fresh specimen would register at room temperature

Fecal Specimens

I. Why collect a fecal specimen?
  A. Look for intestinal infection and to screen for colorectal cancer
II. Types of fecal specimens
  A. Random specimen
    1. Bacterial cultures
    2. O & P
    3. Fats and fibers
  B. Occult blood specimen
    1. Collect 3 days after meat-free diet
    2. Avoid aspirin, vitamin C
  C. Seventy-two hour stool specimen
    1. Quantitative fecal fat
III. Collection procedure for fecal specimens
  A. Appropriate collection container
  B. Proper patient instructions
    1. Directly into container
    2. No urine or water contamination
    3. Room temperature or refrigerated depending on test ordered
  C. Proper specimen transport
    1. Tightly sealed
    2. Wrapped in plastic bag
  D. Prompt specimen delivery

Semen Specimens

I. Why collect a semen specimen?
  A. Used to determine whether viable sperm are present in the semen

II. Collection procedure for semen specimen
  A. Proper patient instructions
    1. Avoid ejaculation 3 days prior
  B. Sterile plastic collection container
  C. Time of specimen collection recorded
  D. Record partial or complete sample
  E. Specimen transported at body temperature
  F. Deliver to lab within 30 minutes

Throat Specimens

I. Why collect a throat specimen?
  A. Used to diagnose throat infection (i.e., Group A *Streptococcus*)
  B. Tests performed include Rapid Strep test and/or culture
II. Collection procedure for throat specimen
  A. Assemble equipment
  B. Collect sample with sterile swab
  C. Avoid tongue
  D. Process and transport sample

Nasopharyngeal Specimens

I. Why collect a nasopharyngeal specimen?
  A. Used to diagnose whooping cough, croup, pneumonia, and other respiratory tract infections
II. Collection procedure for nasopharyngeal specimen
  A. Collect with cotton or Dacron sterile-tipped wire
  B. Swab nostril to reach back of nasopharynx
  C. Rotate swab and remove sample
  D. Process and transport sample in transport or growth media

Nasal Washing

I. Why collect nasal washings?
  A. Used to test for RSV and influenza

Culture and Sensitivity Testing

I. Performed on any body fluid or body tissue or organ
  A. Cerebrospinal fluid (CSF)
  B. Urine
  C. Peritoneal fluid
  D. Synovial fluid
  E. Pericardial fluid
  F. Wound
  G. Eye
  H. Skin
  I. Throat
  J. Etc.
II. Process

A. Body fluid, tissue, or swab is submitted for culture
B. Sensitivity testing performed in order to identify best antibiotic to be used in treatment of infection

Sweat Electrolyte Specimens—Sweat Chloride Test

I. Why collect a sweat (chloride) electrolyte specimen?
A. Used for diagnosis of cystic fibrosis
II. Collection procedure for sweat (chloride) electrolyte specimen
A. Iontophoretic pilocarpine test—iontophoresis
B. Collect sweat using sterile filter paper
C. Cover filter paper with paraffin and use forceps to handle
1. Weighed
2. Analyzed coulometrically—electrical charge to measure conductivity of the electrolyte
3. Amount of chloride in sweat is measured.
a. Values greater than 60 milliequivalents (mEq) are indicative of cystic fibrosis
b. Intermediate values of 35 to 60 mEq require repeat testing

Cerebrospinal Fluid Specimens—STAT Collection

I. Why collect a cerebrospinal fluid (CSF) specimen?
A. To diagnose meningitis or other central nervous system infections
II. Collection procedure for CSF
A. Done only by a physician via lumbar puncture
B. Sample tubes are numbered in order of collection
C. Tubes delivered to appropriate department by number
1. Tube 1—microbiology, room temperature
2. Tube 2—chemistry, room temperature
3. Tube 3—hematology, refrigerate
4. Order and site of delivery may vary by institution's policy
D. Special transport and temperature requirements

Body Fluid Specimens

I. Why draw body fluids?
A. Body fluids are drawn for analysis or therapy and are always collected by the physician
B. Fluid is collected in a sterile container, labeled, and transported STAT
II. Synovial fluid

A. Collected from joint space
B. Diagnose arthritis or for pain reduction
III. Peritoneal fluid
A. Collected from abdominal cavity
B. Diagnose ascites—abnormal accumulation of peritoneal fluid
IV. Pleural fluid
A. Collected from cavity surrounding lungs
B. Diagnose pleural pneumonia
V. Pericardial fluid
A. Collected from area around the heart
B. Diagnose pericarditis

Amniotic Fluid Specimens

I. Why collect amniotic fluid specimens?
A. Reflects what is going on in utero
1. Formed by metabolism of fetal cells
a. Comprised of transfer of water across placenta
b. Comprised of fetal urine during third trimester
B. Analyzed for genetic disorders—Down syndrome
C. Analyzed for fetal lung age
1. Traditional test lethicin/sphingomyelin ratios
2. Newer test fluorescence polarization test (ratio of phospholipids to albumin)
D. Analyzed for hemolytic disease of the newborn—assess bilirubin level
E. Analyzed for spina bifida—assess proteins (i.e., alpha fetal protein)
II. Collection procedure for amniotic fluid specimens
A. Collected by a physician during amniocentesis
B. Fluid collected into sterile container
C. Fluid protected from light
D. Transport to lab immediately

CERTIFICATION PREPARATION QUESTIONS

1. Which of the following specimens provides the physician with a "snapshot" of the inner workings of the body?
a. Throat culture
b. Stool specimen
c. Urine specimen
d. CSF specimen

2. Which of the following urine specimens would be best for urine pregnancy testing?
   a. Random specimen
   b. First morning void
   c. Catheter collection
   d. 24-hour urine collection

3. The physician suspects the patient may have a urinary tract infection (UTI) and orders a UA. Which of the following samples is the *best* collection for screening for obvious abnormalities in urine such as a UTI?
   a. Random specimen
   b. First morning void
   c. Catheter collection
   d. 24-hour urine collection

4. Which of the following specimens is the best to detect low levels of certain compounds, which are excreted in various amounts at different times of the day?
   a. Random specimen
   b. First morning void
   c. Catheter collection
   d. 24-hour urine collection

5. A patient arrives at the lab for a urine C & S (culture and sensitivity). What specimen do you instruct the patient to collect?
   a. Random specimen
   b. Midstream clean catch
   c. First morning void
   d. 24-hour urine collection

6. The phlebotomist is instructing the patient in the collection of a midstream clean-catch urine. The proper order of steps once hands are washed is:
   a. Cleanse; void portion into container; void remainder into toilet
   b. Cleanse; void portion into toilet; void remainder into container
   c. Void portion into toilet; cleanse; collect remainder into container
   d. Cleanse, void portion into toilet; void portion into container; void remainder into toilet

7. Which of the following urine samples is collected using a soft, clear plastic bag with an adhesive strip that fits over the genital area?
   a. Midstream clean catch
   b. First morning void
   c. Catheter collection
   d. Pediatric urine collection

8. You are performing blood draws at the local nursing home and have an order for a urine culture on one of your regular patients who is severely physically challenged. What would the specimen of choice be for the collection of the urine culture from this patient?
   a. Random specimen
   b. Midstream clean catch
   c. Catheter collection
   d. Pediatric urine collection

9. The med-surg unit calls down to say they have an order for a patient suspected of having an anaerobic urinary tract infection. They want to know how it should be collected. What type of specimen would you tell them needs to be collected?
   a. Midstream clean catch
   b. Random
   c. Suprapubic aspiration
   d. Catheter

10. You are involved in the chain of custody for collection of a urine drug screen and have just received the voided specimen. A freshly collected urine sample for urine drug screening should be at what temperature?
    a. Refrigerated
    b. Normal body temperature
    c. Room temperature
    d. None of the above

11. All of the following are a part of chain of custody sampling for urine drug screening, *except*:
    a. Special forms
    b. Specimen seals
    c. Specialized collection containers
    d. Special cleansing pads

12. Which of the following samples is used to test for the presence of intestinal infections and/or to screen for colorectal cancer?
    a. Urine specimen
    b. Stool specimen
    c. Throat culture
    d. Sweat electrolyte

13. A phlebotomist is instructing a patient on how to properly collect a stool sample for occult blood testing. The patient should be instructed to refrain from the consumption of meat for how many days?

a. 1
b. 2
c. 3
d. 5

14. Which type of fecal specimen is used to determine the presence of parasites and their eggs?
    a. Random fecal specimen
    b. Occult blood specimen
    c. 24-hour fecal specimen
    d. 72-hour fecal specimen

15. A patient has an order for collection of fecal fat. Which of the following fecal specimens would the phlebotomist instruct the patient to collect to determine the presence of fecal fat?
    a. Random fecal specimen
    b. Occult blood specimen
    c. 72-hour specimen
    d. Loose stool specimen

16. The phlebotomist is documenting lab receipt of a fecal specimen from a patient. What condition(s) would indicate that the fecal specimen is unacceptable?
    a. Does not contain any urine
    b. Not at room temperature
    c. Collected from the toilet
    d. Refrigerated

17. Before the collection of a semen specimen, the patient must be instructed not to ejaculate for _____ days.
    a. 1
    b. 3
    c. 5
    d. 7

18. In order for a semen sample to be analyzed before the deterioration of the sperm, the patient must be instructed to deliver the semen sample to the lab within _____ minutes of collection.
    a. 10
    b. 20
    c. 30
    d. 45

19. The phlebotomist is giving the patient instructions on the collection of a semen sample for fertility studies. At what temperature should the phlebotomist

clearly emphasize that a semen sample be transported to the laboratory?
    a. Body temperature
    b. Refrigerated
    c. Frozen
    d. Warmed

20. Volume of semen samples submitted for analysis can vary for a number of reasons. In which semen analysis procedure is the volume of the sample an issue?
    a. Success of a vasectomy
    b. Forensic specimen for rape victim
    c. Fertility testing of male
    d. Sample for in vitro fertilization

21. Which of the following specimens is used to diagnose a potential streptococcus infection?
    a. Nasopharyngeal swab
    b. Throat culture swab
    c. Sweat electrolyte
    d. Sputum sample

22. All of the following are reasons to use a tongue depressor during collection of a throat culture, *except*:
    a. To make the throat more visible
    b. To make collection of the sample easier
    c. To prevent contamination of the swab
    d. To keep patient from gagging

23. A throat swab may be used for which of the following tests?
    a. Strep culture
    b. Whooping cough
    c. RSV
    d. Influenza

24. A pediatric patient has an order for a nasopharyngeal culture. A nasopharyngeal culture is used to diagnose all of the following, *except*:
    a. Cystic fibrosis
    b. Whooping cough
    c. Croup
    d. Pneumonia

25. What collection device is used to collect a nasopharyngeal sample?
    a. Sterile collection cup
    b. Nonsterile cotton swab
    c. Sterile cotton tipped wire
    d. None of the above

26. Which of the following diseases may be diagnosed in part by a sweat electrolyte specimen?
    a. Chagas disease
    b. Cystic fibrosis
    c. Down syndrome
    d. Tourette syndrome

27. Which of the following testing mechanisms is necessary for collection of sweat (chloride) electrolyte samples?
    a. Immunoelectrophoresis
    b. Protein electrophoresis
    c. Iontophoretic pilocarpine test
    d. Immunodiffusion

28. The collection device used to obtain a sweat electrolyte sample is a sterile:
    a. Vial
    b. Filter paper
    c. Specimen cup
    d. Cuvette

29. Special precautions must be taken during collection of the sweat chloride sample to preserve the integrity of the specimen. These precautions dictate that:
    a. The patient must not move during collection
    b. The filter paper must be handled without the use of gloves
    c. The filter paper must be wrapped in paraffin during collection
    d. The patient should be kept warm throughout the procedure

30. The phlebotomist is called to the ER to assist the physician with the collection of a CSF specimen. Which of the following procedures will the physician use for collection of a CSF specimen?
    a. Lumbar puncture
    b. Core needle biopsy
    c. Epidural injection
    d. Paracentesis

31. CSF specimens are *most* commonly used to diagnose which of the following diseases?
    a. Meningitis
    b. Paralysis
    c. Seizure disorders
    d. Migraine headaches

32. What is the *most* important procedural step that a phlebotomist must follow when assisting in collection of CSF samples?
    a. Refrigerate the entire sample
    b. Number the tubes in order of collection
    c. Deliver all tubes to the lab within 1 hour of collection
    d. Record sample color when collected

33. Which tube in the CSF collection order should the phlebotomist deliver to the microbiology lab?
    a. Tube 1
    b. Tube 2
    c. Tube 3
    d. Tube 4

34. Which of the following samples is collected from the space between the joints?
    a. Synovial fluid
    b. Peritoneal fluid
    c. Pleural fluid
    d. Pericardial fluid

35. Which of the following samples is collected from the abdominal cavity?
    a. Synovial fluid
    b. Peritoneal fluid
    c. Pleural fluid
    d. Pericardial fluid

36. Which of the following samples is collected from the area that surrounds the heart?
    a. Synovial fluid
    b. Peritoneal fluid
    c. Pleural fluid
    d. Pericardial fluid

37. Which of the following samples is collected from the area surrounding the lungs?
    a. Synovial fluid
    b. Peritoneal fluid
    c. Pleural fluid
    d. Pericardial fluid

38. The process by which amniotic fluid is obtained is known as _____.
    a. Fluidic aspiration
    b. Thoracentesis
    c. Amniocentesis
    d. Electrophoresis

39. Screening tests are available for certain genetic defects of an unborn fetus. All of

the following conditions may be diagnosed using amniotic fluid, *except*:
a. Down syndrome
b. Fetal lung age
c. Hemolytic disease of the newborn
d. Cleft palate

40. The phlebotomist is called up to the unit to pick up an amniotic specimen. Which of the following special precautions must be taken when transporting an amniotic sample?
a. The sample must be refrigerated
b. The sample must be protected from light
c. The sample must be transported on a swab
d. The sample must be centrifuged on collection

ANSWERS AND RATIONALES

1. **Answer: C**
Rationale: The urine specimen can provide the physician with valuable information about multiple body systems and functions by analysis of salts, waste products, and many other molecules that naturally circulate throughout the bloodstream but may be excreted by the body via urine. Prerenal, renal, and postrenal snapshots are provided in analysis of urine.
Text Reference: p. 222

2. **Answer: B**
Rationale: First morning specimens are collected right after the patient awakens and are very concentrated. This sample provides the highest concentration of analyte constituents of any urine sample and therefore has the highest retrieval rate for substances that may not be found in a more dilute or random sample.
Text Reference: pp. 222-223

3. **Answer: B**
Rationale: A UTI can usually be identified by analysis of a random specimen. The random specimen can be collected at any time and can provide the physician with valuable general information regarding the concentration of proteins, glucose, and other significant constituents of urine, but the first morning specimen provides the highest concentration of analyte constituents

and is therefore considered to be the best specimen of choice.
Text Reference: p. 223

4. **Answer: D**
Rationale: The 24-hour urine collection is used to detect low levels of certain proteins and hormones. Timed specimens are used to determine the average value of those substances that are excreted in the urine at various times throughout the day.
Text Reference: p. 223

5. **Answer: B**
Rationale: The midstream clean-catch urine is the preferred sample for performing a culture and sensitivity. The sample is collected using a sterile cup and provides the least likelihood of contamination by external bacterial sources.
Text Reference: p. 223

6. **Answer: D**
Rationale: The purpose of collecting a midstream, clean-catch urine is to collect a urine specimen that will have a lower rate of bacterial contamination external to the urinary tract system when performing C & S testing on the sample. This method will produce a specimen that is free from any external bacteria and bacteria surrounding the urethral opening and any genital secretions. The proper order after the patient washes his or her hands is to cleanse first, void a portion of urine into the toilet, move the container under the stream to collect a portion, remove the container from the stream, and void the remainder into the toilet.
Text Reference: p. 224

7. **Answer: D**
Rationale: Urine sample collection on infants and very small children may be difficult. The easiest way to collect these samples is through the use of a soft, clear plastic bag that is fitted to the genital area via an adhesive strip. This collection is not a sterile collection procedure.
Text Reference: p. 223

8. **Answer: C**
Rationale: The physical disabilities of the patient would make it difficult for the patient

to properly collect a clean-catch specimen. A catheterized specimen is collected by a physician or nurse via a catheter that is inserted through the urethra directly into the bladder to maintain the integrity of the specimen. When a urinary tract infection is suspected and the patient is unable to collect a midstream clean-catch specimen, then catheter collection is the method of choice.
Text Reference: p. 222

9. **Answer: C**
Rationale: UTIs suspected of being anaerobic in nature need to be collected via suprapubic aspiration in order to protect the specimen from exposure to oxygen, which may be detrimental to recovery and survival of the organisms. Urine samples collected by suprapubic aspiration must be collected by the physician. A needle is inserted through the abdominal wall and into the bladder for collection of this sample. This procedure is beyond the scope of practice for a nurse, medical assistant, or a phlebotomist.
Text Reference: p. 223

10. **Answer: B**
Rationale: If a urine sample is freshly voided, it should be near normal body temperature when the sample is collected and presented to the phlebotomist. The collection containers for urine drug screening contain a temperature strip on the outside for verification of the sample temperature. Sample temperature must be recorded at the time of collection.
Text Reference: pp. 223, 225

11. **Answer: D**
Rationale: Collection and handling procedures for specimens for urine drug screens must follow established chain of custody procedures. These procedures include special forms that must be completed by the person collecting the sample, specimen seals, and specialized collection containers.
Text Reference: pp. 223, 225

12. **Answer: B**
Rationale: A stool specimen is the specimen of choice for detecting the presence of parasites and their eggs, fecal fat, and occult blood.
Text Reference: p. 225

13. **Answer: C**
Rationale: The patient must abstain from eating meat for a period of 3 days before collection of stool for occult blood testing. If the patient does not follow these instructions the sample may yield a false-positive result.
Text Reference: p. 225

14. **Answer: A**
Rationale: A random specimen is used for most fecal determinations, including bacterial cultures and ova and parasites.
Text Reference: p. 225

15. **Answer: C**
Rationale: A 72-hour fecal specimen is used for quantitative fecal fat determination. A special large container must be provided to the patient for specimen collection. While not routinely requested, this test is still used to measure the amount of fat that is present in the stool and the percentage of dietary fat that is not absorbed into the body.
Text Reference: pp. 225-226

16. **Answer: C**
Rationale: A fecal specimen should never be retrieved from the toilet as it could be contaminated by cleaning agents and urine. A sample that has been exposed to urine may be falsely contaminated with bacterial agents other than those typically found in feces. Patients should not collect samples that have been contaminated with urine for fecal analysis. Fecal specimens can be kept at room temperature or refrigerated depending on the test.
Text Reference: p. 226

17. **Answer: B**
Rationale: The patient must be instructed to avoid ejaculation for 3 days before collection of a semen sample for analysis to ensure the appropriate sample.
Text Reference: p. 226

18. **Answer: C**
Rationale: Sperm die quickly and therefore must be transported to the laboratory within 30 minutes of collection to ensure viability of the sample.
Text Reference: p. 226

19. **Answer: A**
    Rationale: The sample should be kept as close to body temperature as possible, and transported to the lab within 30 minutes or less to ensure specimen viability.
    Text Reference: p. 226

20. **Answer: C**
    Rationale: Due to the nature of fertility testing, the sample must have an adequate volume to accurately represent the state of the semen in the patient.
    Text Reference: p. 226

21. **Answer: B**
    Rationale: The throat culture swab is used to diagnose throat infections including those most commonly caused by the bacteria streptococcus.
    Text Reference: p. 226

22. **Answer: D**
    Rationale: The use of the tongue depressor serves multiple purposes, including making access to the back of the throat easier. Most important, however, is that the tongue be kept from contaminating the swab. The swab should also not touch the lips or side of the cheek to avoid contamination. Gagging may occur with the use or without the use of a tongue depressor.
    Text Reference: pp. 226-227

23. **Answer: A**
    Rationale: The throat swab is used to perform throat cultures or rapid strep testing. A separate swab must be collected for each test performed. Nasopharyngeal swabs are used for whooping cough and other upper respiratory infections (URIs). Influenza may use nasal washing specimens. RSV specimens include nasal washings, nasal swab and nasal or tracheal aspirate depending upon test methodology.
    Text Reference: p. 226

24. **Answer: A**
    Rationale: The nasopharyngeal swab is used to detect the presence of many types of upper respiratory infections such as whooping cough, croup, pneumonia, and bronchitis.
    Text Reference: p. 226

25. **Answer: C**
    Rationale: Due to the narrow nasal passages and the need for the collection device to reach the back of the nasopharynx, a very small cotton or Dacron-tipped wire is used to collect the mucus sample for a nasopharyngeal sample.
    Text Reference: p. 226

26. **Answer: B**
    Rationale: Sweat electrolyte testing is performed as part of the diagnosis of cystic fibrosis. A person with cystic fibrosis will have elevated levels of chloride in the sweat. This test is often referred to as a sweat chloride test.
    Text Reference: p. 228

27. **Answer: C**
    Rationale: The iontophoretic pilocarpine test administration requires special training. During this test, sweating is induced by producing a weak electrical current which draws the drug pilocarpine into the skin in the testing area.
    Text Reference: p. 228

28. **Answer: B**
    Rationale: The sweat is collected onto a piece of sterile filter paper or gauze, which is then weighed and analyzed coulometrically to determine chloride levels.
    Text Reference: p. 228

29. **Answer: C**
    Rationale: The filter paper must be wrapped in paraffin during the collection procedure to prevent any evaporation of the sweat from occurring during the actual testing process.
    Text Reference: p. 228

30. **Answer: A**
    Rationale: The collection of a cerebrospinal fluid specimen must be performed by a physician during a lumbar puncture, which is also referred to as a spinal tap procedure. During this procedure a needle is placed between the vertebrae at the base of the spine and the CSF sample is aspirated.
    Text Reference: p. 228

31. **Answer: A**
    Rationale: CSF specimens are most commonly obtained to rule out or confirm the presence of meningitis that is either viral or bacterial in nature. CSF can also be used to aid in the diagnosis of other central nervous system infections as well.
    Text Reference: p. 228

32. **Answer: B**
    Rationale: The numbering of the tubes as they are collected is essential to the correct analysis of CSF. Each tube is labeled and delivered to a different laboratory department dependent on the tests that may be ordered by the physician.
    Text Reference: p. 228

33. **Answer: A**
    Rationale: Typically, the first tube collected is delivered to the microbiology lab for analysis for microorganisms. Tubes 2 and 3 are delivered to chemistry and hematology respectively for testing.
    Text Reference: p. 228

34. **Answer: A**
    Rationale: Synovial fluid is the name given to any fluid that is removed from the space between joints, such as the knee, elbow, or shoulder, for example.
    Text Reference: p. 228

35. **Answer: B**
    Rationale: Peritoneal fluid is the name given to any fluid that is drawn from the abdominal cavity.
    Text Reference: p. 228

36. **Answer: D**
    Rationale: The area around the heart may fill with fluid. Fluid samples taken from the area around the heart are known as pericardium or pericardial fluid.
    Text Reference: p. 228

37. **Answer: C**
    Rationale: Pleural fluid is the fluid that is collected from the area surrounding the lungs.
    Text Reference: p. 228

38. **Answer: C**
    Rationale: Amniotic fluid must be collected by a physician during a very risky procedure known as amniocentesis.
    Text Reference: p. 228

39. **Answer: D**
    Rationale: Down sydrome, fetal lung age, and hemolytic disease of the newborn may be diagnosed using amniotic fluid analysis. Cleft palate is prenatally diagnosed using MRI, not amniotic fluid. The fluid may also be used to diagnose or predict the presence of other diseases, such as spina bifida and other genetic disorders.
    Text Reference: p. 228

40. **Answer: B**
    Rationale: Because amniotic samples are analyzed for bilirubin content to aid in the determination of the presence of hemolytic disease of the newborn, the sample must be protected from light.
    Text Reference: p. 228

SPECIMEN TRANSPORT, HANDLING, AND PROCESSING

Tina Lewis

INTRODUCTION

Proper handling of specimens after collection is critical to ensure the accuracy of the test results obtained from them. Analytes may change in composition and concentration over time and with temperature changes or exposure to light. The best drawing technique in the world is meaningless if the sample is not processed according to established guidelines. Transport systems may be as simple as direct delivery to the lab or as complex as motorized carrier systems routed through a central distribution site. In the lab, the central processing station catalogs the sample, centrifuges it, and prepares aliquots for distribution to other departments. Rejection of specimens can be prevented with proper attention to collection techniques, handling, and transport.

CONTENT OVERVIEW

General Guidelines for Specimen Transport

I. General requirements
   A. Additive tubes properly mixed—gently invert 5 to 10 times for proper mixing and to minimize hemolysis
   B. Properly labeled
   C. Place in upright position after collection
      1. Promotes clot formation
      2. Prevents contamination of specimen with stopper
      3. Reduces likelihood of aerosol formation
   D. Transport per institution guidelines (i.e., leak-resistant bag)
   E. Transport outside the institution to other labs requires biohazard labeled, crush-resistant containers with absorbent material inside
II. Time constraints
   A. Glycolysis
      1. The metabolic breakdown of glucose within blood cells
      2. Continues after removal of blood from the body
      3. Preanalytical handling of the specimen greatly impacts specimen quality.
   B. Tests affected by glycolysis
      1. Glucose
      2. Calcitonin

3. Phosphorus
4. Aldosterone
5. Different enzymes
   C. Delivery times to lab depend on type of sample
      1. Routine—within 45 minutes
      2. STAT—immediately
      3. Timed—ASAP after draw
      4. ASAP—ASAP after draw
   D. Separation of cells from plasma or serum should take place within 2 hours per Clinical Laboratory Standard Institute (CLSI) standards
      1. Most specimens remain stable for longer periods after separation
      2. After 2 hours, test values may be erroneous
         a. Glucose falsely decreases
         b. Potassium falsely elevated
         c. Lactate dehydrogenase falsely elevated
      3. Appropriate storage (i.e., room temp, refrigeration, freezing, 37° C depends on sample type and test ordered)
      4. Sodium fluoride inhibits glycolysis— glucose samples collected in gray-stopper tubes are good for long periods
         a. Room temperature: 24 hours
         b. Refrigeration at 2° to 8° C: 48 hours
      5. EDTA specimens
         a. 24 hours
         b. Blood smears from EDTA must be made within 1 hour of collection to prevent distortion of cell morphology
III. Temperature considerations
   A. Temperature extremes can result in hemolysis of specimen.
      1. Keeping specimens warm at 37° C during collection and transport
         a. Prewarm tubes in activated heel-warmer
         b. Transport tubes in activated heel-warmer
         c. Incubation of specimen
            i. Notify lab staff on arrival of specimen
            ii. Place in incubator until testing can be performed (i.e., EDTA

specimen for CBC on patient
with cold agglutinins)
  d. Tests
    i. Cold agglutinins
    ii. Cryofibrinogen
  2. Keeping specimens cool
    a. Slows down metabolic processes
    b. Keeps analytes stable during
       transport and processing
    c. Slurry of crushed ice and water so
       specimen i.e., cells don't freeze
    d. Tests
      i. Blood gases—if glass syringe and
          delayed delivery
      ii. Lactic acid
      iii. Ammonia
  3. Keeping specimens at room temp
    a. Place specimen in transport device
       per institution's protocols
    b. Keep at room temperature
    c. Courier specimens—place in cooler
       to protect from extreme heat or cold
IV. Protecting specimens from light
  A. Light-sensitive analytes need to be
     protected from light exposure
  B. Methods of protecting specimens include
     one of the following:
    1. Amber-colored microtubes
    2. Wrap in aluminum foil
    3. Place in brown envelope or heavy
       paper bag
  B. Tests that require protection from light
    1. Bilirubin
    2. Vitamin B_{12}
    3. Folate
    4. Carotene
    5. Urine porphyrin

Transporting Samples to the Lab
I. Modes of transportation are dependent on
    size of institution and degree of specialization
  A. Factors to consider in determining the
     type of specimen transportation system:
    1. Reliability of system
    2. Speed of delivery
    3. Preservation of specimen
    4. Cost versus alternative
II. Hand carried
  A. Directly to laboratory and received per
     hospital protocol
  B. Drop-off/pick-up station within hospital with
     standards for documentation and tracking
    1. Logbook

    a. Log specimen drop-off—protocol as
       determined by institution
      i.   Date
      ii. Time
      iii. Name
      iv. Hospital number
      v.   Room number
      vi. Type of specimen
      vii. Name of delivery person
    b. Laboratory personnel pick-up
      i. Specimens documented as
          directed above
  2. Delivered and received into lab per
     institution protocol
III. Pneumatic tube system
  A. Uses sealed containers that run through a
     network of tubes
  B. Shock absorbing foam inside carrier
     containers
  C. Samples may be routed to central station
     and then on to lab
  D. Used for paperwork and/or blood
     specimens
IV. Motorized vehicles on tracks
  A. Small, self-contained motorized carriers
     run on tracks from different areas of
     hospital—deliver specimens, etc.
V. Courier delivery
  A. Samples may be picked up at sites
     remote to the hospital (i.e., physician
     offices, small clinics, etc.)
    1. Sample must be processed at collection
       site due to time delay between courier
       pick-ups
    2. Scheduled courier pick-up and delivery
       times
VI. Overnight mail
  A. Requires special packaging for
     specimens to ensure protection and
     integrity of sample and to prevent
     contamination of other materials during
     transport

Processing
I. Safety—OSHA guidelines
  A. PPE worn during sample processing
  B. PPE required
    1. OSHA-approved gown
    2. Gloves
    3. Protective face gear
      a. Goggles and face mask
      b. Chin-length face shield
      c. Countertop safety shield

II. Central processing
   A. Log date and time of arrival
   B. Check accession number
   C. Sort by destination and sample type
   D. Centrifuge specimens if needed—tubes remained capped during centrifugation
      1. Prevents contamination of specimen
         a. Dust
         b. Sweat
         c. Powder from gloves
         d. Other contaminants
      2. Prevents aerosolization
      3. Cap removal may result in alteration of specimen
         a. Increase in pH as CO_2 is released
         b. Evaporation of analytes (i.e., alcohol, ketones, etc.)
   E. Aliquot if needed
III. Clotting
   A. Complete clotting of specimen
      1. Allow 30 to 45 minutes clotting time at room temperature
      2. Clot activator tubes reduce clotting time (i.e., 30–60 minutes depending on tube used; check manufacturer recommendations)
      3. Thrombin reduces clotting time to 5 minutes
      4. Specimens that may require longer clotting time
         a. Specimens from patients on heparin or Coumadin
         b. Chilled specimens
         c. Specimens with high WBC counts
   B. Incomplete clotting of specimen
      1. Sample continues to clot after separation
      2. Interferes with testing
IV. Centrifuging
   A. Process of centrifugation occurs at high speeds
   B. Separates out components of the specimen on the basis of density
      1. Dense cellular elements at bottom
      2. Less dense plasma or serum moves to top layer
   C. Types of centrifuges
      1. Tabletop
      2. Floor models
      3. Refrigerated
   D. Principles of operation
      1. Balance specimens—may need a water balance tube
      2. Centrifuge at speed and time recommended for testing of sample

   3. Unbalanced centrifugation
      a. Rotor damage
      b. Movement during centrifugation— may fall off counter
      c. Direct danger to lab personnel
      d. Breakage of specimens—biohazard
   E. Repeated centrifugation is not recommended
      1. Hemolysis may occur
      2. Analytes may deteriorate
V. Removing a stopper
   A. Major risk—aerosolization on removal of stopper resulting from contamination of stopper with blood during collection and transport
   B. Automated instruments allow for penetration of stopper without the need for removal
   C. Hemaguard stoppers help reduce formation of aerosol
   D. Commercial stopper removers available
   E. Stopper removal process
      1. Behind tabletop safety shield or
      2. Place 4×4-inch gauze over top of stopper
      3. Pull up and twist if necessary
      4. Do *not* rock stopper or pop it off
      5. Use caution on tubes without gel separators to avoid remixing of sample
VI. Preparing aliquots
   A. Do *not* pour aliquot—use disposable pipetting system
   B. Label and cap before delivery
VII. Transport and processing of nonblood specimens
   A. Microbiology samples
      1. Transport immediately to increase chances for recovery of pathogenic organisms
      2. Collected in transport media collection device—no further processing
      3. Refrigerate if required
      4. Room temperature if required
   B. Twenty-four hour urine collection
      1. Measure volume and record
      2. Aliquot as required for test
   C. Stool samples
      1. Room temperature if required
      2. Refrigerate if required
VIII. Specimen rejection
   A. Improper or inadequate identification
   B. Hemolysis
   C. Incorrect tube for test ordered

D. Incorrect tube collected (i.e., EDTA instead of serum separator tubes [SST])
E. Expired tubes
F. Inadequate ratio of blood to additive (i.e., short draw on sodium citrate tube, may clot, results erroneous)
G. Insufficient volume for testing—QNS (quantity not sufficient)
H. Specimen drawn at incorrect time (i.e., therapeutic drug level)
I. Contaminated specimen (i.e., urine C & S in nonsterile container)
J. Improper handling (i.e., cold agglutinins not kept warm)

CERTIFICATION PREPARATION QUESTIONS

1. How many times should a tube of blood containing an anticoagulant be inverted immediately after drawing?
   a. Does not need to be inverted
   b. 5 to 10 times
   c. 15 to 20 times
   d. 25 to 30 times

2. The label printer is malfunctioning and you must hand label the specimens you collected on your inpatient. Of the information listed below, which of the following is *not* required to be on the specimen label?
   a. Patient name
   b. Date of collection
   c. Date of birth
   d. Time of collection

3. You are returning to the lab from performing house calls at the local nursing home. You ensure that your specimen tubes remain in the upright position during specimen transport if at all possible for all of the following reasons, *except*:
   a. It promotes complete clot formation of the sample
   b. Prevents sample contamination due to prolonged contact with the stopper
   c. Reduces the likelihood of aerosol formation during stopper removal
   d. Slows down the metabolic processes of cells during transport

4. What is glycolysis?
   a. The breakdown of sugar

b. The breakdown of cholesterol
c. The breakdown of triglycerides
d. The breakdown of enzymes

5. As a general rule, what is the maximum amount of time that should elapse before a specimen is delivered to the laboratory?
   a. 15 minutes
   b. 30 minutes
   c. 45 minutes
   d. 60 minutes

6. You are in charge of processing specimens at your outpatient drawing center. It has been a busy day and you are ready for lunch. You still have specimens that need processing and must verify those that are in need of processing before you leave. According to the Clinical and Laboratory Standards Institute (CLSI), what is the maximum amount of time that should elapse before cells should be separated from plasma or serum?
   a. 3 hours
   b. 2 hours
   c. 1 hour
   d. 30 minutes

7. Due to the inhibition of glycolysis, which anticoagulated tube may be sustained up to 24 hours at room temperature without separation of cells and plasma?
   a. Sodium citrate
   b. Sodium fluoride
   c. Potassium EDTA
   d. Sodium EDTA

8. Blood smears that are to be made from EDTA whole blood should be made from the tube within what time parameter?
   a. 15 minutes
   b. 30 minutes
   c. 1 hour
   d. 24 hours

9. As a phlebotomist you know the importance of preanalytical factors that can preserve or compromise the integrity of a specimen. Which of the following does *not* result in sample hemolysis?
   a. Vigorous shaking of the collection tube
   b. Extreme temperature changes
   c. Traumatic collection procedures
   d. Exposure to ultraviolet light

10. Hemolysis is defined as:
    a. Destruction of white blood cells
    b. Destruction of red blood cells
    c. Increased lipid content
    d. Increased bilirubin content

11. The phlebotomist has received an order to draw a specimen from a patient known to have a cold agglutinin. The test that has been ordered requires that an EDTA whole blood tube be collected in a prewarmed tube and remain warmed until testing. The test ordered is a:
    a. BUN
    b. CK-MB
    c. CBC
    d. ALT

12. Which of the following tests requires prewarming of the collection tube and transportation of the specimen to the lab in an activated heel-warmer?
    a. Cryoglobulins
    b. C-reactive protein
    c. Rapid plasma reagin
    d. Ammonia

13. You have just been diverted to draw a STAT H & H and electrolytes after completing a draw on your current patient. You will be delayed in the delivery of your specimen but don't know how long the STAT draw will take as the physician is still examining the patient. You decide to place one of your specimens in a slurry of ice. Which of the following samples did you collect that requires chilling of the sample during transportation to the laboratory?
    a. Arterial blood gases
    b. Complete blood count
    c. Prothrombin time
    d. Phosphorus

14. Which of the following tests does *not* require that the collection tube be protected from light during laboratory transport?
    a. Bilirubin
    b. Folate
    c. Calcium
    d. Carotene

15. The phlebotomist is preparing to go to the floor to draw a light-sensitive specimen and must make sure the collect cart has the appropriate transport material available. Which of the transportation techniques is *not* suitable for the transportation of a light sensitive analyte?
    a. Wrap the specimen tube in aluminum foil
    b. Place tube in center rack surrounded by other specimens
    c. Place the sample in a brown envelope or heavy paper bag
    d. Collect the sample in amber-colored microtube

16. The phlebotomist has an order to draw all of the following tests. Which one of the test samples must be protected from light?
    a. Vitamin B_{12}
    b. Aldolase
    c. Potassium
    d. Creatinine

17. Which of the following factors may influence the laboratory's decision to use a pneumatic tube system for specimen delivery?
    a. Reliability of system
    b. Speed of delivery
    c. Specimen damage during transport
    d. All of the above

18. Who regulates the use of personal protective equipment used in laboratory specimen processing?
    a. OSHA
    b. CLIA
    c. TJC
    d. CDC

19. Which of the following is *not* appropriate personal protective equipment for laboratory specimen processing?
    a. Gloves
    b. Scrub jacket
    c. Goggles
    d. Face shield

20. You are responsible for cataloging the specimens being delivered by the courier to the laboratory. Which of the following is a unique identifying number that you will use for cataloging samples in the laboratory?
    a. Patient identification number
    b. Social security number
    c. Accession number
    d. Lot number

21. You are called to assist in central processing. The specimens that you are given to process require the separation of small portions of plasma or serum from cellular elements to individual containers called:
    a. Centrifugation
    b. Aliquots
    c. Accessioning
    d. Sampling

22. All of the following conditions may occur if the stopper of a tube is removed before or comes off during centrifugation *except*:
    a. Carbon dioxide is released
    b. pH of the sample rises
    c. Evaporation of the sample occurs
    d. Lipemia develops

23. The phlebotomist has drawn a series of plain red top tubes (no additives) for immunologic testing. At room temperature, complete clotting of these tubes will occur in what time frame?
    a. 5 to 10 minutes
    b. 15 to 20 minutes
    c. 30 to 45 minutes
    d. 1 hour

24. At room temperature, complete clotting of a tube containing clot activators such as serum separator gels occurs in what time frame?
    a. 10 minutes
    b. 20 minutes
    c. 30 minutes
    d. 1 hour

25. Your lab has just implemented the use of thrombin tubes for some chemistry analytes and you are in charge of processing the tubes on your shift. How long should you wait to centrifuge the thrombin tubes that have been sitting at room temperature to ensure complete clotting of a tube?
    a. 5 to 10 minutes
    b. 15 to 20 minutes
    c. 30 to 45 minutes
    d. 1 hour

26. At room temperature, plasma may be removed from the clot after what time period?
    a. 5 to 10 minutes
    b. 15 to 20 minutes

c. 30 to 45 minutes
d. Not at all

27. Centrifugation separates a sample on the basis of what?
    a. Velocity
    b. Component density
    c. Cell type
    d. Sample size

28. You have just come down from the floor and your samples are ready for centrifugation. What is the most important principle of centrifuging specimens that you must consider?
    a. Specimens must be full draws
    b. Tubes must be balanced
    c. Stopper colors must be matched
    d. All tubes must be clotted

29. You load the centrifuge with specimens, close the lid, turn it on, and begin to walk away when all of a sudden you hear a loud noise and see the centrifuge bouncing on the counter. You must assess the situation after turning off the centrifuge. Which of the following will *not* occur as a result of an unbalanced centrifuge?
    a. The centrifuge may move during operation
    b. Tube breakage may occur during process
    c. Sample may become icteric due to breakage of cells
    d. The rotor of the centrifuge may spin out of the center

30. As a conscientious phlebotomist you are very careful to ensure that you process your specimens only after they have completely clotted and handle plasma specimens with care because you know repeated centrifugation can compromise the specimen. Which of the following will *not* occur as a result of repeated centrifugation?
    a. Hemolysis
    b. Deterioration of analytes
    c. Volume depletion
    d. Erroneous results

31. A microscopic mist of blood that forms droplets that may be released into the atmosphere surrounding the sample is a(n):
    a. Aerosol
    b. Microclot

c. Fume

d. Vapor

32. The phlebotomist was unable to collect two SST tubes to be delivered to two different departments and must now prepare an aliquot so that both departments will have a specimen. Which of the following techniques is recommended for removal of a sample from a collection tube containing a stopper?

   a. Use a needle to aspirate out the sample

   b. Rock the stopper from side to side

   c. Cover the stopper with a 4×4 gauze

   d. Use a serum separator device

33. It is not advisable to pour off serum or plasma when making sample aliquots for all of the following reasons, *except*:

   a. Splashing may occur

   b. Aerosols may form

   c. Plasma samples may remix

   d. Unequal volumes may be aliquoted

34. You were called to the operating room (OR) to pick up a microbiology specimen collected during surgery and hurry back to deliver it to the microbiology department. Why must microbiology specimens be transported to the lab immediately?

   a. To increase the likelihood of recovering pathogenic organisms

   b. Because of increased processing time required for microbiology samples

   c. Due to the instability of the specimen transport media for microorganisms

   d. The physician is waiting for the STAT report on the identification of the organism

35. Before making aliquots of a 24-hour urine sample, what must a phlebotomist do?

   a. Record the patient's delivery time

   b. Measure and record the total sample volume

   c. Sterilize the collection container

   d. Contact the physician

36. You are processing specimens received from the community clinic and write QNS across one of the requisitions. What does the acronym QNS stand for?

   a. Quality not standard

   b. Quality not sufficient

   c. Quantity not standard

   d. Quantity not sufficient

37. The phlebotomist is assigned to assist with specimen processing for a few hours in the morning. In the process of receiving and checking specimens for acceptability the phlebotomist finds an SST tube that is half filled, accepts it, and then finds a sodium citrate tube that is partially full and rejects the specimen. Why would the sodium citrate specimen be rejected?

   a. The quantity of blood is insufficient to perform the test requested

   b. The blood to anticoagulant ratio is altered, yielding erroneous results

   c. The tube was not labeled properly and requires that a new tube be drawn

   d. Both tubes are acceptable for testing and should not be rejected

38. Improper mixing of a tube containing an anticoagulant on blood collection will result in all of the following, *except*:

   a. The patient must be redrawn

   b. Clot formation may occur in the tube

   c. The specimen will be lipemic

   d. The specimen will be rejected

39. All of the following are acceptable modes of specimen delivery to the laboratory, *except*:

   a. Patient delivery

   b. Overnight mail

   c. Pneumatic tube system

   d. First-class mail

40. In the transportation of specimens it is crucial that anyone who must handle the specimen be protected from possible contamination. Which of the following is the safest way to transport samples to the laboratory from within the hospital for the protection of anyone who might come in contact with that sample?

   a. Cardboard box

   b. Sharps container

   c. Leak-resistant biohazard bag

   d. Test tube rack

ANSWERS AND RATIONALES

1. **Answer: B**

   Rationale: A tube of blood that is drawn that contains an anticoagulant should be inverted at least 5 to 10 times immediately

after drawing. Inverting the tube ensures that the anticoagulant is properly mixed with the blood specimen to prevent the formation of clots.
Text Reference: p. 233

2. **Answer: C**
Rationale: The tube label should contain the patient's name, a second identifier that is not the patient's date of birth or social security number, the date and time of collection, and the phlebotomist's initials, at minimum. Second identifiers should be a number that is unique to only that patient. For security purposes social security numbers are not used. The patient's date of birth is not sufficient as a second identifier, there could potentially be two patients with the same name (e.g., John Smith) that have the same birth dates.
Text Reference: pp. 140, 233

3. **Answer: D**
Rationale: Although it is not always feasible to transport blood collection tubes to the laboratory in the upright position, it is recommended for all of the reasons listed above. Any time a specimen can be transported in the upright position, it only further ensures the potential for accurate test reporting.
Text Reference: p. 233

4. **Answer: A**
Rationale: Glycolysis is the metabolic breakdown of sugar within cells. Glycolysis is the primary cause of inaccurate test results, including tests for glucose, calcium, phosphorus, aldosterone, and many enzymes.
Text Reference: p. 233

5. **Answer: C**
Rationale: Routine laboratory tests should be delivered to the lab within 45 minutes of collection. STAT laboratory tests should be delivered to the lab immediately after collection.
Text Reference: p. 233

6. **Answer: B**
Rationale: According to the CLSI, no more than 2 hours should elapse before cells are

separated from plasma or serum. Separation of the cells from the plasma or serum helps maintain the specimen integrity. Once the cells are separated out, the plasma or serum may be kept for longer periods of time. Storage temperatures for the plasma or serum will be dependent on the sample type and the tests ordered.
Text Reference: p. 233

7. **Answer: B**
Rationale: Because fluoride inhibits glycolysis, glucose samples that are collected in sodium fluoride tubes may remain intact without being separated for up to 24 hours at room temperature and 48 hours if refrigerated. If the specimen cannot be analyzed in that time frame, however, the cells must be separated from the plasma.
Text Reference: pp. 233-234

8. **Answer: C**
Rationale: EDTA will eventually begin to distort the cell morphology that is examined on a peripheral blood smear if it remains in contact with those cells for prolonged time periods. The EDTA sample is stable for up to 24 hours for analysis but blood smears should be made within 1 hour of collection.
Text Reference: p. 234

9. **Answer: D**
Rationale: Hemolysis occurs when the samples are exposed to extreme temperature changes, such as heating or cooling inappropriately, shaking of the collection tube, and traumatic collection procedures.
Text Reference: p. 234

10. **Answer: B**
Rationale: Hemolysis occurs when red blood cells are lysed within the sample. Hemolysis causes a discoloration of the plasma or serum from a normal yellow color to a pink or red color dependent on the amount of hemolysis that has occurred.
Textbook Reference: pp. 134, 177-178, 234, 237

11. **Answer: C**
Rationale: Cold agglutinins cause the red blood cells to agglutinate together. This agglutination

can cause problems in whole blood CBC analysis on the instrumentation and on review of the peripheral blood smear if the specimen is not handled appropriately. BUN, CK-MB, and ALT are drawn in clot tubes and are not affected.
Text Reference: p. 234

12. **Answer: A**
Rationale: Both cryoglobulin and cold agglutinin samples must be collected in a prewarmed tube and then transported to the laboratory warm as well. Transportation to the laboratory in a warm condition may be easily accomplished by the use of an activated heel-warmer.
Text Reference: p. 234

13. **Answer: A**
Rationale: Arterial blood gas samples, especially those collected in a glass syringe must be transported immediately after collection to the laboratory in a combination of cold water and ice if there is a delay in delivery. Transporting the sample under any other condition will cause erroneous test results.
Text Reference: pp. 200, 234

14. **Answer: C**
Rationale: Samples collected for the analysis of calcium do not require transportation of the sample in a light-protected collection device. Calcium is, however, affected by glycolysis and the samples must have the serum or plasma removed from the cells as soon as possible to prevent erroneous results. Bilirubin, folate, and carotene must all be protected from light or the analyte will deteriorate.
Text Reference: p. 234

15. **Answer: B**
Rationale: Aluminum foil, brown envelope, heavy paper bag, or amber-colored microcollection tube may be used for protection of a light-sensitive analyte during transportation to the laboratory and would be available per the institution's protocol. It is the phlebotomist's responsibility to make sure that the appropriate transport material is at hand on completion of the draw *before* leaving the lab.
Text Reference: p. 234

16. **Answer: A**
Rationale: Of the samples listed above, only vitamin B_{12} requires that the specimen be

protected from light before analysis during transportation to the lab and specimen processing.
Text Reference: p. 234

17. **Answer: D**
Rationale: The laboratory must assess the efficiency and effectiveness of a pneumatic tube system for the transportation of laboratory specimens before the inception of this type of transport mechanism.
Text Reference: p. 235

18. **Answer: A**
Rationale: The Occupational Safety and Health Administration is responsible for the regulation of personal protective equipment usage in all aspects of laboratory services. TJC may also check for regulation compliance but the actual regulation comes from the OSHA Standards.
Text Reference: p. 236

19. **Answer: B**
Rationale: OSHA requires that laboratory personnel wear full-length lab coats with closed cuffs that button or snap down the front. Surgical scrub jackets do not fit those criteria.
Text Reference: p. 236

20. **Answer: C**
Rationale: The accession number is a number assigned to a particular sample that allows cataloging of that sample by the laboratory for future reference and reporting purposes.
Text Reference: p. 236

21. **Answer: B**
Rationale: Samples are often centrifuged in a central processing area of the laboratory and then small samples of serum or plasma (aliquots) are separated into individual containers and delivered to appropriate areas of the laboratory for testing.
Text Reference: p. 236

22. **Answer: D**
Rationale: Stoppers should remain on all samples that are being centrifuged to prevent release of carbon dioxide, increase in pH of sample, and evaporation of certain analytes. Lipemia is the cloudy appearance of serum or plasma due to the presence of

triglycerides and is not affected by removal of the stopper. In addition, the sample may become contaminated and the likelihood of aerosol formation is increased.
Text Reference: p. 236

23. **Answer: C**
Rationale: Complete clotting of a sample collected in a nonadditive tube may take up to 45 minutes at room temperature.
Text Reference: p. 236

24. **Answer: C**
Rationale: Serum separator gel decreases the clot formation time by activating the clotting process much quicker than tubes containing no additives and usually is achieved in about 30 minutes or so per manufacturer directive.
Text Reference: p. 236

25. **Answer: A**
Rationale: Thrombin is a clot activator that rapidly increases the formation of clotting in any sample. Complete clotting may occur in samples collected in thrombin additive tubes in as little as 5 minutes.
Text Reference: p. 236

26. **Answer: D**
Rationale: Plasma samples can only be obtained from anticoagulated specimens, not clotted specimens. Specimens containing anticoagulants do not clot if properly collected and mixed.
Text Reference: p. 236

27. **Answer: B**
Rationale: Centrifugation separates serum or plasma from the cellular components of the blood based on density. In addition, the cellular components that are denser move to the bottom of the tube and the lighter cells will form layers on top of the heavier cells. The plasma or serum will remain on top of the cellular elements regardless of their orientation in the tube.
Text Reference: p. 236

28. **Answer: B**
Rationale: Balancing of the specimens is critical in centrifugation. If the specimens are of different numbers or volumes, a balance

tube containing water may be used. Not all tubes requiring centrifugation are clot tubes (i.e., coagulation tubes).
Text Reference: p. 236

29. **Answer: C**
Rationale: Icteric samples occur from the presence of bilirubin in the serum or plasma in excess amounts. Centrifugation in an unbalanced centrifuge will not cause the sample to be icteric.
Text Reference: p. 236

30. **Answer: C**
Rationale: Specimens should only be centrifuged one time if at all possible. Repeat centrifuging may result in hemolysis or deterioration of the analyte and produce an erroneous test result. It does not change the sample volume.
Text Reference: p. 236

31. **Answer: A**
Rationale: Aerosols may form during centrifugation. If the stopper of a tube is removed improperly after centrifugation, the aerosols may be released into the laboratory area when the tube is opened.
Text Reference: p. 237

32. **Answer: C**
Rationale: It is recommended that processing personnel use 4 × 4 gauze to cover the stopper and then pull the stopper straight up to remove. It is acceptable to twist the stopper as you pull upward to aid in the removal process. Serum separator devices are not used in any way to aid in stopper removal. Never rock the stopper back and forth as this increases the risk for aerosols.
Text Reference: p. 237

33. **Answer: D**
Rationale: When making sample aliquots, it is recommended to use a disposable pipette or pipetting system to make aliquots. The use of a pipette or pipetting system will decrease the potential for splashing, aerosol production, and the contamination of plasma samples with cellular components due to remixing.
Text Reference: p. 237

34. **Answer: A**
    Rationale: Many pathogenic organisms are very susceptible to collection and transport conditions. To increase the chances of isolating the organism in the sample, the sample should be transported immediately.
    Text Reference: p. 238

35. **Answer: B**
    Rationale: The phlebotomist must always measure and record the total sample volume if the sample will be divided into aliquots before delivery to the laboratory departments. If the phlebotomist is unable to measure and record the volume, then the entire sample must be delivered to the laboratory.
    Text Reference: p. 238

36. **Answer: D**
    Rationale: QNS means that the quantity of the sample provided to the laboratory is not sufficient to perform the requested test.
    Text Reference: p. 238

37. **Answer: B**
    Rationale: If the sodium citrate tube is not completely full, the blood to anticoagulant ratio will be altered and the specimen will be diluted. This alteration will cause test results to be erroneous and therefore the specimen will be rejected.
    Text Reference: p. 238

38. **Answer: C**
    Rationale: The specimen that is collected in a tube containing an anticoagulant that has not been properly mixed will not be accepted by the laboratory. Clot formation can alter various test results. Lipemia is not a result of improper mixing. Hemolysis may occur if the specimen is vigorously inverted. The sample will be rejected and the patient will have to be redrawn before the requested test can be completed.
    Text Reference: p. 233

39. **Answer: D**
    Rationale: Specimens may be delivered to the lab via courier, the phlebotomist, collection staff, overnight mail, a pneumatic tube system, or, on occasion, by the patient. First-class mail would take 2 to 3 days or longer, resulting in deterioration of specimen analytes and erroneous test results.
    Text Reference: p. 238

40. **Answer: C**
    Rationale: Specimens that must be transported to the laboratory should be placed in a leak-resistant biohazard bag. These bags identify the potential hazard associated with the sample contained inside as well as provide a barrier to those handling the specimen should that specimen leak.
    Text Reference: p. 235

QUALITY PHLEBOTOMY

Tina Lewis

INTRODUCTION

Quality phlebotomy is a set of policies and procedures designed to ensure the highest quality patient care, consistent specimen analysis, and reduction of errors, increased efficiency, and cost effectiveness. Continual, gradual improvement in the standard of care delivered is the goal of quality phlebotomy. The phlebotomist is best able to control preanalytical variables, which are those that influence patient care and sample integrity before analysis in the lab. Patient preparation, specimen collection, and transport and processing are critical areas for quality phlebotomy. You have learned the important precautions and techniques designed to maintain both patient comfort and safety and the quality of the sample collected. Those items will be reviewed and the lab procedures that have an impact on the quality of test results will be discussed. Quality assurance programs are not optional. They are required by the The Joint Commission (TJC) (formerly known as The Joint Commission on Accreditation of Healthcare Organizations [JCAHO]).

CONTENT OVERVIEW

Features of Quality Phlebotomy

I. Total quality management (TQM)
  A. Policies and procedures to ensure customer satisfaction
  B. Gradual, continual improvements in the quality of services provided
  C. Includes both quality control and quality assurance
    1. Major goal is continuous quality improvement
    2. No minimum threshold standard only upward improvement
    3. Customers
      a. Patients
      b. Physicians
      c. Other health care providers (i.e., phlebotomists who have direct patient contact and are responsible

for customer satisfaction in area of blood draws).
II. Quality assurance (QA)
  A. Specific program
  B. Sets standards that include policies and procedures
  C. Guarantee quality patient care: technical and non-technical
    1. Procedure performance standards
    2. Documentation
      a. Lab procedure manual
      b. Floor book distributed to nursing stations, other departments (see Floor Book)
        i. Detailed schedules
        ii. Variables affecting patient care and test results
      c. Continuing education of lab personnel
    3. Monitoring of procedural compliance
    4. Track patient outcomes
    5. Monitor resolution of problems
    6. Monitor customer satisfaction and complaints
    7. Scheduled evaluation of all lab activities
III. Quality control (QC)—part of QA
  A. Quantitative methods that are used to monitor the quality of procedures to ensure accuracy of test results
    1. Regular inspection of equipment
    2. Calibration of equipment
    3. Monitor methods or protocol for patient prep, identification, collection procedures and equipment, collection priorities, transportation of specimens
IV. Procedure manual
  A. Protocols
  B. QA relevant to manual
    1. Update of standards and protocols to reflect advances in field
    2. Training of lab personnel in performance of procedure
    3. Testing schedule of standard samples (QC)
    4. Monitoring of results
  C. Test information
    1. Principle of test
    2. Purpose
    3. Type of specimen required

4. Collection method
5. Equipment and supplies
D. Floor book—or directory of services
  1. Laboratory schedules
  2. Sweep times
  3. Written notification of changes
  4. Patient preparation information
  5. Specimen types and handling information
  6. Normal values
E. QA procedures relevant to floor book:
  1. Monitoring number of incomplete or duplicate requests
  2. Collecting statistics
    a. Missed draws
    b. Delayed collections
    c. Turnaround times (TAT)—time between test request and receiving results

V. Monitoring of variables
A. Variables are factors that can be measured
  1. Preanalytical
  2. Analytical
  3. Postanalytical
B. Affect outcome of test results and patient care
C. Controlled via written procedures
D. Monitored to ensure effect on test results is minimized
E. Phlebotomy is mainly concerned with preanalytical variables
F. CLIA waived testing includes all three variables

Preanalytical Variables

I. Requisitions
A. Requisition handling—accurate, complete
B. Variables to be controlled
  1. Duplicate or missing requisitions
  2. Missing information
    a. tests
    b. patient information
    c. physician name
    d. test priority (i.e., routine, STAT, etc.)
C. Delay in collection, processing, and reporting of results
D. QA includes recording and counting number of each type of requisition error

II. Equipment—monitor for defects
A. Tubes
  1. Lot number
  2. Expiration dates
B. Stoppers
  1. Check sealing, cracks

C. Tube vacuum
  1. Check draw volumes
  2. ±10% of stated draw volume for entire shelf life
D. Needles
  1. Blunted points or burrs
  2. Broken seal
E. Syringe plungers
  1. Move freely

III. Patient identification
A. Most important part of phlebotomy procedure
B. Misidentification—injury or death
C. Name and patient number on requisition matches the patient's armband that is attached to patient's arm
D. QA procedure—Delta check, a post-analytical check
  1. Previous patient results checked with current results
  2. Stark difference (delta) between the two results outside of limit that would be expected from random variance
  3. Result is flagged
  4. Lab personnel must investigate

IV. Patient preparation
A. Posture
  1. Erect patient versus supine patient
    a. Sample exhibits higher concentrations of large molecule substance
      i. Enzymes
      ii. Albumin
      iii. WBCs
      iv. RBCs
  2. Result of gravity shift in fluid distribution on standing
  3. Patient should be seated for 15 minutes prior to blood draw.
B. Short-term exercise
  1. Increases several blood constituents:
    a. Muscle enzymes (i.e., creatine kinase)
    b. WBCs
    c. Fatty acids
C. Long-term exercise
  1. Increases sex hormones
  2. Increase in aldolase
  3. Many of the same values increased in short-term exercise
D. Medications and medical treatments
  1. Aspirin increases bleeding times
  2. Radiographic dyes
    a. Increase specific gravity of urines

4. Blood transfusions
   a. Dimorphic blood picture
   b. Improve H & H if bleeding controlled, etc.
5. IV fluids
   a. Difference between pretest and posttest results after IV administration
   b. Drawing from same arm as IV
6. Anticoagulants
   a. Coumadin, heparin—require extra time to stop bleeding after phlebotomy

E. Alcohol consumption
1. Glucose values may be elevated
2. Liver enzymes may be elevated
3. Platelet aggregation studies affected

F. Smoking
1. Increases catecholamines
2. Increases cortisol
3. Increases WBCs
4. May result in increased MCV
5. Increases Hgb
6. Decreases eosinophils
7. Affects ABG results

G. Stress
1. Anxiety, crying, hyperventilating
   a. Increases WBCs
   b. Alters ABGs
   c. Affects adrenal cortex stress hormone levels

H. Diurnal variation—see previous discussion in Chapter 14 Content Overview

I. Fasting
1. Prolonged fasting increases bilirubin and fatty acids
2. Overnight fast concentrates most analytes
3. Fasting specimen requires 8- to 12-hour fast
   a. No food—alters many constituents (i.e., glucose, triglycerides)
   b. No caffeine, such as coffee, tea, soda—transient rise in blood sugar, increases metabolism
   c. Nonfasting specimen may appear *lipemic*—turbid due to increase in triglycerides that interfere with photometric tests (i.e., passage of light through specimen)
   d. High-speed centrifugation—pretreatment of specimen to remove lipemia

J. Age
1. Tests reference ranges may vary with age depending on test so age, date of birth important information on requisitions
2. Test results may vary with age—organ function declines (i.e., liver and kidney function)
3. Cholesterol and triglyceride values increase
4. Sex hormones increase then decrease
5. RBCs higher in infants versus adults

K. Altitude
1. Higher altitudes have higher RBC mass due to lower O_2 levels
2. Values increased at higher altitudes
   a. RBCs
   b. Hgb
   c. Hct

L. Dehydration
1. Hemoconcentration due to loss of plasma fluids
2. Causes—prolonged diarrhea and/or vomiting
3. Falsely increased values
   a. RBCs
   b. Enzymes
   c. Calcium
   d. Sodium

M. Sex
1. Reference ranges vary for males and females for certain tests
2. Higher values for the following
   a. RBCs
   b. Hgb
   c. Hct

N. Pregnancy
1. Physiologic changes in body affect test results
2. Increased retention of water
3. Leads to dilution effect
4. Falsely lower results
   a. RBCs
   b. Hgb
   c. Other analytes

V. Specimen collection—phlebotomists control the variables that can arise during the specimen collection process. Choosing a site that is healthy and easily accessible is important.
A. Site selection
1. Problem sites
   a. Hematoma
      i. Not freshly drawn blood
      ii. Fluid contamination
      iii. Erroneous results

b. Edema
   i. Fluid contamination
   ii. Erroneous results
c. Arm on mastectomy side
   i. Fluid contamination due to edema
   ii. Risk of infection
   iii. Erroneous results
d. Burns
   i. Painful
   ii. Risk of contamination
   iii. Fluid contamination
   iv. Erroneous results
e. Scars
   i. Difficult to penetrate
   ii. Painful
f. Previous puncture sites
   i. Painful
   ii. Contamination of fluids
   iii. Erroneous results
g. Sites near arteriovenous (AV) shunts
   i. Used for dialysis only
h. Fistulas
   i. Need physician approval
i. Heels
   i. Back of heel or other regions in bone proximity
   ii. Risk of osteomyelitis
j. Use of an artery
   i. Higher risk of infection
   ii. Some results vary from venous blood results
k. Arm with IV
   i. Erroneous results
   ii. May use if IV turned off 2 minutes before draw
   iii. Draw below IV site

B. Tourniquet application
  1. Do not leave on for more than 1 minute to reduce hemoconcentration
  2. Application too long can cause petechiae
  3. Too tight—pain and/or injury to patient

C. Site cleansing
  1. Reduces risk of infection—refer to Chapter 9 Content Overview
  2. Blood cultures require special cleaning procedure—refer to Chapter 14 Content Overview
  3. Iodine
    a. Must be completely removed from site after collection to prevent irritation
    b. Not used on heels—impossible to keep from contaminating sample

    c. Interferes with bilirubin, uric acid, and phosphorus tests

D. Specimen collection
  1. Right tube—size and additive
  2. Correct order of draw—refer to Chapter 8 Content Overview
  3. BC → Lt Blue → Red or Gold → Green → Lavender → Gray
  4. Adequate sample volume for test or tube
  5. Specimen adequately and properly mixed

E. Labeling
  1. Label immediately after the draw in presence of patient
  2. Complete information—Refer to Chapter 9 Content Overview
  3. Note any special conditions on requisition

VI. Patient's perception—level of care received directly related to performance of the phlebotomist and is also reflection of the laboratory
  A. Skill
  B. Professionalism
  C. Care

VII. Accidental puncture with contaminated needle
  A. Perform first aid immediately
  B. Report to a supervisor on completion of first aid
  C. Follow-up testing blood-borne pathogens
  D. Counseling
  E. QA procedures
    1. Monitor number of needlesticks
    2. Implement training
    3. Implement equipment modifications

VIII. Transportation—refer to Chapter 16 Content Overview
  A. Method of delivery
  B. Sample treatment during transportation
  C. Temperature requirements of samples
  D. Timing of delivery (i.e., Stats, etc.)
  E. QA procedures monitor
    1. Delivery times of various timed collections
    2. Turnaround times (TATs)
    3. Pneumonic tube system effects on samples (i.e., excessive agitation resulting in hemolysis)

IX. Processing
  A. Separation times—within 2 hours
    1. Glucose falsely decreases
    2. Potassium falsely elevated

3. Lactate dehydrogenase falsely elevated
4. Other tests—refer to Chapter 16
   Content Overview

B. Centrifuge maintenance
1. Every 3 months
2. Speed—to ensure proper separation of sample components
3. Rotors
4. Cups and cushions checked according to lab protocol
5. Cleaned according to lab protocol

C. Evaporation and contamination
1. Keep specimen caps on to prevent evaporation
   a. Plasma or serum
   b. Analytes (i.e., ABGs, alcohol, ammonia)
2. Keep specimen cap on to prevent contamination with dust, pollen, talc

D. Refrigerators and freezers
1. Monitor daily manually or electronically

E. Aliquot handling and labeling
1. Adequate volume
2. Complete label to include source and additive
3. Never combine specimens from different additive tubes

Analytical Variables
I.   Refers to any variables that affect the testing process
II. Bad reagents
III. Pipetting errors
IV. Instrument malfunction, etc.

Postanalytical Variables
I.   Test results
     A. Transmission of results to appropriate venue
     B. Mode of delivery
        1. Phone call
        2. Fax
        3. Computer transmission
     C. Results
        1. Interpretation
        2. Follow-up
        3. Need for retesting
     D. Delta checks—refer to previous discussion in III. D.

CERTIFICATION PREPARATION QUESTIONS

1. Which of the following terms describes the quantitative methods used to monitor the quality of procedures?
   a. Quality phlebotomy
   b. Quality control
   c. Quality enhancement
   d. Quality assurance

2. Patient preparation, collection, and specimen transportation protocols are all part of which of the following?
   a. Quality phlebotomy
   b. Quality control
   c. Quality enhancement
   d. Quality assurance

3. Quality assurance programs are mandated by which of the following organizations?
   a. OSHA
   b. COLA
   c. TJC
   d. CDC

4. "Customers" of the clinical laboratory include all of the following, *except*:
   a. The physicians
   b. The patients
   c. The families
   d. Other health care providers

5. Which of the following contain protocols and other information about tests performed in the lab, the reason for test performance, specimen requirements, collection methods, and required equipment and supplies?
   a. Floor book
   b. Procedure manual
   c. Maintenance logs
   d. QA manual

6. Which of the following contains information pertinent to coordination of nursing staff and laboratory staff?
   a. Floor book
   b. Procedure manual
   c. Maintenance logs
   d. QA manual

7. The phlebotomist receives a request to perform a sweat chloride test on a 2-year-old child and wants to refresh her memory before performing the test. The phlebotomist consults the _____ before going to the child's room.
   a. Physician
   b. Procedure manual

c. Floor book

d. Delta check

8. As a phlebotomist you are responsible for monitoring and controlling variables that impact your scope of practice in the collection of quality specimens. Which of the following variables is the phlebotomist most responsible for controlling?
   a. Preanalytical variables
   b. Analytical variables
   c. Postanalytical variables
   d. None of the above

9. Which of the following is *not* a preanalytical variable?
   a. Requisition handling
   b. Patient preparation
   c. Specimen analysis
   d. Specimen collection

10. The phlebotomist is working in the outpatient department and is informed by the patient that the physician forgot to mark one of the tests. What should the phlebotomist do?
    a. Add it to the requisition based on information from the patient
    b. Perform the venipuncture drawing only those tests ordered
    c. Send the patient back to the physician's office to have the test added
    d. Call the physician's office to confirm the tests to be performed

11. The phlebotomist is preparing to perform a venipuncture on the patient. All of the following preanalytical procedures can be performed, *except*:
    a. Check tube lot and expiration date
    b. Inspect needle for any defects
    c. Check Vacutainer tubes for vacuum leaks
    d. Check syringe plunger to make sure it moves freely

12. The phlebotomist must check the patient's ID before drawing blood. Which of the following statements is true regarding patient identification?
    a. Proper identification is made when the patient number on the requisition matches the number on the patient's ID band.
    b. Proper identification is made when the patient's birth date on the requisition

    matches the number on the patient's ID band.
    c. Proper identification is made when the patient's social security number on the requisition matches the number on the ID band.
    d. Proper identification is made when the patient's name on the requisition matches the name on the ID band.

13. A patient must have blood redrawn because a delta alert came up when the MLS ran a test on the blood that the phlebotomist just drew. What is a delta check?
    a. A change in patient identification that is identified by the phlebotomist when collecting a specimen
    b. A procedure used to help spot identification errors by comparison of current patient results with previous patient results
    c. An internal alert system used by the laboratory to notify the phlebotomist of a change in a patient's status
    d. A procedure for patient identification that involves physical identification of the patient by two health care professionals

14. All of the following variables may adversely affect patient test result values, *except*:
    a. Patient posture
    b. Exercise
    c. Medication intake
    d. Basal state

15. The patient informed the phlebotomist that he or she has been taking aspirin. You check your labels and see that aspirin may affect several of the tests ordered. Which of the following laboratory results would *not* be affected by the patient's consumption of aspirin?
    a. Bleeding times
    b. Prothrombin time
    c. Occult blood
    d. Glucose

16. The following tests are ordered to be drawn on an inpatient in a fasting state. The patient tells the phlebotomist that she ate some leftover cookies during the night that her family had brought. It was approximately 1:30 AM when she finished eating them and it is now 5 AM. Which of the following tests can the phlebotomist draw?

a. Cholesterol profile
b. Arterial blood gases
c. Glucose
d. Triglycerides

17. Which of the following conditions may affect laboratory results for white blood cells and arterial blood gases?
    a. Smoking
    b. Stress
    c. Diurnal variation
    d. Both a and b

18. An ER patient tells you as you are drawing his blood that he is visiting from Leadville, CO, which has the highest elevation of any city in the country. You make a note on the label to inform the tech who will be performing the test because you know that altitude can affect some of the complete blood count (CBC) test results for this patient. Which of the following results is *not* affected by altitude?
    a. Hemoglobin
    b. Red cell count
    c. White cell count
    d. Hematocrit

19. A patient comes into the emergency room (ER) suffering from several days of vomiting and diarrhea. All of the following results for this patient may be affected by prolonged diarrhea or vomiting, *except*:
    a. Red blood cells
    b. Enzymes
    c. ABO/Rh
    d. Sodium

20. Which of the following conditions causes increased water retention by the patient and therefore a dilution effect, causing a false decrease in hemoglobin and red cell counts?
    a. Sex of the patient
    b. Age of the patient
    c. Pregnancy
    d. Smoking

21. Which of the following preanalytical variables does the phlebotomist *not* have complete control of?
    a. Site selection
    b. Posture
    c. Tourniquet application
    d. Site cleansing

22. The phlebotomist is having trouble finding a patient's vein and is reluctant to remove the tourniquet once it is located. The phlebotomist checks to see if the time limit of _____ minute(s) has been exceeded.
    a. 5
    b. 3
    c. 2
    d. 1

23. You are performing a dermal puncture on a newborn to collect a bilirubin and glucose and find you are out of alcohol wipes but you do have iodine swabs. You know that iodine is unacceptable as an antiseptic on dermal punctures for all of the following reasons, *except*:
    a. Antiseptic qualities are inferior for newborns
    b. Contaminates dermal puncture sample
    c. Interferes with bilirubin testing
    d. Interferes with uric acid

24. Why should the patient's age be recorded on the specimen requisition?
    a. To be a second identifier for the patient in addition to the name
    b. To document the patient's age since age can affect lab values
    c. To document the patient's age for insurance purposes
    d. To comply with OSHA regulations for patient data collection

25. As a phlebotomist you take extreme care when labeling your specimens because you know that incorrect labeling can:
    a. Render the specimen useless
    b. Cause patient to be redrawn
    c. Lead to patient misdiagnosis
    d. All of the above

26. A phlebotomist comes in direct contact with many patients and could potentially be a link in the chain of infection. What is the number one way to prevent disease transmission?
    a. Antiseptic cleaning of the puncture site
    b. Handwashing before and after each patient
    c. Use of sterile equipment during procedures
    d. Use of safety devices such as a sharps container

27. Which of the following should the phlebotomist avoid when making a site selection?
    a. Veins in the back of the hand
    b. The median antecubital vein
    c. The arm nearest a mastectomy
    d. The brachial antecubital vein

28. The phlebotomist had difficulty collecting a routine blood draw and a hematoma developed before collecting a second tube SST tube. The order was for a metabolic panel and rapid plasma reagin (RPR) test. How will the phlebotomist resolve this situation?
    a. Divide the specimen into aliquots to be delivered to each department
    b. Since it is was ordered as a routine test, just put it back in the draw pile for later
    c. Have another phlebotomist redraw the patient to collect the second tube
    d. Apologize to the patient and attempt to re-stick the patient for the second tube

29. The phlebotomist is processing specimens received from a physician's office and notes that the following hand-labeled specimens have been delivered:
    Requisition for Jenny Collins for CBC and chem profile. Tubes received:
    Chem profile—Jenny Collins
    CBC—tube missing
    Requisitions for Judy Connors for CBC and glucose. Tubes received:
    2 CBC tubes—one 4 mL tube, one 2 mL tube—each labeled Judy Connors
    Glucose tube—labeled Judy Connors
    To resolve this situation, the phlebotomist should:
    a. Check the time on each tube and match the tubes and names to the corresponding times
    b. Call the physician's office to have the nurse stop on her way home to relabel the tube
    c. Relabel the 2 mL to read Jenny Collins per physician's office confirmation she had small veins
    d. Call the physician's office for a redraw on both patients per laboratory protocol

30. If the phlebotomist incurs an accidental needle puncture, the phlebotomist must report the injury to a supervisor as soon as possible. What is the standard protocol for accidental needlesticks?
    a. The site is cleaned and an incident report is completed
    b. The site is cleaned, a report completed, and follow-up testing performed
    c. The site is cleaned, a report completed, follow-up testing performed, and counseling by a health care professional is required
    d. The site is cleaned, a report is completed, and counseling by a health care professional is required

31. If a serum sample is not separated from the formed elements within 2 hours from the time of collection, which of the following may occur?
    a. The specimen will show a falsely lowered glucose and a falsely elevated potassium.
    b. The specimen will show a falsely elevated glucose and a falsely lowered potassium.
    c. The specimen will show a falsely lowered glucose and a falsely lowered potassium.
    d. The specimen will show a falsely elevated glucose and a falsely elevated potassium.

32. The nurse delivers an ammonia level to the laboratory that was drawn by the physician 45 minutes ago. The phlebotomist should:
    a. Put the specimen in an ice slurry and deliver to chemistry for immediate testing
    b. Reject the specimen because it must be kept on a slurry of ice and delivered immediately to the lab
    c. Accept the specimen as is and deliver to chemistry for immediate testing
    d. Tell the nurse to check the nursing station's lab manual for specimen requirements

33. The phlebotomist is centrifuging and processing the samples collected in the morning sweep. Which of the following tubes does *not* require the serum to be transferred to another labeled tube within 2 hours to avoid falsely increased or decreased laboratory values?
    a. Sodium citrate tube
    b. EDTA tube
    c. Serum separator tube
    d. Plain red top tube

34. Which of the following tests may be altered if the specimen is allowed to remain open to the air and evaporation occurs?
    a. Arterial blood gases
    b. Alcohol
    c. Ammonia
    d. All of the above

35. The phlebotomist is responsible for controlling variables that occur at the preanalytical stage so that samples of the highest integrity are presented for testing. Which of the following conditions can degrade the sample quality?
    a. Balancing of specimens during centrifugation
    b. Fluctuations in temperature while in cold storage
    c. Diurnal variation of the analyte being tested
    d. 12-hour basal fasting state

36. During specimen processing the phlebotomist must follow the protocols regarding the uncapping of specimens for several reasons, one being contamination of the specimen. All of the following are potential contaminates of specimen that is left uncovered, *except*:
    a. Dust
    b. Glove powder
    c. Aerosols
    d. Evaporation

37. In general, any factor that can be measured or counted that affects the outcome of results and therefore patient care is known as a:
    a. Variable
    b. Preanalytical factor
    c. Postanalytical factor
    d. Delta check

38. The patient just informs the phlebotomist that they are coming from their early morning workout at the gym. The phlebotomist checks the requisition to see if there are any tests that may be affected by exercise. Which of the following test results may *not* be affected by *short-term* exercise?
    a. Creatine kinase
    b. White blood cells
    c. Sex hormones
    d. Fatty acids

39. Which of the following does *not* affect the patient's perception of the phlebotomist?
    a. Professionalism in appearance and action
    b. Certification as a phlebotomist
    c. Skill in performing venipuncture
    d. All of the above affect patient perception

40. When should the phlebotomist wash his or her hands?
    a. When entering the patient's room
    b. When leaving the patient's room
    c. When entering and leaving the patient's room
    d. When all patients have been drawn on each floor

ANSWERS AND RATIONALES

1. **Answer: B**
   Rationale: Quality control refers to the quantitative methods used to monitor the quality of procedures, such as regular inspections and calibration of equipment to ensure accurate test results.
   Text Reference: p. 243

2. **Answer: D**
   Rationale: Quality assurance is a larger set of methods used to guarantee quality patient care. These protocols include patient preparation, collection, and specimen transportation.
   Text Reference: p. 243

3. **Answer: C**
   Rationale: TJC standards require that processes be in place to monitor and evaluate the quality of patient care on an ongoing basis.
   Text Reference: p. 243

4. **Answer: C**
   Rationale: Total quality management is a process by which the goal is continued improvement in every area regardless of current performance status to provide better customer service. The customer in the laboratory includes not only patients, but also physicians, and other health care providers.
   Text Reference: p. 243

5. **Answer: B**
   Rationale: Procedure manuals provide specific information regarding all aspects of a given test protocol. Procedures must be updated to comply with advances in the field, training for lab members, scheduled testing of standard samples, and monitoring of results.
   Text Reference: p. 244

6. **Answer: A**
   Rationale: Floor books include laboratory schedules, sweep times, and written notification of any changes, plus information on patient preparation, specimen types and handling, and normal values.
   Text Reference: p. 244

7. **Answer: B**
   Rationale: The procedure manual contains all protocols and other information about all tests performed by the laboratory. Included in the manual is information regarding the test principle, purpose, type of specimen, volume, collection method, equipment, and supplies.
   Text Reference: p. 244

8. **Answer: A**
   Rationale: The phlebotomist is most responsible for controlling preanalytical variables, which occur before analysis of the specimen.
   Text Reference: pp. 244-249

9. **Answer: C**
   Rationale: Specimen analysis is an analytical variable. Preanalytical variables include all requisition handling, patient preparation, and specimen collection in addition to equipment and patient identification.
   Text Reference: p. 245

10. **Answer: D**
    Rationale: Any time information is missing from a requisition, the phlebotomist must make every effort to get the necessary information before performing the procedure. A simple phone call to the physician's office can confirm the tests that the physician wanted ordered on the patient. To draw the tests ordered without confirming whether or not there is a missing test could delay test results and diagnosis and insurance reimbursement. In addition, the patient may need to come back for a second venipuncture in the event that a patient indicated an incorrect test and the wrong tube was drawn.
    Text Reference: p. 245

11. **Answer: C**
    Rationale: Tubes may lose vacuum without any visible sign of defect; therefore, there is no way that the phlebotomist could check this before specimen collection. The phlebotomist should be aware of incomplete filling of a tube during collection due to vacuum loss so that if it does occur a new tube can be drawn from the same venipuncture and the patient does not have to be stuck again.
    Text Reference: p. 245

12. **Answer: A**
    Rationale: Each patient will be assigned a unique patient identification number. The number should appear on the requisition exactly as it does on the patient arm band for proper identification to take place. Date of birth and social security number should not be used for identification purposes. Social security numbers are not written on the patient's ID band for security purposes.
    Text Reference: p. 245

13. **Answer: B**
    Rationale: A delta check compares current patient test results with previous results for the same patient for the same test. If there is a notable difference between the two results outside the expected variation, it will alert the laboratory personnel so that they can investigate the potential of a laboratory error.
    Text Reference: p. 245

14. **Answer: D**
    Rationale: Many variables may affect a patient's test results that the phlebotomist may be unable to control. The phlebotomist should note these variables on the requisition whenever possible to aid the laboratory in evaluation of results. Basal state is the body's state after 12 hours of fasting and abstention from strenuous exercise and is representative of the best time to draw blood.
    Text Reference: pp. 245-248

15. **Answer: D**
    Rationale: The patient's regular use of aspirin may impact the patient's ability to clot and thereby affect the bleeding time. Excessive aspirin use has been shown to increase PT results. Occult blood tests may be positive due to gastric bleeding that can result from aspirin intake. The phlebotomist should be aware of the potential for excess bleeding from the puncture site as well and be prepared to apply pressure to the site for a longer period of time. The phlebotomist should also make sure to enter all drugs the patient is taking into the system as required at their facility.
    Text Reference: p. 245

16. **Answer: B**
    Rationale: The length of time a patient is fasting affects glucose, cholesterol profile, and triglyceride results. Fasting is not required for total cholesterol and HDL level but is for an LDL, HDL, cholesterol, and triglyceride panel. The patient's fasting time should be recorded by the phlebotomist for use by laboratory personnel in result interpretation. Arterial blood gases are not affected by the patient's fasting status.
    Text Reference: p. 247

17. **Answer: D**
    Rationale: Both smoking and stress can cause alterations in white blood cell and arterial blood gas values. Stress on the body by prolonged crying can alter the patient's arterial blood gases and white blood cell count, as will smoking.
    Text Reference: p. 247

18. **Answer: C**
    Rationale: Patients living at higher altitudes have less oxygen available in the atmosphere. Therefore, the patient's body will learn to compensate by increasing red cell mass. This increase will affect red blood cell, hemoglobin, and hematocrit values.
    Text Reference: p. 247

19. **Answer: C**
    Rationale: Prolonged diarrhea and vomiting can cause dehydration of the patient. Dehydration can affect plasma volumes and cause an increase in RBCs, enzymes,

sodium, and calcium. A patient's blood type does not change.
Text Reference: p. 247

20. **Answer: C**
    Rationale: Pregnancy causes many changes in the body. The presence of the fetus and increased water retention can cause a dilution effect, which will lead to a false decrease in hemoglobin and red blood cells.
    Text Reference: p. 248

21. **Answer: B**
    Rationale: The phlebotomist may not be able to control the posture of the patient. Not all patients will be able to lie flat or sit up in a seated position. The phlebotomist can only record the posture of the patient at the time of draw when patient posture is a consideration for the tests ordered.
    Text Reference: p. 248

22. **Answer: D**
    Rationale: The tourniquets should be left on for no longer than 1 minute to reduce hemoconcentration and prevent the risk of nerve and tissue damage.
    Text Reference: p. 248

23. **Answer: A**
    Rationale: Iodine may contaminate the sample and also may be interfere with various test results such as bilirubin, uric acid, phosphorus, and potassium. Iodine should not be used for dermal puncture.
    Text Reference: p. 248

24. **Answer: B**
    Rationale: The patient's age can affect patient test result values and also is necessary for the laboratory to report appropriate age-dependent reference ranges for the tests ordered.
    Text Reference: p. 247

25. **Answer: D**
    Rationale: Incorrect or mislabeling can lead to many complications in the testing. The specimen that has been identified as mislabeled can no longer be used and the patient must be redrawn. If the labeling error is not caught the results may be reported erroneously and could lead to patient misdiagnosis.
    Text Reference: p. 248

26. **Answer: B**
    Rationale: Handwashing is the number one way to prevent disease transmission. Antiseptic cleaning of the site and use of sterile equipment can reduce the risk of disease as well, but handwashing is universal for all patients in all situations as a means to prevent the spread of disease.
    Text Reference: p. 249

27. **Answer: C**
    Rationale: The site selection by the phlebotomist is one of the most crucial steps in a good specimen collection process. A patient should not be drawn from the arm nearest a mastectomy because this could cause pain or injury to the patient. Lymphostasis if present could result in erroneous results as well.
    Text Reference: p. 248

28. **Answer: A**
    Rationale: Ideally, a tube should be collected for each department for which a test is ordered. However, when problems arise in the drawing process, knowledge of tube requirements for each test is very helpful in salvaging a draw that has gone bad. A metabolic panel and an RPR can both be drawn in an SST tube. Therefore, making two aliquots from the SST tube will prevent an unnecessary redraw of the patient for a second tube.
    Text Reference: p. 251

29. **Answer: D**
    Rationale: A mislabeled tube should never be relabeled on assumption of what the label should read. The mislabeling of names on tubes draws into question the proper labeling of all tubes involved. If the person labeling the tubes confuses names during the labeling process and puts the wrong sticker or hand writes an incorrect name, then both patient specimens are called into question and should be redrawn to ensure accurate testing and diagnosis for both patients.
    Text Reference: p. 248

30. **Answer: C**
    Rationale: When an accidental needlestick occurs, the puncture must be reported to the supervisor as soon as the wound site

is cleaned. An incident report is completed and follow-up testing completed on the phlebotomist and the patient if possible. Counseling sessions must be completed with the injured employee and a qualified health care professional.
Text Reference: p. 249

31. **Answer: A**
    Rationale: If the serum is allowed to remain on the formed elements for a period longer than 2 hours, the serum levels of glucose will begin to decrease due to cell metabolic processes, and the potassium begins to increase as it moves out of the RBCs. Potassium, ammonia, cortisol, and ACTH can also be affected in less than 2 hours.
    Text Reference: p. 250

32. **Answer: B**
    Rationale: Ammonia levels are time and temperature sensitive and must be kept in a slurry of ice and capped before testing to preserve the integrity of the specimen and generate accurate test results. The nurse should have checked the floor book at the nursing station for information pertaining to the ammonia test.
    Text Reference: pp. 214, 249

33. **Answer: C**
    Rationale: Once centrifuged, the serum separator tube forms a gel barrier between the cells and the serum. The gel separator keeps the metabolic process of the cells from altering the contents of the serum. Sodium citrate and EDTA tubes are anticoagulated tubes, which render plasma rather than serum.
    Text Reference: p. 250

34. **Answer: D**
    Rationale: Arterial blood gases are especially altered by exposure to the air. Alcohol and ammonia can evaporate quickly and samples should be kept capped until analysis begins. All samples should remain covered and not be exposed to the air whenever possible.
    Text Reference: pp. 250-251

35. **Answer: B**
    Rationale: Proper specimen processing, fasting, and diurnal variation will not degrade the quality of the specimen. Fluctuations

in temperature can, however, degrade the sample, and temperatures in refrigerators and freezers used for specimen storage must be monitored daily.
Text Reference: p. 249

36. **Answer: D**
    Rationale: Any specimen that is left uncovered in the laboratory area may have the potential to be contaminated by dust, glove powder, aerosols, or even splashing of other samples or liquids into the specimen. Evaporation is not a contaminant but a consequence of leaving a sample uncapped.
    Text Reference: p. 250

37. **Answer: A**
    Rationale: A variable is a factor that can be measured or counted that affects the outcome of results and ultimately patient care. The laboratory has a responsibility to monitor these variables and control or eliminate them whenever possible.
    Text Reference: p. 244

38. **Answer: C**
    Rationale: Short-term exercise can affect CK, WBCs, and fatty acids and creatinine levels. Long-term exercise affects sex hormones and aldolase in addition to those results affected by short-term exercise.
    Text Reference: p. 245

39. **Answer: D**
    Rationale: The patient is often reassured by a professional person who is highly skilled. If the patient observes evidence of the phlebotomist's credentials and certification (i.e., on ID badge), it is often reassuring to the patient before the collection procedure.
    Text Reference: p. 249

40. **Answer: C**
    Rationale: The phlebotomist should wash their hands immediately on entering the patient's room. Neither the equipment for collection nor the patient should be touched before the washing of hands. Also, the phlebotomist should clean their hands before leaving the patient's room to avoid transferring infectious materials outside of that room.
    Text Reference: p. 249

LEGAL ISSUES IN PHLEBOTOMY

Tina Lewis

INTRODUCTION

Legal and ethical considerations form an important underpinning to the practice of medicine, and phlebotomy is no exception. An increasingly complex and litigious health care environment has made instruction in legal issues an important part of the phlebotomist's training. Medical malpractice is the most common legal claim in the health care field. Injuries that arise from failure to follow the standard of care may be grounds for a finding of malpractice. Careful observance of the standard of care, and documentation of that practice, is the best defense against malpractice. New and comprehensive federal regulations governing the privacy of medical information have affected every sector of health care delivery. In addition to the legal requirement to protect patient confidentiality, there is an ethical duty to do so. Although full consideration of all the relevant legal issues is beyond the scope of this review, some important legal and ethical concepts that have impact on the profession will be discussed.

CONTENT OVERVIEW

Why Study Legal Issues?
I. Complexity of the health care system—interplay of three areas
   A. Technologic advances
   B. Associated costs of delivering care
   C. Fear of litigation
II. Rising cost of health care system
   A. Gradual inflation of price of goods and services
   B. Growing sophistication of medical technology
      1. Higher costs for equipment, maintenance
      2. Highly trained operators at all levels of health care
   C. Drug development—increased costs for treatment of patients
   D. Cost of more stringent regulations to protect health care providers, patients, etc.

E. Availability of sophisticated technology—level of the standard of care has risen
   1. Physicians order more tests—to supplement clinical judgment
   2. Patients expect more tests
F. Defensive medicine
   1. Due to increased fear of litigation
   2. Order multiple tests when may not be necessary

The Legal System
I. Laws
   A. Statutory law
      1. Created by legislative body
   B. Case law
      1. Determined by court decisions
   C. Administrative law
      1. Created by administrative agencies
      2. Examples: OSHA, IRS
   D. Public law
      1. Criminal action prosecuted by the public in the person of the government's attorney—the district attorney
      2. Examples
         a. Assault—unjustifiable attempt or threat to touch
         b. Battery—intentional touching without consent
   E. Private law—civil action
      1. Tort
         a. Intentional or unintentional injury
         b. Injury to one person by another who is legally responsible for the injury
      2. Unintentional torts
         a. Basis for most medical malpractice suits
      3. Intentional torts
         a. May be subject to criminal action
      4. Sue for monetary damages
   F. Plaintiff
      1. Person claiming to have been harmed
   G. Defendant
      1. Person being prosecuted for criminal action, civil action, or both
      2. In Medical malpractice, usually includes:
         a. Person identified as causing injury—defendant
         b. Other professionals
         c. Institution

II. Settlement and judgment
   A. Most civil and criminal actions are settled out of court
   B. Parties reach agreement without intervention by judge or jury
   C. Gag order on settlement—cannot discuss amount of settlement
   D. Trial—when agreement cannot be reached to determine damages to be paid out in compensatory or punitive fines
   E. Damages
      1. Monetary compensation awarded in compensation for legal costs, pain, suffering
      2. Civil case—fine imposed
         a. *Compensatory fine*—fine imposed due to injury inflicted in an attempt to replace what was lost
         b. *Punitive fine*—punishment on top of compensatory fine for gross violations of accepted standards of care
      3. Criminal case—may result in prison sentence and/or monetary fine

Professional Liability
I. Acts of commission and omission
   A. Liable for actions as a phlebotomist
      1. Legally responsible
      2. Accountable for consequences
   B. Acts of commission
      1. Perform procedure incorrectly
      2. Perform procedure outside scope of practice
   C. Acts of omission
      1. Fail to perform a procedure according to protocol
      2. Fail to perform procedure that is responsibility of phlebotomist
II. Scope of practice
   A. Refers to phlebotomy procedures, practices, and processes
   B. Permitted to perform based on education, training, and demonstrated competency
   C. Each state has legislation that defines laws and regulations overseeing the roles of individuals in health care in certain professions (i.e., nursing, respiratory therapists, MLS, phlebotomists, EMTs, etc.)

III. Standard of care
   A. Refers to the consensus of medical opinion
      1. What is considered accepted practice for patient care
      2. Applied to a particular situation
   B. Failure to perform an action or procedure that is consistent with the accepted standard of care
      1. Negligence
      2. Subject to criminal and/or civil action
         a. Depends on the intent of the defendant
         b. Depends on whether an injury ensued
   C. Example
      1. Standard of care in phlebotomy at most institutions
         a. Allows for two attempts at a routine venipuncture
         b. After two misses, seek assistance of a senior phlebotomist
      2. Violation of that policy with resultant harm to a patient
         a. Phlebotomist liable
         b. Hospital/lab liable
IV. Medical malpractice
   A. Delivery of care that is substandard
   B. Results in harm to a patient
   C. Medical malpractice charges can ensue when all four elements of negligence have been met
      1. Duty
         a. Defendant owes a duty of care to plaintiff
         b. Phlebotomist expected to draw blood from patient as directed by physician and expected by supervisor
      2. Dereliction/Breach
         a. Defendant breached the duty of care to plaintiff
         b. Based on standard of care for expected action or inaction of plaintiff
         c. Phlebotomist labels specimen with incorrect patient label
      3. Injury
         a. Legally recognizable injury occurred
         b. Based on test result from mislabeled tube
         c. Wrong patient received improper care and suffered injury

4. Direct cause
   a. Injury was a direct result of defendant's acts or omissions
   b. Mislabeling of tube led to improper treatment of patient
   c. Injury would not have been sustained otherwise

V. Other examples of potential malpractice in phlebotomy
   A. Standard of care when drawing blood—no more than two unsuccessful attempts
      1. Duty
         a. Phlebotomist is to adhere to the standard
      2. Dereliction/Breach
         a. Continued attempts by same person results in pain and swelling in patient's arm
      3. Injury
         a. Pain and swelling in patient's arm
      4. Direct cause
         a. Repeated attempts by phlebotomist were the direct cause of the pain and swelling
   B. Standard of care when drawing at patient's bedside—tray does *not* go on patient's bed
      1. Duty
         a. Phlebotomist to adhere to standard of care
      2. Dereliction/Breach
         a. Places tray on patient's bed
      3. Injury
         a. Patient is exposed to bloodborne pathogens when patient movements cause the tray to fall to the floor
         b. Injury established only if patient tests positive for bloodborne pathogen according to postexposure protocols
      4. Direct cause
         a. Infection occurs as a result of this exposure
         b. Not exposure from a different source at a different time
   C. Standard of care when leaving a patient's bedside—raise the bed rail if it was lowered for the draw
      1. Duty
         a. Phlebotomist to perform this action
      2. Dereliction/Breach
         a. Leaves the bed rail lowered
      3. Injury
         a. Patient falls from bed and is injured

      b. Mitigating factors may include whether patient had been visited by a nurse in the meantime
      4. Direct cause
         a. Injury caused by fall
   D. Other standards of care—a few examples of liability issues for phlebotomy
      1. Proper identification of patient
      2. Follows protocol for entire blood collection process in all procedures
      3. Follows institution's protocol for policies and procedures for phlebotomists
      4. Adheres to HIPAA

VI. Defense against malpractice
   A. Meet standard of care
      1. Practice of good care and complete documentation of medical records
      2. If questionable situation arises
         a. Document the incident describing what happened, who did what when, date, time, witnesses, etc.
      3. Follow institution's protocol for documenting and reporting incidents
   B. Patient communication
      1. Clear communication
      2. Informed consent before proceeding with procedure
      3. Requires explaining procedures and assessing patient comprehension and understanding
      4. May need an interpreter
   C. Assessing patient status—ask:
      1. Medications (e.g; Coumadin, heparin)
      2. Mastectomy, etc.

VII. Liability insurance
   A. Covers monetary damages if defendant loses liability suit
   B. May be required to show proof of coverage
   C. Phlebotomists usually covered by institution's liability insurance but not always

Confidentiality
I. Confidentiality is a legal and ethical responsibility
II. HIPAA—Health Insurance Portability and Accountability Act
   A. Set of standards for protection and privacy of health information
III. Protected health information—PHI
   A. Any part of the patient's health information that is linked with identity information

B. Includes: name, address, date of birth, test results, etc.

C. Under HIPAA, patients have right to control their PHI

D. Need patient's consent to disclose any PHI
   1. Federal offense to disclose PHI without patient's permission
   2. Can result in both civil and criminal action depending on state law

E. On admission a patient's privacy rights are discussed and signature secured to release information as necessary under the law
   1. Never discuss patient information with someone not directly involved in the patient's care
   2. Protect conversations about patient to ensure privacy—don't discuss patient in hallway, elevator, cafeteria/café, etc.
   3. Never release medical information concerning a patient to anyone who is not specifically authorized to acquire it
   4. Never leave patient records out where other patients or visitors can view them
   5. Maintain the integrity of the doctor-patient relationship
      a. Do not release test results to patient unless directed by physician or institution policy

IV. The Patient Care Partnership
   A. Developed by the American Hospital Association
   B. Encompasses the right to patient confidentiality and other aspects of ethical patient care
      1. High quality of hospital care
      2. Clean and safe environment
      3. Involvement in your care
      4. Protection of your privacy
      5. Help when leaving the hospital
      6. Help with your billing claims

CERTIFICATION PREPARATION QUESTIONS

1. Which of the following factors have led to the rise in health care costs?
   a. Inflation of the price of goods and services
   b. Growing sophistication in medical technology

   c. Need for higher qualified individuals
   d. All of the above

2. Which of the following laws is created by a legislative body such as Congress?
   a. Statutory law
   b. Case law
   c. Public law
   d. Administrative law

3. Which of the following laws is created as a result or determination of a court decision?
   a. Statutory law
   b. Case law
   c. Public law
   d. Administrative law

4. Which of the following laws is created by an agency such as the Internal Revenue Service or the Occupational Safety and Health Administration?
   a. Statutory law
   b. Case law
   c. Public law
   d. Administrative law

5. Which of the following laws is prosecuted by a district attorney representing the people?
   a. Statutory law
   b. Case law
   c. Public law
   d. Administrative law

6. Which of the following terms describes an unjustifiable attempt to touch another person or a threat to do so?
   a. Assault
   b. Battery
   c. Felony
   d. Liability

7. Which of the following terms describes the intentional touching of another person without consent?
   a. Assault
   b. Battery
   c. Felony
   d. Liability

8. Which of the following may a phlebotomist be held liable for if a dirty needle is used on a patient?
   a. Assault

b. Battery
c. Assault and battery
d. Criminal action

9. Which of the following types of law violation may lead to a civil action?
   a. Public
   b. Assault
   c. Battery
   d. Private

10. Which of the following terms describes the person in a court proceeding who is claiming to have been harmed by the person accused?
    a. Plaintiff
    b. Defendant
    c. Prosecutor
    d. Bailiff

11. Which of the following terms describes the person in a court proceeding being accused of a harmful action?
    a. Plaintiff
    b. Defendant
    c. Prosecutor
    d. Bailiff

12. A patient files a lawsuit for violation of HIPAA that resulted in denial of insurance coverage. The type of lawsuit the patient can file is:
    a. Civil action
    b. Criminal action
    c. Civil and criminal action
    d. Unintentional tort

13. As a phlebotomist you are legally responsible for your actions and can be held accountable for consequences resulting from those actions. The term referring to this legal responsibility is:
    a. Damages
    b. Liable
    c. Duty
    d. Dereliction

14. Which of the following is considered an example of damages?
    a. Injury a patient suffers due to negligence
    b. Jail time of defendant for negligent action
    c. Monetary compensation to the plaintiff for injury
    d. A breach of contract between the plaintiff and defendant

15. The phlebotomist was in a hurry to complete the STAT arterial blood gas (ABG) so he or she could leave work on time and did not perform the Allen test on the patient. The patient developed a thrombus in the artery and it was later determined that the patient had poor collateral circulation in the area that would have been identified by performing the Allen test. The phlebotomist can be charged with which of the following terms that describes delivery of substandard care that results in harm to the patient?
    a. Assault
    b. Malpractice
    c. Damages
    d. Dereliction

16. A patient filed a civil suit against the phlebotomist. In order for a phlebotomist to be found guilty of malpractice, which of the following must be proven by the plaintiff?
    a. Duty, dereliction, damages, direct cause
    b. Duty, dereliction, damages, injury
    c. Duty, direct cause, injury, damages
    d. Duty, dereliction, injury, direct cause

17. An elderly, confused inpatient suffered a severe hematoma after a venipuncture. The patient's husband noted that the phlebotomist did not apply pressure to the site but simply bent the woman's arm upward and left the room shortly thereafter. The phlebotomist breached the duty of care to ensure proper pressure was applied and bleeding had stopped before leaving the room. Which of the following terms means the defendant breached the duty of care of the patient?
    a. Duty
    b. Dereliction
    c. Injury
    d. Direct cause

18. The phlebotomist and hospital were found guilty of negligence in the care of a patient and must now pay damages. Damages could be awarded for all the following *except*:
    a. Lost wages
    b. Legal costs
    c. Pain and suffering
    d. Medical bill for entire stay

19. The four elements of negligence include duty, direct cause, dereliction, and
    _____.
    a. Malpractice
    b. Liability
    c. Injury
    d. Incidence

20. Who may carry liability insurance for the phlebotomist?
    a. The ordering physician
    b. The phlebotomist
    c. The health care facility
    d. Both b and c
    e. Both a and b

21. What is the primary defense to charges of malpractice?
    a. Deny the action ever occurred
    b. Show that the standard of care was followed
    c. Show the incompetence of the plaintiff
    d. Demonstrate negligence instead of malpractice

22. What is the best way to prove standard of care?
    a. Have another health care worker witness the action
    b. Document any incidents that occur
    c. Have expert witnesses give testimony during trial
    d. Do not do any task that is outside your scope of practice

23. All of the following are important aspects of preventing malpractice litigation, *except*:
    a. Documentation
    b. Patient communication
    c. Getting the patient food or water
    d. Getting informed consent

24. Which of the following defines a set of standards and procedures for the protection of privacy of health information?
    a. CLIA
    b. HIPAA
    c. OSHA
    d. TJC

25. Private health information includes all of the following, *except*:
    a. Any health information that is linked to information that identifies the patient

    b. Any health information containing the patient's diagnosis and treatment
    c. Any health information containing the patient's date of birth
    d. Only a and b
    e. All of the above

26. Which of the following scenarios could lead to a potential breach of standard of care?
    a. Raising a bed rail after blood collection
    b. Placing the phlebotomy tray on the patient's bed
    c. Applying a gauze pad and bandage on venipuncture site
    d. Sticking a patient twice for blood collection

27. Which of the following is not a violation of HIPAA?
    a. Discussion of information concerning a patient with someone not directly involved in that patient's care
    b. Release of information concerning the patient to anyone not specifically authorized to acquire it
    c. Leaving patient information out where others can see it as they wait at the nursing station
    d. Avoiding the use of a patient's name in telephone conversations that may be overheard by passersby

28. Test results can be given to the patient by all of the following, *except*:
    a. Phlebotomist
    b. Patient's physician
    c. Nurse
    d. Resident doctor

29. Which of the following protects the patient's right to privacy out of ethical consideration?
    a. The Health Information Portability and Privacy Act
    b. The Patient Care Partnership
    c. The Patient Advocacy Act
    d. The Occupational Safety and Health Act

30. The Patient Care Partnership was developed by the American Hospital Association and it:
    a. Carries the weight of the law
    b. Does not carry the weight of the law
    c. Is part of HIPAA
    d. Is part of PHI

31. The phlebotomist was clearly negligent in their duty to the patient and the hospital wanted to come to a swift agreement quickly with the patient's lawyers. Which of the following represents an agreement made by two parties in a legal matter without the intervention of a judge or a jury?
    a. Tort action
    b. Damages awarded
    c. Out-of-court settlement
    d. Deliberation

32. The phlebotomist exhibited gross negligence in performing a venipuncture procedure and the court awarded two types of damages to be paid. Damages awarded to the plaintiff to punish the defendant are known as:
    a. Punitive damages
    b. Civil damages
    c. Criminal damages
    d. Restitution damages

33. Before proceeding with *any* collection procedure the phlebotomist should always:
    a. Obtain a positive informed consent
    b. Have the patient sign a release form
    c. Have the patient sign an advanced beneficiary notice
    d. Make sure the insurance information is logged in the CIS

34. As a matter of ethics, a patient should expect all of the following from a health care facility and the providers employed by that facility, *except*:
    a. A clean and safe environment
    b. Protection of privacy
    c. High quality care
    d. One-on-one nursing care

35. The phlebotomist instructed the patient to have a seat while she went to find her supervisor. On her return she found another patient waiting at the desk with a clear view of the first patient's requisition. Leaving a patient's record open out on a desk where other patients register to be seen is a violation of what?
    a. FERPA
    b. HIPAA
    c. OSHA
    d. CLIA

36. In which of the following areas is it permitted to discuss a patient's private health care information?
    a. The hallway with a nurse
    b. The elevator with a physician
    c. The exam room with the patient
    d. An eating area with co-workers

37. Which of the following would *not* be a basis for legal malpractice proceedings?
    a. Intentional tort
    b. Unintentional tort
    c. Negligence
    d. Informed nonconsent

38. If the defendant in a case feels that some part of the legal proceeding was in error, then the defendant has the right to:
    a. Call a mistrial
    b. File an appeal
    c. Refuse the fine
    d. Have a second trial

39. Who is legally responsible for injuries resulting from a venipuncture?
    a. The physician
    b. The laboratory
    c. The phlebotomist
    d. The health care institution

40. You are drawing an outpatient who suddenly goes into convulsions during the draw. You quickly remove the needle, apply pressure, and try to protect the patient from injury as you call for assistance. When any incident occurs during the collection of blood or body fluids, as the phlebotomist performing the procedure, you should immediately:
    a. Document the incident
    b. Complete an incident report
    c. Report the incident to the supervisor
    d. All of the above

ANSWERS AND RATIONALES

1. **Answer: D**
   Rationale: The prices of goods and services have increased dramatically in the health care industry. Technologic advances have brought about more sophisticated

equipment and the need for highly trained individuals to run that equipment.
Text Reference: p. 255

2. **Answer: A**
   Rationale: Statutory law is created by a legislative body such as Congress at the federal level. State legislative bodies typically follow the federal model.
   Text Reference: p. 256

3. **Answer: B**
   Rationale: Case law is usually an interpretation of an existing statutory law that is created by the determination of a court proceeding.
   Text Reference: p. 256

4. **Answer: D**
   Rationale: Administrative laws are created by administrative agencies such as the IRS or OSHA. The regulations are then enforced by these agencies via statutory laws that originally created the agencies themselves.
   Text Reference: p. 256

5. **Answer: C**
   Rationale: Laws are classified as either public or private. Public law violations lead to criminal action and the violator is prosecuted by the government's attorney (the district attorney).
   Text Reference: p. 256

6. **Answer: A**
   Rationale: To commit assault by legal standards, a person must only threaten to touch or harm another individual, or attempt to touch them in any way.
   Text Reference: p. 256

7. **Answer: B**
   Rationale: Battery is the actual intentional touching of another person without consent.
   Text Reference: p. 256

8. **Answer: C**
   Rationale: A phlebotomist can be held liable for assault and battery if they actually complete the collection process on a patient using a dirty needle. The intentional use

of a dirty needle or nerve damage caused by improper technique may lead to the phlebotomist being brought up on charges for assault and battery. Criminal action is the prosecution of someone who violates public law.
Text Reference: p. 256

9. **Answer: D**
   Rationale: Private law offenses may lead to civil or tort action. Public law offenses lead to criminal action. Both assault and battery are public law offenses.
   Text Reference: p. 256

10. **Answer: A**
    Rationale: The plaintiff is the person in a court proceeding that is claiming to be harmed by the accused.
    Text Reference: p. 256

11. **Answer: B**
    Rationale: A person in the court proceeding that is being accused of a harmful action and must defend those actions is known as the defendant.
    Text Reference: p. 256

12. **Answer: C**
    Rationale: A patient has the right to bring about civil action in addition to criminal action for HIPAA violations that result in adverse consequences. The injury may not necessarily be physical in nature but can be economic loss as well.
    Text Reference: pp. 259-260

13. **Answer: B**
    Rationale: The term liable means that a person is legally responsible for their actions and can be held accountable for its consequences.
    Text Reference: p. 257

14. **Answer: C**
    Rationale: In a civil suit, the plaintiff can ask for damages as a result of the defendant's violation. Damages are usually monetary compensation awarded to cover the actual cost of the injury, including lost wages and medical care.
    Text Reference: p. 257

15. **Answer: B**
    Rationale: Malpractice is a term used to describe care that does not meet the current health care standard for that type of health care and as a result causes harm to a patient.
    Text Reference: p. 258

16. **Answer: D**
    Rationale: In order for the phlebotomist to be found guilty of malpractice the plaintiff must prove duty, dereliction, injury, and direct cause.
    Text Reference: p. 258

17. **Answer: B**
    Rationale: Dereliction must be proven by the plaintiff. Dereliction is the breach in the duty of care.
    Text Reference: p. 258

18. **Answer: D**
    Rationale: Damages can be awarded for lost wages, legal costs, pain and suffering, and medical care costs that would be in EXCESS of the cost had there NOT been an injury. In a malpractice case the burden of proof is on the plaintiff. The plaintiff is only awarded damages if the defendant is found guilty of the four elements of negligence.
    Text Reference: p. 258

19. **Answer: C**
    Rationale: The plaintiff must show the four elements of negligence: duty, dereliction, injury, and direct cause in order for the defendant to be found guilty of malpractice.
    Text Reference: p. 258

20. **Answer: D**
    Rationale: The health care facility usually carries the liability insurance for the phlebotomist; however, phlebotomists may choose to carry insurance of their own to protect them if they should lose a liability suit.
    Text Reference: p. 259

21. **Answer: B**
    Rationale: In order to defend against the charge of malpractice, the defendant must show that the standard of care for the care or procedure in question was followed.
    Text Reference: pp. 258-259

22. **Answer: B**
    Rationale: Proper documentation of all procedures and incidences is the best way to defend against legal action. Remember, if it is not documented it did not happen.
    Text Reference: pp. 258-259

23. **Answer: C**
    Rationale: While documentation is the best way to prevent malpractice claims, patient communication is also very important. Clear communication between the patient and the phlebotomist is essential for obtaining informed consent for medical procedures. Getting the patient food or water is not within the scope of practice for a phlebotomist. Patients may be on fluid and/or food restriction. Giving a patient food or water may compromise the patient's condition and result in a lawsuit.
    Text Reference: pp. 258-259

24. **Answer: B**
    Rationale: HIPAA is the Health Insurance Portability and Accountability Act, which was designed to protect the privacy of health information.
    Text Reference: p. 259

25. **Answer: E**
    Rationale: Since a patient's diagnosis and date of birth could be personally identifying and private to the patient, they could be linked to that patient's health information. Any health information that identifies the patient is protected by HIPAA.
    Text Reference: p. 259

26. **Answer: B**
    Rationale: A phlebotomist should always replace a bed rail when completing blood collection and leaving a patient's room. Placing the tray on the bedside table out of the reach of the patient should not compromise the patient's health or welfare. Placing the tray on the bed could potentially lead to patient injury for which the phlebotomist could be held liable. Applying a gauze pad and bandage is appropriate after venipuncture. Although sticking a patient twice is not desired, it is standard protocol for specimen collection if collection is not completed on the first attempt.
    Text Reference: p. 258

27. **Answer: D**
    Rationale: In compliance with HIPAA, it is always a good idea to avoid the use of the patient's name when discussing private health information over the phone, with other health care professionals, or when other bystanders may overhear your conversation.
    Text Reference: pp. 259-260

28. **Answer: A**
    Rationale: It is the responsibility of the phlebotomist to protect the integrity of the doctor-patient relationship. In doing so, it is the physician's responsibility to give out test results to the patient and they should not be divulged by the phlebotomist. A resident doctor who is covering for physicians or assisting physicians is also authorized to release patient test results to the patient. The patient's nurse is also authorized to give the patient results as directed by the physician.
    Text Reference: p. 260

29. **Answer: B**
    Rationale: Patients have the right to have their private health information protected by law and it is the ethical responsibility of all health care professionals to see to it that all the rights of the patient are protected.
    Text Reference: p. 260

30. **Answer: B**
    Rationale: Although the Patient Care Partnership does not carry the total force of the law, it does represent an ideal that health care institutions use to evaluate their own practices.
    Text Reference: p. 260

31. **Answer: C**
    Rationale: An out-of-court settlement is an agreement made between the two parties in a legal proceeding (criminal or civil in nature) in which no judge or jury intervenes and the issue is resolved under agreeable conditions.
    Text Reference: p. 257

32. **Answer: A**
    Rationale: Punitive damages are awarded to the plaintiff by the judge or jury to punish the defendant for his or her wrongdoing.

These damages are above and beyond the usual restitution for lost income, medical care, injury, etc.
Text Reference: p. 257

33. **Answer: A**
    Rationale: The patient is not required to sign a consent or release form each time a phlebotomist performs blood collection. However, the phlebotomist must be sure that the patient completely understands and agrees to the procedure before proceeding with the collection.
    Text Reference: p. 259

34. **Answer: D**
    Rationale: A patient has the right to expect from any quality health care facility and the providers employed therein to receive high quality health care, a clean and safe environment, involvement in their care, protection of their privacy, help when leaving the hospital, and help with billing of their claims. A hospital or health care provider is not legally obligated to do all these things; however, they have an ethical responsibility to the patient to do so. One-on-one nursing care is typically not provided for in the general population of patients. Having dedicated nurses for one-on-one nursing care usually occurs when a private duty nurse is hired by the patient's family.
    Text Reference: p. 260

35. **Answer: B**
    Rationale: HIPAA deals with a patient's right to have all private health information protected. Any information relating to patients or their records should not be left out and visible to any other person not directly involved in that patient's care.
    Text Reference: pp. 259-260

36. **Answer: C**
    Rationale: In an exam room, the patient's private health information may be discussed with them provided there are no other parties present in the room without the patient's permission. It is never permissible to discuss private patient information in public access areas.
    Text Reference: p. 260

37. **Answer: D**
    Rationale: Unintentional torts are the basis for most malpractice suits. Intentional torts would, of course, also be grounds for legal malpractice proceedings. Most malpractice cases are fought over unintentional occurrences that led to the health care provider not following the standard of care. Informed nonconsent occurs when the patient refuses a medical treatment with full knowledge of the harm that may ensue by not having the test or treatment performed.
    Text Reference: p. 256

38. **Answer: B**
    Rationale: If the defendant believes that there was some error in the legal proceeding that rendered the guilty finding, the defendant has the right to file an appeal. Filing an appeal does not automatically guarantee a new trial for the defendant. The appeal will be considered but only the courts can decide whether or not the trial will be reheard or a mistrial will be called. A second trial is not guaranteed.
    Text Reference: p. 257

39. **Answer: C**
    Rationale: Although a patient has the right to sue any member of the health care institution, it is the phlebotomist who is ultimately responsible for any injury resulting from venipuncture.
    Text Reference: pp. 257-258

40. **Answer: D**
    Rationale: Whenever there is any incident that occurs during blood or body fluid collection, whether involving the patient or the employee, the phlebotomist should contact their immediate supervisor and appropriately document the incident on an incident report.
    Text Reference: pp. 258-259

POINT-OF-CARE TESTING

Tina Lewis

INTRODUCTION

Point-of-care testing (POCT) is the performance of analytical tests at the "point of care," which may be at the bedside in an intensive care unit (ICU) or the emergency room (ER), in the clinic, or even in the patient's home. The lab is brought to the patient. Tests are done with small portable instruments that offer significant time and cost savings in many situations. POCT instruments are easy to use, require simple training to operate, and can be used by a variety of health care professionals. Manufacturers' instructions *must* be adhered to for each specific instrument. Blood tests typically performed as point-of-care testing include many in chemistry and in hematology, and are clinical laboratory improvement amendments (CLIA)-waived tests. The FDA decides which tests fall into the CLIA-waived category on the basis of ease of performance and interpretation of the test result. Additionally, the multiskilled phlebotomist may perform electrocardiography, occult blood analysis, urinalysis, pregnancy testing, and rapid group A streptococcus (strep) testing.

CONTENT OVERVIEW

Advantages of Point-of-Care Testing
I.   Simple and accurate
II. Shorter turnaround times
III. Faster diagnosis and treatment
IV. Decreased recovery time
V.   Decreased cost
VI. CLIA-waived tests

Important Points to Remember
I.   Follow manufacturer instructions
   A. Some are calibrated to use the first drop of blood while others are not
   B. Erroneous results and negative consequences for patients if strict adherence to instructions are not met
II. Train all persons in use of instruments
III. Adhere to guidelines for:
   A. Calibrating equipment
   B. Running controls
   C. Performing maintenance
   D. Keeping records

Common Tests Performed at the Point-of-Care
I.   Hematology
   A. H & H
      1. Hemoglobin—anemia, polycythemia
      2. Hematocrit—anemia, polycythemia
      3. Specimen
         a. Whole blood
         b. Heparinized capillary tube
         c. Non-heparinized capillary tube is occasionally used to check automated hematocrits
   B. Coagulation
      1. Prothrombin time (PT)—monitors Coumadin/warfarin therapy
      2. Activated partial thromboplastin time (APTT)—monitors heparin therapy
      3. Activated coagulation time (ACT)—monitors heparin therapy
         a. Also known as the "tilt tube test"
      4. Specimen: whole blood or citrated whole blood
II. Chemistry
   A. Glucose
      1. Most commonly performed POCT
      2. Dermal puncture
      3. Specimen: whole blood
   B. Cardiac troponin T (TnT)
      1. Aids in interaction of actin and myosin of cardiac muscle
      2. Released by damaged cardiac muscle and rises within 4 hours of myocardial infarction (MI)
      3. Stays elevated for 2 weeks
      4. Monitor levels for damage and prognosis
      5. Specimen: whole blood
   C. Cholesterol
      1. Part of routine examination
      2. Monitor therapy with cholesterol-lowering drugs
      3. Specimen: whole blood or heparinized venous sample

D. Blood gases and electrolytes
   1. P_{O_2}, P_{CO_2}, pH
   2. Na^+, Cl^-, HCO_3^-
   3. POCT but not a waived test
   4. Specimen: whole blood
E. B-type natriuretic peptide (brain natriuretic peptide)
   1. Hormone made by heart in response to expansion of ventricular volume and pressure overload
   2. Elevated in congestive heart failure (CHF)
   3. Differentiate between CHF and chronic obstructive pulmonary disease (COPD)
   4. Monitor effectiveness of CHF therapy
   5. Specimen: whole blood EDTA sample

Electrocardiography
I. The cardiac cycle
   A. Sinoatrial node—pacemaker of the heart
      1. Triggers and coordinates contractions by electrical impulses
   B. Depolarization—contraction
   C. Repolarization—recovery and relaxation
II. Electrocardiogram (ECG or EKG) equipment
   A. Records the electrical activity of the heart
   B. Electrodes (sensors)—a standard 12 lead with 10 electrodes are placed in defined locations
      1. Chest
      2. Arms
      3. Legs
   C. Lead—wire connected to each electrode
   D. ECG machine
III. Performing an electrocardiogram—measurements
   A. P wave—atrial depolarization
   B. P-R interval—time between artrial depolarization (contraction) and ventricular repolarization (contraction)
   C. QRS complex—ventricular depolarization
   D. ST segment—time between ventricular depolarization and the beginning of repolarization
   E. T waves—ventricular repolarization
   F. Q-T interval—time between ventricular depolarization and completion of repolarization

Other CLIA-Waived Tests
I. Occult blood
   A. Stool/feces specimen
   B. Instruct patient to refrain from eating meat for 3 days before collection
   C. Screen for digestive diseases (i.e., gastric ulcers, colon cancer)
II. Urinalysis—dipstick testing only
   A. Urine at room temperature
   B. Thoroughly mixed urine
   C. Perform "dipstick" testing
      1. pH, protein, glucose, ketones, bilirubin, urobilinogen, blood, leukocyte esterase, nitrite, and specific gravity
      2. Must adhere to reaction time for accurate interpretation of color change
   D. Microscopic is *not* a waived portion of the test
III. Pregnancy
   A. Detect HCG
      1. Human chorionic gonadotropin is a hormone
      2. Produced by placenta after implantation of fertilized egg
   B. Urine or serum test kits available
IV. Rapid group A streptococcus
   A. *Streptococcus pyogenes*
   B. Throat culture
      1. Usually a double swab is collected
      2. One swab for rapid strep screening test
      3. Other swab for culture if indicated
   C. Test kits produce results in 3 to 5 minutes
   D. Negative test not conclusive
      1. Some physicians request culture to be performed on negative screens

CERTIFICATION PREPARATION QUESTIONS

1. What does the phrase "point of care" mean?
   a. Performance of the test when the patient is undergoing treatment by the physician
   b. Performance of the test immediately after obtaining the sample usually in the same room
   c. Performance of the test as a point of documentation of patient status
   d. Both a and c

2. All of the following are advantages of POCT (point of care testing), *except*:
   a. Decreased turnaround times
   b. Faster diagnosis
   c. Prompt medical attention
   d. Increased recovery time

3. Who decides which tests are considered "waived" tests?
   a. CLIA
   b. OSHA
   c. JCAHO
   d. FDA

4. The phlebotomist was collecting a sample for an ACT test. She removed the blue top tube from the holder and laid it down while she prepared the instrument for testing. She then inverted the tube five times before filling the cartridge. The test result will be:
   a. Unaffected
   b. Decreased
   c. Increased
   d. Valid

5. The phlebotomist should always wipe away the first drop of blood when performing a dermal puncture for _____.
   a. All waived testing
   b. Waived testing calibrated for the second drop of blood
   c. Any POCT performed at the bedside
   d. Both a and c

6. Which of the following point-of-care tests may be used to assess the presence of anemia?
   a. Hematocrit
   b. Hemoglobin
   c. Both a and b
   d. Erythrocyte sedimentation rate

7. You are assigned to cover the open-heart recovery unit and will be monitoring heparin therapy on several patients. Which of the following POCT tests will you perform to monitor heparin therapy?
   a. ACT
   b. PT
   c. APTT
   d. Both a and c

8. The phlebotomist is performing a test that will monitor current therapy for a patient who had been treated with heparin for multiple thrombi and is now taking warfarin. Which of the following POCT tests will be used to monitor warfarin therapy?
   a. ACT
   b. PT
   c. APTT
   d. Both a and c

9. The most commonly performed POCT is the _____.
   a. Hematocrit
   b. PT
   c. Glucose
   d. Cholesterol

10. Which of these POCT analytes is a part of a protein complex in the cardiac muscle that aids the interaction of actin and myosin?
    a. Cardiac TnT
    b. Creatine kinase
    c. Creatinine
    d. B-type natriuretic peptide

11. The phlebotomist draws a TnT on an ER patient experiencing acute chest pain that began about an hour ago and may return for a second draw later. How long after an acute myocardial infarction (MI) will it take for serum levels of cardiac TnT to rise to levels that are indicative of an MI?
    a. No repeat necessary, first one is diagnostic
    b. 2 hours
    c. 4 hours
    d. 8 hours

12. The phlebotomist arrives at the ER to draw blood for a cardiac TnT. What is the sample type needed to perform a cardiac TnT for point-of-care testing?
    a. Anticoagulated whole blood
    b. Plasma
    c. Serum
    d. Urine

13. The phlebotomist needs to perform an ACT test. Which of the following samples will be collected to perform ACT testing?
    a. EDTA
    b. Sodium citrate

c. Dermal puncture whole blood
d. Both b and c

14. POCT for cholesterol includes which of the following:
    a. One-step disposable color card test
    b. Automated instrument
    c. Dipstick
    d. Both a and b

15. To ensure accuracy of test results, users of POCT instruments must strictly adhere to manufacturer guidelines for any calibration and quality control measures that would apply to the individual instruments. Which of the following POCT instruments require calibration?
    a. Arterial blood gas instruments
    b. Electrolyte instruments
    c. Hemoglobin analyzers
    d. All of the above

16. Which of the following tests measures a hormone made by the heart in response to expansion of ventricular volume and pressure overload?
    a. Cardiac troponin T
    b. Creatine kinase
    c. Creatinine
    d. B-type natriuretic peptide

17. What is the medical terminology given to the heart's pacemaker?
    a. Sinoatrial node
    b. Cardiac cycle
    c. Stylus
    d. Aorta

18. Which of the following terms refers to one complete heartbeat consisting of depolarization and repolarization of both the atria and the ventricles?
    a. Sinoatrial node
    b. Cardiac cycle
    c. Stylus
    d. Myocardial event

19. What does the EKG POCT most accurately monitor?
    a. Electrical activity of the heart
    b. One cardiac cycle
    c. Atrial depolarization
    d. Ventricular repolarization

20. How many electrodes are needed to perform a standard EKG?
    a. 8
    b. 10
    c. 12
    d. 15

21. Which of the following waived tests is used to aid in the diagnosis of gastric ulcers and/or colon cancers?
    a. Rapid group A streptococcus
    b. Occult blood
    c. Cholesterol
    d. B-type natriuretic peptide (BNP)

22. The phlebotomist must instruct the patient on collection of a specimen for occult blood and tells the patient to collect a _____ specimen because it is the specimen of choice for occult blood.
    a. Urine
    b. Stool
    c. Sputum
    d. Peritoneal fluid

23. The patient must adhere to dietary restrictions before collection of feces for an occult blood test. What is the most important patient preparation necessary before occult blood testing?
    a. Patient must be fasting for 12 hours
    b. Patient must eat a high-fat diet 3 days before testing
    c. Patient must refrain from eating meat 3 days before testing
    d. Patient must eat a high-carb diet 3 days before testing

24. Which portion of a complete urinalysis is considered "waived" testing?
    a. Microscopic evaluation of casts
    b. Microscopic evaluation and chemical analysis
    c. Microscopic evaluation of bacteria only and chemical evaluation
    d. Chemical evaluation by dipstick

25. The phlebotomist is performing a dipstick analysis on a urine specimen. When examining a urine dipstick for the color change of the reagent pads what is the most important factor the phlebotomist should observe?
    a. Viscosity of the urine
    b. Reaction time

c. Sample volume

d. Color change

26. Pregnancy tests detect the presence of which of the following hormones?
    a. Estrogen
    b. Progesterone
    c. Human chorionic gonadotropin (HCG)
    d. Testosterone

27. All of the following samples can be used for HCG determination *except*:
    a. Urine
    b. Serum
    c. Sputum
    d. Plasma

28. When testing for the presence of rapid group A streptococcus, what is the specimen of choice?
    a. Throat culture swab
    b. Sputum sample
    c. Vaginal swab
    d. Nasal washings

29. Which of the following tests is not a POCT?
    a. BNP
    b. HCG
    c. ALT (alanine aminotransferase)
    d. ABG (arterial blood gas)

30. Which of the following tests is not a "waived" test?
    a. BNP
    b. HCG
    c. Glucose
    d. ABG

31. Hematocrit is a determination of which of the following?
    a. Packed red cell volume
    b. Mean cell volume of RBCs
    c. Mean corpuscular hemoglobin
    d. Red cell size variation

32. Which of the following tests *cannot* be used to monitor heparin therapy?
    a. ACT
    b. Tilt tube test
    c. PT
    d. APTT

33. Which of the following waived tests would be used to monitor a diabetic patient?
    a. Cholesterol
    b. Glucose
    c. HCG
    d. BNP

34. Which of the following tubes would be the specimen of choice used to collect a sample for hematocrit testing?
    a. EDTA
    b. Sodium citrate
    c. Sodium heparin
    d. Lithium heparin

35. What is the color of the stopper of a collection tube containing sodium citrate?
    a. Purple
    b. Red
    c. Green
    d. Blue

36. All of the following samples can be used to determine a patient's cholesterol level, *except*:
    a. Whole blood
    b. Serum
    c. Plasma
    d. Cells

37. Which of the following POCT tests could be performed on whole blood?
    a. Cholesterol
    b. Glucose
    c. Prothrombin time
    d. All of the above

38. The phlebotomist had just removed the dipstick from a patient's urine specimen when she was paged to assist with a STAT draw. She returned 10 minutes later and proceeded to:
    a. Compare the test pads with the reference color chart on the bottle
    b. Resubmerge the dipstick into the urine to get a fresh reading
    c. Recap, remix, and repeat the chemical analysis
    d. Get a new dipstick to repeat the chemical analysis

39. The normal ECG consists of tracing _____ prominent points where the graph changes directions equating to a particular portion of the cardiac cycle.
    a. 5
    b. 8
    c. 10
    d. 12

40. The phlebotomist is performing alternate site testing in the patient's home and needs to make sure he follows all required steps to ensure safe specimen collection. All of the following steps should be taken by the phlebotomist to ensure safe specimen collection, *except*:
    a. Carry a cell phone for emergencies when going on house calls
    b. Preserve the integrity of all specimens by transporting them on ice
    c. Carry a biohazard container on the house call tray
    d. Have the patient sit or recline during specimen collection

ANSWERS AND RATIONALES

1. **Answer: B**
   Rationale: Point-of-care testing is testing that is performed at the place where the specimen is collected, often in the same room as the specimen is collected.
   Text Reference: p. 265

2. **Answer: D**
   Rationale: POCT testing has significantly decreased turnaround times, leading to more prompt medical attention and faster diagnosis and treatment. In many instances this can decrease the patient's recovery time.
   Text Reference: p. 265

3. **Answer: D**
   Rationale: The Food and Drug Administration is responsible for deciding which tests are CLIA-waived tests based on the ease of performing and interpreting of the test.
   Text Reference: p. 265

4. **Answer: C**
   Rationale: ACT testing requires whole blood or citrated blood. Improper mixing of the tube with anticoagulant will result in clotting of the specimen and a prolonged clotting time.
   Text Reference: p. 267

5. **Answer: B**
   Rationale: Many of the manufacturers of waived testing equipment follow the traditional method of wiping away the first drop of blood before beginning testing. However, several of the waived test procedures now use the first drop of blood. The phlebotomist should carefully read the manufacturer's instructions before beginning the collection procedure.
   Text Reference: p. 266

6. **Answer: C**
   Rationale: The microhematocrit and hemoglobin tests are now performed in the POCT method and are both good tests to aid in the assessment of anemia.
   Text Reference: p. 266

7. **Answer: D**
   Rationale: The activated coagulation time (ACT) and the activated partial thromboplastin time can be used to monitor heparin therapy and are available now as POCT.
   Text Reference: p. 267

8. **Answer: B**
   Rationale: The prothrombin time is used to monitor warfarin (Coumadin) therapy and is available as a POCT.
   Text Reference: p. 267

9. **Answer: C**
   Rationale: Glucose monitoring is the most common POCT performed. Glucose testing is performed by capillary puncture and the use of a small hand-held instrument and reagent strips.
   Text Reference: p. 267

10. **Answer: A**
    Rationale: Cardiac troponin T (cardiac TnT) is a protein complex that is released by damaged cardiac muscle.
    Text Reference: p. 268

11. **Answer: C**
    Rationale: Cardiac TnT levels will rise within 4 hours following an acute MI. Levels may remain elevated for up to 2 weeks. TnT levels begin to rise within 1 hour of onset of symptoms and can be detected at the point of care (i.e., in the ambulance for a minority of patients). However, sensitivity increases at 4 hours and has greater diagnostic value for patients at admission.
    Text Reference: p. 268

12. **Answer: A**
    Rationale: Anticoagulated whole blood is used to perform cardiac TnT testing at the bedside and results are available within 15 minutes.
    Text Reference: p. 268

13. **Answer: D**
    Rationale: The ACT test can be performed using whole blood from a dermal puncture or blood collected in a blue sodium citrate tube.
    Text Reference: p. 267

14. **Answer: D**
    Rationale: Some POCT for cholesterol determination are one step methods. Other cholesterol POCT methods use instrumentation.
    Text Reference: p. 268

15. **Answer: D**
    Rationale: All point-of-care instruments require calibration on a schedule specified by the manufacturer along with control assays. Due to the complexity of arterial blood gas and electrolyte testing, these instruments require careful calibration and more training than simpler POCT procedures.
    Text Reference: pp. 266-268

16. **Answer: D**
    Rationale: BNP (B-type natriuretic peptide) production increases in patients with congestive heart disease and the measurement of the BNP allows the physician to quickly differentiate between chronic obstructive pulmonary disease (COPD) and congestive heart disease (CHD).
    Text Reference: p. 268

17. **Answer: A**
    Rationale: The sinoatrial node is located in the upper wall of the right atrium and is the pacemaker for the heart.
    Text Reference: p. 269

18. **Answer: B**
    Rationale: The term that indicates one complete heartbeat is the cardiac cycle.
    Text Reference: p. 269

19. **Answer: A**
    Rationale: The EKG monitors the entire electrical activity of the heart. Cardiac cycles are monitored over and over and atrial depolarization and ventricular repolarization are both parts of the cardiac cycle that is monitored in the overall electrical activity of the heart.
    Text Reference: p. 269

20. **Answer: B**
    Rationale: The electrical activity of the heart is monitored using a 12-lead EKG. There are 10 electrodes that are placed in defined locations on the patient's chest, arms, and legs. It should be noted that the terms lead and electrode are not interchangeable. The 12 leads are derived from the signals obtained from the 10 electrodes.
    Text Reference: p. 269

21. **Answer: B**
    Rationale: Occult blood testing is used to aid in the diagnosis of gastric ulcers and colon cancers by testing. Special patient preparation is required before specimen collection.
    Text Reference: pp. 270-271

22. **Answer: B**
    Rationale: Occult blood tests are performed on stool samples only.
    Text Reference: pp. 270-271

23. **Answer: C**
    Rationale: There are several dietary restrictions that must be given and observed by the

patient before occult blood testing to ensure that the test results are valid and that there are no false-negative or more commonly false-positive results. Refraining from the consumption of meat for 3 days before testing is one of several dietary restrictions the patient must observe. The phlebotomist should be sure to instruct the patient clearly on these restrictions and it is a good idea to provide them with written instructions as well.
Text Reference: pp. 270-271

24. **Answer: D**
Rationale: Chemical evaluation of urine by the "dipstick" plastic strip containing embedded reagents is considered a waived test. A complete urinalysis consists of the examination of physical, chemical, and microscopic properties of urine. Both the physical and chemical evaluations are considered waived. Microscopic evaluation of urine is considered moderate complexity and is therefore not a waived test.
Text Reference: pp. 271

25. **Answer: B**
Rationale: It is essential that the reagent pads are read against the reference color chart at exactly the right time. Allowing the reaction to go past the allotted time frame could cause a false-positive result. If the reaction is not allowed to proceed to completion, however, and the test pad is read too quickly, the result may be a false-negative or decreased value.
Text Reference: p. 271

26. **Answer: C**
Rationale: Pregnancy is determined by the presence of HCG. HCG is produced by the placenta after implantation of a fertilized egg.
Text Reference: p. 271

27. **Answer: C**
Rationale: Urine, plasma, and serum can be tested for the presence of HCG. HCG testing kits are available for both specimen types. The phlebotomist must be familiar with the type of testing kit available to ensure proper test collection.
Text Reference: p. 272

28. **Answer: A**
Rationale: The presence of group A streptococcus is determined using waived testing methods on specimens collected on a throat culture swab. During collection the phlebotomist must be careful not to contaminate the swab on the tongue or sides of mouth.
Text Reference: p. 272

29. **Answer: C**
Rationale: ALT is a liver enzyme that is not yet available as a POCT. All of the other tests listed above are POCT.
Text Reference: pp. 266-272

30. **Answer: D**
Rationale: Arterial blood gases, although available as POCT, are not yet classified by the FDA as waived tests due to the complexity of testing and the critical nature of the test results.
Text Reference: p. 268

31. **Answer: A**
Rationale: Hematocrit represents the level of red blood cells in the blood. The red cell level can be determined by the hematocrit, which is a packed red cell volume. Mean cell volume and mean corpuscular hemoglobin are indices that indicate specific characteristics of the individual red cells and not the total volume of red cells in their entirety.
Text Reference: pp. 266-267

32. **Answer: C**
Rationale: The prothrombin time (PT) is used to monitor warfarin (Coumadin) therapy. The ACT, also known as the tilt tube test, as well as the APTT are used to monitor heparin therapy.
Text Reference: p. 267

33. **Answer: B**
Rationale: Glucose monitoring is a good mechanism by which to monitor diabetic patients. Many diabetic patients have home testing devices that are similar to those used in health care facilities as waived testing instruments.
Text Reference: p. 267

34. **Answer: A**
    Rationale: A hematology test such as hematocrit will be completed on whole blood collected in an EDTA tube, in a non-heparinized capillary tube with blood from an EDTA tube, or via heparinized capillary tube from dermal puncture.
    Text Reference: pp. 266-267

35. **Answer: D**
    Rationale: A collection tube containing sodium citrate has a stopper that is light blue in color.
    Text Reference: pp. 122, 267

36. **Answer: D**
    Rationale: Whole blood, serum, or plasma could be used for cholesterol determination. The type of sample collected is dependent on the instrument and methodology is used by the laboratory.
    Text Reference: p. 268

37. **Answer: D**
    Rationale: Cholesterol, glucose, or prothrombin time could be performed using whole blood if using a POCT instrument. If alternative equipment is used for testing the sample type may vary.
    Text Reference: pp. 266-268

38. **Answer: C**
    Rationale: Timing is critical in reading the urine dipstick for chemical analysis of a urine. Ten minutes exceeds all time limits for reading results. The phlebotomist must recap and remix the specimen before repeating the analysis with a new dipstick.
    Text Reference: p. 271

39. **Answer: A**
    Rationale: The normal ECG consists of tracing 5 prominent points where the graph changes directions. These are arbitrarily known as P, Q, R, S, and T.
    Text Reference: p. 269

40. **Answer: B**
    Rationale: When performing a venipuncture or other collection procedure in the patient's home the phlebotomist should have the patient recline or sit for specimen collection, carry antiseptic towelettes for handwashing, carry a cell phone for emergencies, bring biohazard and sharps containers, verify the patient has stopped bleeding before leaving, recheck the phlebotomy area to ensure nothing is left behind, and preserve the specimen at the proper temperature for transport. Not all specimens require chilling when there is a delay in testing. Specimens should not be put directly on ice but rather in an ice slurry if required.
    Text Reference: p. 265

MOCK EXAM

1. A number of states have enacted legislation requiring that phlebotomists be _____ before working in the state as a phlebotomist.
   a. Registered
   b. Certified
   c. Approved
   d. Licensed

2. The department that uses radiant energy to treat cancers is:
   a. Nuclear medicine
   b. Radiology
   c. Oncology
   d. Respiratory therapy

3. OSHA Hazardous Communication Standard (HAZCOM):
   a. Requires manufacturers to supply MSDS
   b. Displays the type of hazard on their label
   c. Warns of the location of hazardous materials
   d. Describes all safety procedures for using chemicals

4. Gloves should be changed and hands washed:
   a. After each patient contact
   b. Only when gloves become soiled
   c. Only when there is a tear in the glove
   d. Only if patients are in isolation precautions

5. Hyperinsulinemia can result in:
   a. Diabetes mellitus
   b. Diabetes insipidus
   c. Hypoglycemia
   d. Graves' disease

6. Circulation through the heart and rest of the body's tissues is referred to as:
   a. Systemic circulation
   b. Visceral circulation
   c. Pulmonary circulation
   d. Semilunar circulation

7. All of the following equipment may be used in performing a venipuncture on small, fragile veins, except a:
   a. Syringe
   b. 21-gauge needle
   c. Blood transfer device
   d. Winged infusion set

8. The phlebotomist touches the needle to the skin, hesitates, and moves it over slightly to the left and then proceeds to:
   a. Gently insert the needle and collect the blood
   b. Release the tourniquet and start over
   c. Explain to the patient that the vein moved slightly
   d. Pick up the alcohol pad to reclean and insert the needle

9. Potassium levels can be collected by dermal puncture but it is not the method of choice for all of the following reasons, except:
   a. There is a greater risk for sample hemolysis
   b. Potassium levels are lower in capillary blood
   c. A larger sample volume is required for testing
   d. Venous blood reference ranges are higher

10. Drawing blood from a foot or leg requires:
    a. Assistance from the nurse
    b. Permission from the physician
    c. Specialized venipuncture equipment
    d. Giving the patient a dose of heparin first

11. The maximum amount of blood to be drawn on newborns and infants in a 24-hour period is based on:
    a. Baby's age
    b. Body weight
    c. Physician's orders
    d. Patient's condition

12. Which test that measures the gas exchange ability of the lungs and the buffering capacity of the blood?
    a. Pulmonary function test
    b. Bicarbonate assay
    c. Arterial blood gases
    d. O_2 saturation

13. Pretest preparation for the oral glucose tolerance test includes:
    a. Consuming a high-protein meal the day before the test
    b. Fasting for 8 hours immediately before the test
    c. Eating high-carbohydrate meals 3 days before testing
    d. Performing light exercise daily the week before testing

14. Which urine specimen is used to screen for protein or glucose abnormalities:
    a. Random
    b. Timed
    c. First morning
    d. 24 hour

15. Professionalism is evidenced in a phlebotomist who exhibits all of the following, *except:*
    a. Well-groomed appearance
    b. Knowledge and skill
    c. Aggressiveness
    d. Professional detachment

16. The classification of fire extinguisher that can be used on electrical fires is:
    a. Type A
    b. Type B
    c. Type C
    d. Type K

17. In the chain of infection, the source is represented by all of the following, *except:*
    a. Fomite
    b. Asymptomatic person
    c. Symptomatic person
    d. Vector

18. The word root cubit- means:
    a. Tail
    b. Elbow
    c. Head
    d. Vein

19. The only vein to carry oxygenated blood is the:
    a. Superior vena cava
    b. Aorta
    c. Pulmonary vein
    d. Brachial vein

20. You need to collect a CBC, blood culture, and metabolic panel. The tube stoppers and order of draw that you will use are:
    a. Lavender, gold, yellow
    b. Gold, yellow, lavender
    c. Green, lavender, yellow
    d. Yellow, gold, lavender

21. Identification of an inpatient requires that the phlebotomist:
    a. Ask the patient to state their name and date of birth
    b. Ask the patient their name and have them sign the label
    c. Ask the patient to state their name and check the armband
    d. Ask the patient to verify the information on the label

22. When performing daily glucose monitoring on inpatients, the phlebotomist selects the following dermal puncture device:
    a. 1 mm depth, 2.5 mm width
    b. 2 mm depth, 1.5 mm width
    c. 0.85 mm depth, 1.75 mm width
    d. 2.25 mm depth, 23-gauge puncture lancet

23. Blood should not be drawn from the arm on the side of a mastectomy because of:
    a. Lymphostasis due to lymph node removal
    b. Edematous fluids that may hemolyze the blood
    c. Hemoconcentration of analytes in the arm
    d. Veins that are sclerosed or occluded in the arm

24. The physician orders a STAT CBC and glucose on a child who has been crying excessively in the waiting room and during the draw. The phlebotomist should note this on the requisition, because excessive crying can:
    a. Elevate WBCs
    b. Lower hemoglobin
    c. Lower glucose
    d. Increase RBCs

25. Arterial sites in an adult include all of the following, *except:*
    a. Femoral
    b. Dorsalis pedis
    c. Scalp
    d. Brachial

26. Which substance exhibits diurnal variation with levels twice as high in the morning versus the late afternoon?
    a. Estradiol
    b. Cortisol
    c. Glucose
    d. Serum iron

27. Which type of fecal specimen is ordered on a patient suspected of having salmonella?
    a. Random
    b. 72 hour
    c. O & P
    d. Fats

28. Certification of a phlebotomist:
    a. Grants permission to perform a service or procedure
    b. Documents evidence of proficiency in practice
    c. Grants permission to perform services and documents proficiently
    d. Documents updates on new skills of the phlebotomist

29. A test for immunology includes:
    a. CBC
    b. ANA
    c. BUN
    d. ALT

30. An example of a percutaneous exposure is:
    a. Blood splash in the eye
    b. Blood exposure by needlestick
    c. Blood splashes on the intact skin
    d. Blood exposure on lab coat

31. The virus that is viable outside of the host organism for 1 to 3 days is:
    a. HBV
    b. HIV
    c. HAV
    d. HCV

32. Which of the following volumes is needed to yield 2 mL of serum?
    a. 2 mL
    b. 4 mL
    c. 7 mL
    d. 10 mL

33. Sodium citrate functions to:
    a. Promote faster clotting of the specimen
    b. Coat tube walls to prevent RBC adherence
    c. Prevent clotting of the specimen
    d. Provide surface area for platelet activation

34. The correct prioritization of collection for a routine, timed, ASAP test is as follows:
    a. Timed, routine, ASAP
    b. ASAP, timed, routine
    c. Timed, ASAP, routine
    d. Routine, timed, ASAP

35. The phlebotomist is performing a dermal puncture on a newborn for a glucose and proceeds to collect the blood in a(n):
    a. Gold top microtainer
    b. Microhematocrit
    c. Amber-colored bullet
    d. Natelson pipette

36. While drawing an early morning outpatient, the phlebotomist noticed that the patient was turning pale, cold, and damp as she put on the second of three tubes. The correct course of action is to:
    a. Give the patient an emesis basin and a cold cloth
    b. Withdraw the needle and have the patient lower her head
    c. Proceed to complete the draw with smelling salts ready
    d. Tell the patient to breathe deeply and slowly

37. All of the following precautions must be considered when collecting blood for bilirubin testing, *except:*
    a. Light sensitive
    b. Hemolysis lowers result
    c. Collections are timed
    d. Do not turn off bili-light

38. When performing the Allen test on a cardiac patient, the phlebotomist notes that no color appeared after blanching. She proceeds to:
    a. Check the other arm
    b. Perform the arterial puncture
    c. Massage the arm and redo the test
    d. Apply a heat pack to the site

39. A potential donor may be rejected if they do not meet the standard requirements for all of the following, *except:*
   a. Weight
   b. Temperature
   c. Height
   d. Hemoglobin

40. A urine C & S is used to diagnose:
   a. Illicit drug use
   b. Urinary tract infection
   c. Ova and parasites
   d. Proteins and hormones

41. Requires medical institutions to have procedures in place that actively protect confidentiality of medical information:
   a. CLIA
   b. TJC
   c. HIPAA
   d. NAACLS

42. The division of the laboratory that analyzes blood and body fluids:
   a. Clinical microscopy
   b. Anatomic and surgical pathology
   c. Clinical pathology
   d. Clinical laboratory

43. Used by all health care employees to prevent the spread of HIV and HBV during patient care:
   a. Expanded precautions
   b. Standard Precautions
   c. Isolation precautions
   d. Contact precautions

44. The following term is synonymous with heart attack:
   a. Bradycardia
   b. Myocardial infarct
   c. Cardiopathy
   d. Tachycardia

45. All of the following are common lab tests for digestive disorders, *except:*
   a. Ammonia
   b. Amylase
   c. Gastrin
   d. Glucose

46. In general, patients who have an illness caused by a highly transmissible and epidemiologically important pathogen require what type of precautions:
   a. Isolation precautions
   b. Universal precautions
   c. Expanded precautions
   d. Contact precautions

47. A white blood cell that exhibits phagocytic activity is:
   a. Lymphocyte
   b. Eosinophil
   c. Neutrophil
   d. Basophil

48. All of the following can elevate potassium levels of the blood specimen, *except:*
   a. Incorrect order of draw
   b. Hemolysis of the specimen
   c. Use of the incorrect anticoagulant
   d. Using a 21-gauge needle

49. Methods to enhance venipuncture location include all of the following, *except:*
   a. Slapping the site
   b. Applying a warm towel
   c. Dangling the arm downward
   d. Gentle upward massage

50. Puncture of the bone during a dermal puncture could potentially result in osteochondritis, which is:
   a. Inflammation of the bone or bone marrow
   b. Inflammation of the calcaneus
   c. Inflammation of the bone or cartilage
   d. Inflammation of the phalanx

51. The angle of needle insertion depends on all of the following, *except:*
   a. Depth of the vein
   b. Width of the vein
   c. Antecubital vein
   d. Hand vein

52. When collecting blood for a neonatal screen, the phlebotomist should:
   a. Apply blood to both sides of the circles
   b. Fill the circle with one large drop of blood
   c. Perform either a dermal or venous puncture
   d. Place the card in a vertical position to dry

53. Performing an arterial puncture on geriatric patients poses increased risk for:
    a. Air bubbles in the syringe
    b. Formation of a hematoma
    c. Hemolysis of the sample
    d. Puncturing a vein not an artery

54. Blood culture site preparation requires all of the following, except:
    a. Cleaning 1.5 to 2 inches beyond the intended puncture site
    b. Scrubbing the site with 2% iodine or povidone-iodine
    c. Allowing iodine or the povidone-iodine to dry for 1 minute
    d. Removing the iodine with alcohol before the stick

55. NAACLS is an agency that grants:
    a. Approval of phlebotomy programs
    b. Certification of phlebotomists
    c. Accreditation of hospitals and laboratories
    d. State licensure of phlebotomists

56. When processing specimens for the morning run, the phlebotomist notes that there are several specimens exhibiting cloudy serum referred to as:
    a. Hemolysis
    b. Lipemia
    c. Icteric
    d. Hazy

57. All of the following are general rules of electrical safety that apply to health care employees, except:
    a. Know the location of the circuit breaker box for equipment
    b. Avoid contact with electrical equipment while drawing blood
    c. Unplug equipment before performing any maintenance on it
    d. Open equipment with an electrical warning with extreme caution

58. The phlebotomist prepares to enter the room of a patient in contact isolation and will don:
    a. Mask and gloves
    b. Gown and gloves
    c. N95 respirator and gloves
    d. Gloves only

59. All of the following can be used to assess whether or not a patient has suffered a heart attack, except:
    a. Creatine kinase
    b. Protein
    c. Troponin
    d. Myoglobin

60. After assessing the patient's small veins, the phlebotomist decides to use a 23-gauge needle and which of the following tube volumes to draw a glucose, BUN, and potassium?
    a. 3 mL light green
    b. 7 mL green
    c. 8 mL PST
    d. 10 mL red plastic

61. The phlebotomist noticed that the patient's arm was developing petechiae while selecting the puncture site. The correct course of action is to:
    a. Perform the venipuncture with no tourniquet
    b. Use a blood pressure cuff instead of a tourniquet
    c. Ask the patient if they are on anticoagulant therapy
    d. Follow the procedure for routine venipuncture

62. When performing a bilirubin dermal puncture on a newborn, the phlebotomist should never use this antiseptic:
    a. Zepharin chloride
    b. Povidone-iodine
    c. 70% isopropyl alcohol
    d. Benzalkonium chloride

63. Fluid shifts can result in patients who are in upright positions for an extended period of time and may produce erroneous test results for all of the following, except:
    a. H & H
    b. Calcium
    c. Enzymes
    d. Glucose

64. Techniques used to perform a venous puncture on a geriatric patient include:
    a. Probing to find the vein
    b. Using a 21-gauge butterfly
    c. Applying pressure longer
    d. Applying a tight tourniquet

65. Arterial blood gas specimens may be rejected for which of the following reasons:
    a. Use of a heparin anticoagulant
    b. Delivering the sample 20 minutes after collection
    c. Air bubbles in the syringe
    d. Using the computer label

66. Time-sensitive specimens are:
    a. Drawn at a specified time
    b. Peak and trough draws
    c. Tested immediately after collection
    d. Drawn in the AM versus PM

67. Nasal washings are used to test for the presence of which of the following:
    a. MRSA
    b. RSV
    c. HBV
    d. CRP

68. The physician's office prepares specimens for courier transport to the laboratory by:
    a. Placing all blood specimens on a slurry of ice
    b. Putting blood specimens in a sealed biohazard bag
    c. Separating serum and cells into transport tubes
    d. Keeping all blood specimens at body temperature

69. To prevent aerosolization when removing the tube stopper, the phlebotomist can do all of the following, *except:*
    a. Cover stopper with a 4 × 4 gauze and pull straight up
    b. Rock the stopper gently side to side to pop the top
    c. Use tubes with special Hemagard stoppers
    d. Remove stopper behind countertop safety shield

70. Preparation of aliquots includes all of the following, *except:*
    a. Pouring aliquots into labeled transfer tubes
    b. Prelabeling aliquot tubes before filling
    c. Centrifuging tubes for 10 to 15 minutes
    d. Capping all tubes before delivery to departments

71. OSHA requires all of the following PPE when processing specimens, *except:*
    a. Full-length lab coat
    b. Utility gloves
    c. Goggles
    d. Mask

72. A special number used to catalog samples in the laboratory is a:
    a. Medical record number
    b. Barcode number
    c. Accession number
    d. Patient number

73. All of the following specimen tubes must be centrifuged, *except:*
    a. SST
    b. Red
    c. Gray
    d. Lavender

74. A balanced centrifuge requires tubes be placed in the same or diagonal positions across from each other that are of:
    a. Equal weight
    b. Equal height
    c. The same color
    d. The same additive

75. Which of the following microbiologic specimens must be refrigerated?
    a. Throat
    b. Blood culture
    c. Ova and parasite
    d. Urine

76. Requirements for patient preparation and specimen handling for chain of custody specimens are established by:
    a. CLIA
    b. TJC
    c. NIDA
    d. HIPAA

77. Warm collection and storage are required for all of the following specimens, *except:*
    a. Cryoglobulin
    b. Cold agglutinins
    c. C-reactive protein
    d. Cryofibrinogen

78. Identification of the patient for a chain of custody specimen requires:
    a. A picture identification
    b. Signature of the patient
    c. Verbal and written verification
    d. Police identity verification

79. Which of the following specimens must be protected from light?
    a. Synovial fluid
    b. Amniotic fluid
    c. Peritoneal fluid
    d. Pericardial fluid

80. Characteristics of an acceptable blood smear include all of the following, *except:*
    a. Free of holes
    b. Feathered edge
    c. Thick smear
    d. Even distribution

81. Which of the following is an example of quality assurance:
    a. Logging incidences of mislabeled specimens
    b. Measuring the draw volume on collection tubes
    c. Calibrating centrifugation times every 3 months
    d. Monitoring temperatures of refrigerators and freezers

82. Preanalytical variables that a phlebotomist can control include all of the following, *except:*
    a. Inversion of the specimen
    b. Right tube, right order
    c. Right volume of test reagents
    d. Labeling of the specimen

83. Under HIPAA, confidentiality can be described as being all of the following, *except:*
    a. A legal responsibility
    b. A right of the patient
    c. An ethical responsibility
    d. Flexible in an emergency

84. The phlebotomist is legally bound to do all of the following, *except:*
    a. Discuss the patient's tests to gain informed consent
    b. Adhere to phlebotomy standards of care
    c. Perform duties within their scope of practice
    d. Protect confidentiality of patient's records

85. Chemistry tests that can be performed as POCT include all of the following, *except:*
    a. ABGs
    b. CBC
    c. BUN
    d. Electrolytes

86. The POCT used to assess congestive heart disease is:
    a. BNP
    b. ACT
    c. Cholesterol
    d. Cardiac TnT

87. An instrument used to assess anemia is a(n):
    a. Glucometer
    b. Cardiac reader
    c. Hemoglobin analyzer
    d. ACT tester

88. Waived testing analyzers that are calibrated for the second drop of blood require:
    a. Two drops of blood for analysis
    b. A puncture depth of 0.85 mm
    c. Cleansing using tincture of Betadine
    d. The first drop of blood be wiped off

89. A CLIA-waived test that can be performed by a phlebotomist is:
    a. Prothrombin time
    b. Urine microscopic
    c. Arterial blood gas
    d. CBC differential

90. Another name for the occult blood test is:
    a. Hidden blood test
    b. Guaiac test
    c. Hemastix test
    d. Hemoglobin test

91. ECG testing requires all of the following equipment and supplies, *except:*
    a. 12 electrodes
    b. 18-gauge needle
    c. Alcohol pads
    d. Disposable razor

92. Required billing information includes all of the following, *except*:
    a. Insurance information
    b. ICD-9 code
    c. CPT code
    d. State code

93. Mom brings her 12-year-old daughter to the outpatient laboratory for preoperative blood work. The proper course of action for the phlebotomist is to:
    a. Explain the procedure to the mom and the child
    b. Talk to the mom about the venipuncture procedure
    c. Tell the girl that if she does not move it will not hurt at all
    d. Discuss the purpose of the tests and the procedure with the girl

94. A 4-year-old child is screaming and thrashing as the phlebotomist tries to look for a vein. Mom is upset and is not helpful in restraining the child. The best course of action the phlebotomist should take is to:
    a. Instruct the mom in the importance of restraining the child
    b. Reason with the child about the importance of the blood draw
    c. Offer the child a reward if they hold still for the draw
    d. Seek the assistance of another phlebotomist to restrain the child

95. After explaining to the patient the importance of drawing blood, the patient still refuses and tells the phlebotomist to leave. The proper course of action is to:
    a. Tell the patient that he or she has no choice and proceed to do the procedure
    b. Call the lab and ask for assistance in getting the patient to cooperate
    c. Inform the patient's nurse of the situation and let the nurse talk to the patient
    d. Put the lab request back in the stack to be drawn on the next shift

96. The phlebotomist arrives in the ER to draw a patient who does not speak English. To gain informed consent the phlebotomist should:
    a. Get a nurse to witness the conversation with the patient
    b. Speak slow and loud while using exaggerated enunciation
    c. Assume the patient has given consent by virtue of being in the ER
    d. Wait until the hospital translator comes and explains the procedure

97. Additive tubes include all of the following, *except*:
    a. Green
    b. Red glass
    c. Light blue
    d. Red/gray

98. Tube additive that inhibits complement and phagocytosis:
    a. SPS
    b. EDTA
    c. Silicone
    d. Thixotropic gel

99. While performing a venipuncture, the needle becomes disengaged from the adapter. The proper course of action is to:
    a. Stabilize the needle with the index finger and complete the draw
    b. Immediately stop the procedure and carefully withdraw the needle
    c. Grasp the needle with one hand and reattach the adapter with the other
    d. Grasp the needle hub, remove the adapter, and pop tubes directly onto the needle

100. A heparinized syringe is used in the collection of which of the following tests:
    a. Electrolytes
    b. CBC
    c. ABGs
    d. ALT

MOCK EXAM ANSWERS

Note: Page numbers from Warekois and Robinson: *Phlebotomy: Worktext and Procedures Manual,* second edition.

1. **Answer: D**
   Text Reference: pp. 6-8; Licensure

2. **Answer: B**
   Text Reference: p. 13; Hospital Organization

3. **Answer: A**
   Text Reference: p. 26; Chemical Hazards

4. **Answer: A**
   Text Reference: p. 36; Breaking the Chain of Infection: Hand Hygiene

5. **Answer: C**
   Text Reference: p. 85; Pancreas

6. **Answer: A**
   Text Reference: p. 94; Circulatory System

7. **Answer: B**
   Text Reference: pp. 118-119; Safety Syringes and Safety Syringe Needles; Winged Infusion Sets or Butterflies

8. **Answer: B**
   Text Reference: p. 137; Routine Venipuncture

9. **Answer: C**
   Text Reference: pp. 149, 154; Differences between Venous and Capillary Blood; Dermal Puncture

10. **Answer: B**
    Text Reference: p. 170; Use of an Alternative Site

11. **Answer: B**
    Text Reference: pp. 184-185; Special Physiologic Considerations

12. **Answer: C**
    Text Reference: p. 196; Arterial Blood Gas Testing

13. **Answer: C**
    Text Reference: p. 208; Oral Glucose Tolerance Test

14. **Answer: A**
    Text Reference: p. 222; Types of Urine Specimens

15. **Answer: C**
    Text Reference: pp. 3-5; Job Skills, Personal Characteristics

16. **Answer: C**
    Text Reference: p. 29; Classes of Fires

17. **Answer: D**
    Text Reference: p. 34; Chain of Infection

18. **Answer: B**
    Text Reference: p. 54; Word Roots

19. **Answer: C**
    Text Reference: pp. 95-97; Circulation through the Heart

20. **Answer: D**
    Text Reference: p. 124; Order of Draw

21. **Answer: C**
    Text Reference: p. 131; Routine Venipuncture

22. **Answer: D**
    Text Reference: p. 151; Puncture Depth and Width; Content Overview: Equipment for Dermal Puncture

23. **Answer: A**
    Text Reference: p. 170; Problems in Site Selection: Mastectomies

24. **Answer: A**
    Text Reference: p. 185; Special Physiological Considerations

25. **Answer: C**
Text Reference: p. 198; Arteries Used for Arterial Puncture

26. **Answer: B**
Textbook Reference: p. 209; Diurnal Variation

27. **Answer: A**
Text Reference: p. 225; Types of Fecal Specimens

28. **Answer: B**
Text Reference: p. 6; Certification

29. **Answer: B**
Text Reference: p.18; Serology or Immunology

30. **Answer: B**
Text Reference: p. 46; Contact with Blood-Borne Pathogens

31. **Answer: B**
Text Reference: pp. 46-47; Viral Survival; Content Overview

32. **Answer: B**
Text Reference: p. 101; Blood

33. **Answer: C**
Text Reference: p. 121; Anticoagulants

34. **Answer: C**
Text Reference: p. 129; Requisitions; Content Overview

35. **Answer: A**
Text Reference: p. 150; Microsample Containers

36. **Answer: B**
Text Reference: p. 171; Complications During Collection: Changes in Patient Status; Syncope

37. **Answer: D**
Text Reference: p. 187; Special Derma Puncture Procedures: Neonatal Bilirubin

38. **Answer: A**
Text Reference: p. 199; Modified Allen Test

39. **Answer: C**
Text Reference: p. 211; Blood Donor Collection

40. **Answer: B**
Text Reference: p. 223; Collection Procedures for Urine Specimens

41. **Answer: C**
Text Reference: p. 9; Confidentiality

42. **Answer: C**
Text Reference: pp. 13-14; Clinical Laboratory

43. **Answer: B**
Text Reference: p. 40; Standard Precautions

44. **Answer: B**
Text Reference: pp. 53-54, 97; Prefixes; Word Roots; Blood Vessels—Arteries

45. **Answer: D**
Text Reference: pp. 79, 88; Common Lab Tests for Digestive Disorders

46. **Answer: C**
Text Reference: p. 45; Isolation Control Measures

47. **Answer: C**
Text Reference: pp. 102-103; White Blood Cells

48. **Answer: D**
Text Reference: pp. 124, 178; Order of Draw; Tests Affected by Hemolysis

49. **Answer: A**
Text Reference: p. 135; Routine Venipuncture Procedure

50. **Answer: C**
Text Reference: p. 151; Site Selection General Considerations

51. **Answer: B**
Text Reference: pp. 137, 173; Routine Venipuncture: Perform the Procedure; Hand Collection Using a Winged Infusion Set: Insert the Needle

52. **Answer: B**
    Text Reference: p. 188; Neonatal Screening

53. **Answer: B**
    Text Reference: p. 200; Arterial Puncture Complications

54. **Answer: D**
    Text Reference: p. 212; Blood Culture Collection

55. **Answer: A**
    Text Reference: p. 6; Accreditation

56. **Answer: B**
    Text Reference: pp. 16-17; Specimen Collection for Chemistry

57. **Answer: D**
    Text Reference: p. 28; Electrical Hazards

58. **Answer: B**
    Text Reference: p. 45; Contact Precautions

59. **Answer: B**
    Text Reference: p. 88; Summary of Common Lab Tests by Body System

60. **Answer: A**
    Text Reference: p. 133; Routine Venipuncture: Assemble Your Equipment

61. **Answer: D**
    Text Reference: p. 141; Attend the Patient

62. **Answer: B**
    Text Reference: pp. 117, 153-154; Cleaning the Puncture Site; Dermal Puncture; Select and Clean the Site

63. **Answer: D**
    Text Reference: p. 178; Factors That Affect Sample Integrity: Tests Affected by Patient Position

64. **Answer: C**
    Text Reference: pp. 190-191; Special Considerations for Blood Collection

65. **Answer: C**
    Text Reference: p. 200; Specimen Rejection

66. **Answer: C**
    Text Reference: p. 214; Time-Sensitive Specimens

67. **Answer: B**
    Text Reference: p. 226; Nasopharyngeal Specimens; Nonblood Specimens

68. **Answer: B**
    Text Reference: pp. 235-236; Transporting Specimens to the Lab

69. **Answer: B**
    Text Reference: p. 237; Removing a Stopper

70. **Answer: A**
    Text Reference: p. 237; Preparing Aliquots

71. **Answer: B**
    Text Reference: p. 236; Processing: Safety

72. **Answer: C**
    Text Reference: p. 236; Central Processing

73. **Answer: D**
    Text Reference: pp. 122-123; Color-Coded Tops

74. **Answer: A**
    Text Reference: p. 236; Centrifuging

75. **Answer: D**
    Text Reference: p. 238; Transport and Processing of Nonblood Specimens

76. **Answer: C**
    Text Reference: p. 215; Legal and Forensic Specimens

77. **Answer: C**
    Text Reference: p. 214; Cryofibrinogen and Cryoglobulin

78. **Answer: A**
    Text Reference: p. 215; Legal and Forensic Specimen

79. **Answer: B**
    Text Reference: p. 228; Amniotic Fluid Specimens

80. **Answer: C**
Text Reference: pp. 216-218; Blood Smear Preparation

81. **Answer: A**
Text Reference: p. 243; Features of Quality Phlebotomy

82. **Answer: C**
Text Reference: p. 248; Specimen Collection

83. **Answer: D**
Text Reference: p. 259; Confidentiality—HIPAA

84. **Answer: A**
Text Reference: pp. 257-260; Professional Liability

85. **Answer: B**
Text Reference: p. 266; Common Tests Performed at the Point of Care

86. **Answer: A**
Text Reference: p. 268; B-Type Natriuretic Peptide

87. **Answer: C**
Text Reference: p. 267; Hematology: Anemia and Polycythemia Evaluation

88. **Answer: D**
Text Reference: pp. 265-266; Advantages of Point of Care Testing

89. **Answer: A**
Text Reference: p. 267; Coagulation Monitoring

90. **Answer: B**
Text Reference: p. 270; Occult Blood; Content Overview: Occult Blood

91. **Answer: B**
Text Reference: p. 270; Performing an Electrocardiogram

92. **Answer: D**
Text Reference: Content Overview: Billing/Coding

93. **Answer: A**
Text Reference: pp. 185-186; Special Psychological Considerations

94. **Answer: D**
Text Reference: p.186; Involvement of Parents and Siblings

95. **Answer: C**
Text Reference: p. 169; Patient Refusal

96. **Answer: D**
Text Reference: p. 169; Language Problems

97. **Answer: B**
Text Reference: p. 122; Color-Coded Tops

98. **Answer: A**
Text Reference: p. 123; Color-Coded Stoppers: Yellow Sterile

99. **Answer: B**
Text Reference: p. 138; Routine Venipuncture

100. **Answer: C**
Text Reference: p. 196; Arterial Blood Gases: Heparinized Syringe and Needle

INDEX

Entries followed by t denote tables.